T0319365

BACE

BACE
Lead Target for Orchestrated Therapy of Alzheimer's Disease

Edited by

VARGHESE JOHN

Buck Institute for Age Research
Novato, California

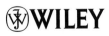

WILEY

A JOHN WILEY & SONS, INC., PUBLICATION

The cover design was done by Loretta Sheridan, design specialist at the Buck Institute for Age Research. It models the symbolic "tangled web" that BACE – whose 3D structure is shown – weaves around the brain resulting in loss of neurons, brain shrinkage, and Alzheimer's disease.

For general information on our other products and services or for technical support, please contact our Customer Care Department within the United States at (800) 762-2974, outside the United States at (317) 572-3993 or fax (317) 572-4002.

Wiley also publishes its books in a variety of electronic formats. Some content that appears in print may not be available in electronic formats. For more information about Wiley products, visit our web site at www.wiley.com.

Library of Congress Cataloging-in-Publication Data:

BACE : lead target for orchestrated therapy of Alzheimer's disease / [edited by] Varghese John.
    p. ; cm.
  Includes bibliographical references and index.
  ISBN 978-0-470-29342-3 (cloth)
  1. Alzheimer's disease–Chemotherapy. 2. Aspartic proteinases–Inhibitors–Therapeutic use. 3. Amyloid beta-protein precursor. I. John, Varghese, 1958–
    [DNLM: 1. Alzheimer Disease–drug therapy. 2. Amyloid Precursor Protein Secretases–pharmacology. 3. Amyloid Precursor Protein Secretases–therapeutic use.
WT 155 B117 2010]
  RC523.B24 2010
  618.97'6831–dc22
                                2009037093

Printed in the United States of America.

10 9 8 7 6 5 4 3 2 1

*Mind's underground moths
grow filmy wings
and take a farewell flight
in the sunset sky.*

*Leave out my name from the gift
if it be a burden
but keep my song.*

*April, like a child,
writes hieroglyphs on dust with flowers,
wipes them away and forgets.*

*Memory, the priestess,
kills the present
and offers its heart to the shrine of the dead past.*

From *Fireflies* by Rabindranath Tagore

CONTENTS

PREFACE   xi

ACKNOWLEDGMENTS   xiii

CONTRIBUTORS   xv

CHAPTER 1   *BACE, APP PROCESSING, AND SIGNAL TRANSDUCTION IN
ALZHEIMER'S DISEASE*   1

Dale E. Bredesen and Edward H. Koo

1.1   Introduction   **1**
1.2   BACE Cleavage of APP as a Molecular Switching Mechanism   **2**
1.3   AD: An Imbalance in Cellular Dependence?   **3**
1.4   BACE Cleavage, Caspase Cleavage, and Neuronal Trophic
      Dependence   **4**
1.5   BACE Cleavage of APP, Dependence Receptors, and Alzheimer
      Pathology   **5**
1.6   Key Mutations Proximal of APP Processing to Aβ   **9**
1.7   Final Remarks   **10**

CHAPTER 2   *IDENTIFICATION OF BACE AS A TARGET IN
ALZHEIMER'S DISEASE*   15

Robert L. Heinrikson and Sukanto Sinha

2.1   Introduction   **15**
2.2   The Search for β-Secretase   **17**
2.3   Validation of the BACE Target   **27**
2.4   Final Remarks   **28**

CHAPTER 3   *BACE BIOLOGICAL ASSAYS*   35

Alfredo G. Tomasselli and Michael J. Bienkowski

3.1   Introduction   **35**
3.2   Clinical and Physiological Hallmarks of Alzheimer's Disease (AD)   **36**
3.3   APP Processing   **36**
3.4   Aspartyl Protease Classification   **37**
3.5   BACE Structure   **38**
3.6   Mechanism, Kinetics, Inhibition, and Specificity   **39**
3.7   Assay Strategies for Inhibitor Finding and Development   **45**
3.8   Common Assays Used to Identify and Study Inhibitors   **48**
3.9   BACE Assays   **50**
3.10 Final Remarks   **54**

CHAPTER 4 *PEPTIDIC, PEPTIDOMIMETIC, AND HTS-DERIVED BACE INHIBITORS*   59

James P. Beck and Dustin J. Mergott

4.1   Introduction   **59**
4.2   Elan/Pharmacia (Pfizer)   **59**
4.3   Oklahoma Medical Research Foundation (OMRF)/Multiple Collaborators   **70**
4.4   Eli Lilly   **72**
4.5   Merck   **74**
4.6   GlaxoSmithKline   **80**
4.7   Schering Plough   **82**
4.8   Bristol-Myers Squibb   **85**
4.9   Novartis   **87**
4.10   Amgen   **88**
4.11   Wyeth   **90**
4.12   Final Remarks   **94**

CHAPTER 5 *FRAGMENT-BASED APPROACHES FOR IDENTIFICATION OF BACE INHIBITORS*   107

Andreas Kuglstatter and Michael Hennig

5.1   Introduction   **107**
5.2   Biophysical Methods Applied to BACE Fragment Screens   **108**
5.3   BACE Inhibitors Identified by Fragment Screening   **110**
5.4   Final Remarks   **119**

CHAPTER 6 *STRUCTURE-BASED DESIGN OF BACE INHIBITORS: TECHNICAL AND PRACTICAL ASPECTS OF PREPARATION, 3-DIMENSIONAL STRUCTURE, AND COMPUTATIONAL ANALYSIS*   123

Felix F. Vajdos, Veerabahu Shanmugasundaram, and Alfredo G. Tomasselli

6.1   Introduction   **123**
6.2   Preparation of BACE for Structural Studies   **126**
6.3   Crystallographic Studies of BACE   **130**
6.4   Structural Studies with BACE Inhibitors: Peptidomimetics and Nonpeptidomimetics   **135**
6.5   Computational Approaches   **145**
6.6   Final Remarks   **150**

CHAPTER 7 *PHARMACOLOGICAL MODELS FOR PRECLINICAL TESTING: FROM MOUSE TO DOG TO NONHUMAN PRIMATES*   159

Jason L. Eriksen, Michael Paul Murphy, and Elizabeth Head

7.1   Introduction   **159**
7.2   BACE1 and Mouse Models of AD   **161**
7.3   Testing BACE Inhibitors in the Canine Model of Human Aging and AD   **163**
7.4   BACE Inhibitors and Nonhuman Primates   **167**
7.5   Final Remarks   **168**

CHAPTER 8 *ADSORPTION, DISTRIBUTION, METABOLISM, EXCRETION
(ADME), EFFICACY, AND TOXICOLOGY FOR BACE INHIBITORS* **177**

Ishrut Hussain and Emmanuel Demont

8.1 Introduction **177**
8.2 Development of BACE Inhibitors with Optimized ADME Properties **180**
8.3 *In Vivo* Efficacy of BACE Inhibitors **188**
8.4 Toxicology of BACE Inhibitors **192**
8.5 Final Remarks **193**

CHAPTER 9 *CLINICAL TRIALS FOR DISEASE-MODIFYING DRUGS SUCH
AS BACE INHIBITORS* **197**

Henry H. Hsu

9.1 Introduction **197**
9.2 Update on Beta-Amyloid Therapies in Clinical Development **198**
9.3 Clinical Development of BACE Inhibitors and Other Disease-Modifying
Drugs **203**
9.4 Final Remarks **212**

CHAPTER 10 *FUTURE STRATEGIES FOR DEVELOPMENT OF NOVEL
BACE INHIBITORS: ANTI-APP β-SITE ANTIBODY AND APP BINDING
SMALL MOLECULE APPROACHES FOR ALZHEIMER'S DISEASE* **217**

Beka Solomon, Michal Arbel-Ornath, Clare Peters-Libeu, and Varghese John

10.1 Introduction **217**
10.2 β-Secretase: Discovery, Function, and Inhibitors **218**
10.3 Generation of Aβ Peptides via the Endocytic Pathway **220**
10.4 Generation of Anti-APP β-Site Antibodies **221**
10.5 Antibody Interference with Aβ Production in Cellular Model **223**
10.6 Antibody Interference with Aβ Production in Animal Models **226**
10.7 Identification of APP Binding Small Molecules that Block β-Site
Cleavage of APP **228**
10.8 Final Remarks **230**

AFTERWORD **235**

Ruth Abraham

Introduction **235**
Artwork as a Measure of the Progression of AD **236**

INDEX **243**

PREFACE

Alzheimer's disease (AD) now afflicts over 5.0 million people in the United States. As the population ages, AD may become the most devastating disease of our time, for which there is no effective therapy currently available. A recent Hollywood movie, *Away from Her*, directed by Sarah Polley based on a true story, highlights the steep decline in memory that occurs in AD that makes this disease so devastating.

A number of targets have been identified for therapeutic intervention in the treatment of AD of which the enzyme BACE (beta-site APP cleaving enzyme) is considered a critical component. BACE is a rapidly evolving target for drug discovery in the treatment of AD. Since its isolation and cloning in 1999, the understanding of BACE has advanced rapidly. Now both academic groups and pharmaceutical companies are actively working to identify BACE inhibitors that could advance into the clinic.

BACE has been shown to be the first step in the aberrant processing of neuronal amyloid precursor protein (APP) leading to the formation of Aβ peptide found in the amyloid plaques, which are hallmarks of the disease. BACE is an aspartyl protease much like the HIV protease that is the target of a number of AIDS drugs. As in AIDS where effective control of the disease first was achieved with HIV protease inhibitors, it is hoped that potent BACE inhibitors would provide the way to effectively treat AD. An advantage of BACE as a drug discovery target is that it has been crystallized and its 3D structure has been solved, and this means that medicinal chemists have a greater possibility of designing potent BACE inhibitors. However, unlike HIV protease inhibitors, BACE inhibitors have the additional hurdle of crossing the blood–brain barrier for treatment of AD.

This book discusses the development of BACE inhibitors as therapeutics for AD and the research that led to the identification of BACE and new BACE inhibitors that have advanced to the clinic – the work described here will be useful to all scientists involved in this field. In addition, the book provides insights into new mechanisms for the APP-based memory dysfunction in AD besides its role as a precursor of Aβ. The detailed story of the discovery of BACE and its potential role in AD, the biochemical assays used in the development of BACE inhibitors, the structural biology work that resulted in greater insights into the enzyme activity and inhibitor binding, and the use of X-ray fragment-based approaches in the development of new BACE inhibitors are outlined in this book. The structure–activity relationships of different series of BACE inhibitors along with the absorption, distribution, metabolism, and excretion (ADME) characteristics of various BACE inhibitors and their contribution to brain bioavailability and efficacy are also outlined. Various animal models available for testing BACE inhibitors and the clinical testing pathway for a first-in-man class BACE inhibitor that is currently in clinical trials are also described. Finally, the last chapter of the book delves into alternative approaches to BACE inhibition based on binding to precursor protein APP.

The intended audience for this book includes chemists, biologists, and clinicians involved in AD research. The book comprehensively covers various aspects of the current drug discovery efforts for BACE inhibitors as potential therapeutics for AD and is envisioned to also have utility as a supplemental text in a medicinal chemistry course. Understanding the various aspects of the BACE drug-discovery process hopefully will facilitate teamwork and enhance productivity among the scientists already working in this area, and potentially could lead to new approaches to treatment of AD. The book also would be informative to AD patients and their families who are trying to understand the various treatment options that may become available in the future. A list of current clinical trial enrollment options for AD is included. The Afterword section of the book illustrates another aspect of the disease that is not well-known but may be relevant to disease progression and therapy – the changes in artistic ability of AD patients as a function of the disease progression.

The BACE story as described in this book – from isolation of the enzyme, to inhibitor development, to structural biology, to *in vivo* testing and development in the clinic, represents a unique drug discovery and development story for a central nervous system (CNS) target. Despite the many research teams involved in the drug discovery efforts, the number of BACE inhibitors reaching the clinic has been scarce. Given that BACE is a key enzyme in APP processing and the production of Aβ peptide in AD, the need for development of effective drugs that block this enzyme is critical in development of new AD therapeutics. This book was written to cover virtually all aspects of this rapidly developing field, both the successes and failures, and to provide members of the diverse drug-discovery team with a global understanding of key aspects of the field essential for productive and successful drug discovery, as well as to offer researchers and clinicians an overview of the groundbreaking progress that has been made to develop inhibitors of BACE for treatment of AD.

Varghese John, PhD

Color figures can be accessed at ftp://ftp.wiley.com/public/sci_tech_med/BACE

ACKNOWLEDGMENTS

The editor gratefully acknowledges the contributions of all the authors of the chapters of this book, and is grateful for their time and their dedication in putting together an informative update on BACE inhibitors and the search for effective therapies for Alzheimer's disease. The editor is very thankful to Molly Susag for the administrative assistance and Loretta Sheridan for the book cover design and artwork. The editor is also thankful to the members of the Alzheimer's Drug Discovery Network (ADDN) at the Buck Institute for discussions of the book. Finally, the author would like to acknowledge the support of his family in this effort.

CONTRIBUTORS

Ruth Abraham, MA, Herzlia Pituach, Israel

Michal Arbel-Ornath, PhD, Department of Molecular Microbiology & Biotechnology, George S. Wise Faculty of Life Sciences, Tel-Aviv University, Tel Aviv, Israel

James P. Beck, PhD, Discovery Chemistry Research & Technology, Lilly Research Laboratories, Eli Lilly and Company, Indianapolis, IN

Dale E. Bredesen, MD, Buck Institute for Age Research, Novato, CA; Department of Neurology, University of California, San Francisco, CA

Michael J. Bienkowski, PhD, Pfizer Inc., Saint Louis, MO

Emmanuel Demont, PhD, GlaxoSmithKline R&D, Hertfordshire, United Kingdom

Jason L. Eriksen, PhD, Department of Pharmacological and Pharmaceutical Sciences, University of Houston, Houston, TX

Elizabeth Head, PhD, Department of Molecular and Biomedical Pharmacology, Department of Molecular and Cellular Biochemistry and the Sanders-Brown Center on Aging, University of Kentucky, Lexington, KY

Robert L. Hendrickson, PhD, Proteos, Inc., Kalamazoo, MI

Michael Hennig, PhD, F. Hoffmann-La Roche Ltd, Basel, Switzerland

Henry H. Hsu, MD, CoMentis, Inc., South San Francisco, CA

Ishrut Hussain, PhD, GlaxoSmithKline R&D, Harlow, United Kingdom

Varghese John, PhD, Buck Institute for Age Research, Novato, CA

Edward H. Koo, MD, Department of Neurosciences, University of California at San Diego, La Jolla, CA

Andreas Kuglstatter, PhD, Roche Palo Alto LLC, Palo Alto, CA

Clare-Peters Libeu, PhD, Buck Institute for Age Research, Novato, CA

Dustin J. Mergott, PhD, Discovery Chemistry Research & Technology, Lilly Research Laboratories, Eli Lilly and Company, Indianapolis, IN

Michael Paul Murphy, PhD, Department of Molecular and Cellular Biochemistry and the Sanders-Brown Center on Aging, University of Kentucky, Lexington, KY

Veerabahu Shanmugasundaram, PhD, Pfizer Global Research and Development, Groton, CT

Sukanto Sinha, PhD, Active Site Pharmaceuticals, Inc., Berkeley, CA

Beka Solomon, PhD, Department of Molecular Microbiology & Biotechnology, George S. Wise Faculty of Life Sciences, Tel-Aviv University, Tel Aviv, Israel

Alfredo G. Tomasselli, PhD, Pfizer Inc., Saint Louis, MO

Felix F. Vajdos, PhD, Pfizer Global Research and Development, Groton, CT

CHAPTER 1

BACE, APP PROCESSING, AND SIGNAL TRANSDUCTION IN ALZHEIMER'S DISEASE

Dale E. Bredesen[1,2] *and Edward H. Koo*[3]

[1]Buck Institute for Age Research, Novato, [2]Department of Neurology, University of California, San Francisco, and [3]Department of Neurosciences, University of California at San Diego, La Jolla, CA

1.1 INTRODUCTION

Alzheimer's disease (AD) is a remarkably, and to date inexplicably, common disease, affecting over five million Americans at a national cost of approximately $150 billion annually – a cost that does not begin to address the impact of the disease on families, individuals, and society. With the graying of America, the prediction is for approximately 13 million cases by 2050 and, given the late appearance of symptoms in the pathogenic process, many more pre-Alzheimer's cases, including both mild cognitive impairment (MCI) and pre-MCI conditions. Thus, AD is unfolding as one of the most important global health concerns.

Since the first description of the disease just over 100 years ago, extensive clinical, pathological, genetic, and biochemical data have been accumulated, implicating the amyloid-beta (Aβ) peptides, especially Aβ1-42, as key mediators in the pathogenesis of this disorder, the so-called amyloid cascade hypothesis. However, the physiological role of these peptides remains unknown, as does the mechanism(s) of their neurodegenerative effect.

The Aβ peptides are derived proteolytically from the β-amyloid precursor protein (APP) by β-site APP cleaving enzyme (BACE) (or β-secretase) cleavage of the extracellular domain, followed by γ-secretase cleavage of the transmembrane domain. However, APP is also cleaved at other sites, for example, at the α-site by α-secretase (with ADAM10 being the most likely candidate) and at the cytosolic caspase site by caspases (with caspase-8 and caspase-6 being the most likely candidates, given their P4 preference along with co-immunoprecipitation and kinetic data). With four major cleavage sites, theoretically 14 peptides could be produced, and it is becoming more apparent that other APP-derived peptides beyond Aβ also play critical roles in elements of the Alzheimer's phenotype [1–3]. Therefore, Aβ may turn out to be one part of a much larger pathogenetic scenario, and thus, BACE may ultimately be one target of a cocktail of drugs that modulates APP processing at more than one site, as well as affecting targets other than APP.

In neurodegenerative diseases such as AD, neurons in various nuclei are lost in disease-specific distributions. However, the neuronal loss is a relatively late event, typically following synaptic dysfunction, synaptic loss, neurite retraction, and the appearance of other abnormalities such as axonal transport defects. This progression argues that cell death programs may play at best only a secondary role in the neurodegenerative process. However, emerging evidence from several laboratories has suggested an alternative possibility: that although cell death itself occurs late in the degenerative process, the pathways involved in cell death *signaling* do indeed play critical roles in neurodegeneration, both in sub-apoptotic events such as synapse loss and in the ultimate neuronal loss itself [3–6].

Although initial comparisons of the intrinsic suicide program in genetically tractable organisms such as the nematode *Caenorhabditis elegans* failed to disclose obvious relationships to genes associated with familial AD – for example, presenilin-1 and the β-APP do not bear an obvious relationship to any of the major *C. elegans* cell death genes (ced-3, ced-4, or ced-9) – more recent studies suggest a fundamental relationship between developmental and degenerative processes [3, 4, 7–10]. For example, Nikolaev et al. recently found that in a culture model of trophic factor withdrawal in developing neurons, one pathway involved in neurite retraction is mediated by a cleavage product of sAPPβ [3], the latter released after BACE cleavage of APP. A detailed understanding of the interrelationship between fundamental cell death programs and neurodegenerative processes is still evolving, and it promises to offer novel approaches to the treatment of these diseases. In this review, we will discuss BACE cleavage of APP and how it might be involved in certain aspects of Alzheimer's pathology.

1.2 BACE CLEAVAGE OF APP AS A MOLECULAR SWITCHING MECHANISM

Neurons, as well as other cells, depend for their survival on stimulation that is mediated by various receptors and sensors, and programmed cell death may be induced in response to the withdrawal of trophic factors, hormonal support, electrical activity, extracellular matrix support, or other trophic stimuli [11]. For years, it was generally assumed that cells dying as a result of the withdrawal of required stimuli did so because of the loss of a positive survival signal, for example, mediated by receptor tyrosine kinases [12]. While such positive survival signals are clearly critical, data obtained over the past 15 years argue for a complementary effect that is pro-apoptotic, activated by trophic stimulus withdrawal, and mediated by specific receptors dubbed "dependence receptors" [13, 14]. Over a dozen such receptors have now been identified, and examples include DCC (deleted in colorectal cancer), Unc5H2 (uncoordinated gene 5 homologue 2), neogenin, rearranged during transfection (RET), Ptc, and APP [14–24]. These receptors interact in their intracytoplasmic domains with caspases, including apical caspases such as caspase-9, and may there-fore serve as sites of induced proximity and activation of these caspases. Caspase activation leads in turn to receptor cleavage, producing pro-apoptotic fragments [15, 22]; however, caspase cleavage site mutation of dependence receptors suppresses the cell death signals mediated by the receptors [13, 22]. A striking example of this effect was obtained in studies of neural tube development: withdrawal of Sonic hedgehog from the developing chick spinal cord led to apoptosis mediated by its receptor, Patched, preventing spinal cord development; however, transfection of a caspase-uncleavable mutant of Patched blocked apoptosis and restored significant development, even in the absence of Sonic hedgehog [25].

Thus, cellular dependence on specific signals for survival is mediated, at least in part, by specific dependence receptors that induce apoptosis in the absence of the required stimulus – when unoccupied by a trophic ligand, or when bound by a competing, anti-trophic ligand – but block apoptosis following binding to their respective ligands [11, 14, 23]. Expression of these dependence receptors thus creates cellular states of dependence on the associated trophic ligands. These states of dependence are not absolute, since they can be blocked downstream in some cases by the expression of anti-apoptotic genes such as bcl-2 or p35 [11, 20, 26]; however, they result in a shift of the apostat [27, 28] toward an increased likelihood of triggering apoptosis. In the aggregate, these receptors may serve as part of a molecular integration system for trophic signals, analogous to the electrical integration system composed of the dendritic arbors within the nervous system.

Although cellular dependence on trophic signals was originally described in the developing nervous system, neurodegeneration may also utilize the same path-ways, since APP exhibits several features characteristic of dependence receptors: an intracytoplasmic caspase cleavage site (Asp664) [18, 29], co-immunoprecipitation with an apical caspase (caspase-8), caspase activation, derivative pro-apoptotic peptides (including the Aβ peptide; see below), and suppression of apoptosis induc-tion by mutation of the caspase cleavage site [18, 30].

These findings raise several questions: first, does BACE cleavage of APP play a role in APP's putative dependence-related pro-apoptotic function? Second, does the caspase cleavage of APP occur in human brain and, if so, is this increased in patients with AD and coordinated with BACE cleavage? Third, if this cleavage is prevented, is the Alzheimer's phenotype affected? These questions are addressed below.

1.3 AD: AN IMBALANCE IN CELLULAR DEPENDENCE?

Although cellular dependence on trophic signals was originally described in mole-cules and pathways critical for the developing nervous system, degeneration in neurons of the aged organism may also utilize the same pathways. For example, APP, a molecule holding a central position in AD pathogenesis because of its inti-mate relationship to Aβ peptides, exhibits several features characteristic of depen-dence receptors: a caspase cleavage site (Asp664) [1, 29], interaction with an apical caspase (caspase-8), derivative pro-apoptotic peptides released after caspase activation, and suppression of apoptosis induction by mutation of the caspase cleavage site [1, 30, 31]. Although APP demonstrates many of the characteristics of a dependence receptor, what is unclear is whether there is a physiological ligand that maintains the balance of APP in favor of survival rather than neuronal death, as has been seen with other trophic factor receptors.

In this context, BACE may hold a surprising central position. This is because cleavage of APP by BACE generates not only the C-terminal fragment of APP that is the direct precursor of Aβ, but this cleavage also releases sAPPβ, which can interact with DR6 to effect neuronal damage (see below). What is unclear is whether BACE cleavage of APP plays a role in APP's putative dependence-related pro-apoptotic function. And second, whether caspase cleavage of APP occurs in human brain and, if so, is this increased in patients with AD and coordinated with BACE cleavage? And lastly, if this cleavage is prevented, is the Alzheimer's phenotype affected? These questions are addressed below.

Extensive genetic and biochemical data have implicated the Aβ peptide as a central mediator of AD, but the mechanism(s) of action remains controversial: the ability of Aβ to generate a sulfuranyl radical involving methionine 35 has been implicated, and so have its direct effects on postsynaptic structures, the metal-binding property of Aβ, as well as its aggregating property, and its ability to form pore-like structures in membranes, just to list a few of the mechanisms proposed [32]. These proposed mechanisms share a focus on the chemical and physical properties of the Aβ peptide. However, cellular signaling is emerging as a complementary mechanism by which Aβ exerts its critical effects, and multiple candidates have surfaced as key downstream mediators, including APP itself, the insulin receptor, and tau, among others [30, 33, 34]. These cellular signals may also mediate neuronal dependence on trophic support, as described below.

1.4   BACE CLEAVAGE, CASPASE CLEAVAGE, AND NEURONAL TROPHIC DEPENDENCE

Neoepitope antibodies directed against residues 657–664 of human APP disclosed the presence of caspase-cleaved APP fragments in human brain, especially in the hippocampal region [8], with an approximately fourfold increase in Alzheimer's patients over age-matched controls. However, in brains without Alzheimer's pathology, there was an inverse relationship between age and immunohistochemical detection of APPneo, with a different distribution from AD brains: in the Alzheimer brains, the staining was primarily in neuronal somata and peri-neuronally, whereas in the non-Alzheimer brains, the staining was observed predominantly in the processes. These findings suggest that the caspase cleavage of APP occurs physiologically and is reduced with age, but that this process remains more active and perhaps aberrant in cellular distribution in association with AD.

To test whether preventing the caspase cleavage of APP has any consequences on the Alzheimer's phenotype, a transgenic mouse model of age-associated amyloid pathology was generated in which APP containing the Swedish and Indiana familial AD mutations were combined with a mutation of the caspase site (D664A) was expressed under the control of the neuronal-specific platelet-derived growth factor-B (PDGF-B) promoter. Although the caspase mutation (D664A) had no effect on amyloid production or plaque formation, these animals did not exhibit any overt synapse loss, early p21-activated kinase (PAK) phosphorylation, dentate gyral atrophy, electrophysiological abnormalities (including reductions in excitatory post-synaptic potentials [EPSPs] and long-term potentiation [LTP]), neophobia, or memory deficits that frequently characterize these APP overexpressing mice [4, 6, 35]. These findings indicate that key features of the Alzheimer's associated phenotype in a standard transgenic mouse model depend on the presence of the caspase cleavage site within APP. This finding, when combined with the extensive previous work showing that the Alzheimer's phenotype is critically dependent on Aβ, suggests that the APP caspase site may lie downstream from the Aβ accumulation and that cleavage of this site is one pathway that contributes to neuronal injury [30, 33]. This possibility has received support from studies showing that Aβ interacts directly with APP in the Aβ region itself, leading to APP multimerization, caspase cleavage at Asp664, and cell death signaling [30, 33].

1.5   BACE CLEAVAGE OF APP, DEPENDENCE RECEPTORS, AND ALZHEIMER PATHOLOGY

The above model of caspase cleavage of APP focuses primarily on the cytosolic region of APP where the caspase site is situated. Experimental evidence suggested that Aβ-induced multimerization and subsequent caspase cleavage of APP can take place with either APP or the BACE-cleaved C99 APP fragment. However, there did not appear to be any preference between these two substrates. How, then, might BACE cleavage of APP relate to the caspase cleavage of APP? Recent work from the Tessier-Lavigne lab [3] provides surprising new insight into this question: following trophic factor withdrawal from developing neurons in culture, BACE was apparently activated, resulting in the shedding of sAPPβ. Following further processing near the amino-terminus of sAPPβ by an unidentified protease, the resulting amino-terminal peptide of the APP ectodomain was able to interact with death receptor 6 (DR6). This binding led to caspase-6 activation and subsequent neurite retraction, which is of interest given previous studies showing that APP is cleavable by caspase-6, and that its caspase site (VEVD) is indeed most compatible with a caspase-6 site [1]. This is a surprising observation because the large sAPP ectodomain (mainly sAPPα) has traditionally been thought to play a neurotrophic rather than toxic role. Nonetheless, increased BACE cleavage of APP should lead to the production of more Aβ peptide, and this in turn will result in more Aβ–C99 interaction and potentially more caspase cleavage of APP. Thus, BACE cleavage of APP results in two downstream pathways that damage neurons: through the sAPPβ fragment interacting with DR6 receptor (via N-APP production) and through Aβ-induced caspase cleavage of APP C99 fragment.

If APP does indeed function as a dependence receptor, AD may be considered a "state of altered dependence." What then is/are the trophic ligand/s for APP? Several candidate APP interactors have been described, such as collagen (types I and IV), heparan sulfate proteoglycan, glypican, laminin, and F-spondin [36–38]. F-spondin's interaction with APP leads to a reduction in β-secretase activity. Lourenco et al. have recently shown that netrin-1, a multifunctional axon guidance and trophic factor, also binds APP [9]. Furthermore, netrin-1 also interacts with Aβ itself, and Aβ is capable of interfering with netrin-1 binding to APP. The binding of netrin-1 to APP results in enhanced interaction of APP with intracytoplasmic mediators Fe65 and Dab, upregulation of KAI1, and a marked reduction of net Aβ production [9].

These findings suggest a model in which the Aβ peptide functions as an "anti-trophin," first by blocking netrin's guidance and trophic effects and then through

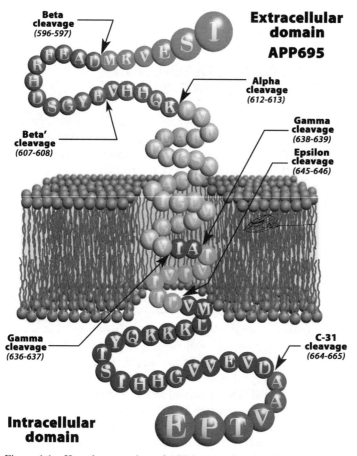

Figure 1.1   Key cleavage sites of APP by proteases involved in normal and aberrant processing. (See color insert.)

binding to and facilitating APP oligomerization, recruiting and activating caspase-8 (and possibly caspase-6), engendering the processing of APP at Asp664, and inducing neurite retraction, then, ultimately, neuronal cell death [4, 30, 33]. Whether the D664A mutation of APP exerts effects beyond the prevention of caspase cleavage (e.g., an alteration of the intracytoplasmic structure of APP) is not yet known. However, regardless of the mechanism, the results suggest that APP signal transduction may be important in mediating AD [39], at least in the transgenic mouse model, possibly downstream from Aβ oligomerization and binding of APP. The results also suggest that BACE cleavage and caspase cleavage of APP may work in concert to lead to neurite retraction, and potentially other aspects of the AD phenotype.

The results obtained in the transgenic mouse model of AD also suggest an alternative to the classic models of AD. As noted above, chemical and physical properties of Aβ have been cited as the proximate cause of AD pathophysiology. However, these theories do not explain why Aβ is produced ubiquitously and constitutively, nor do they offer a physiological function for the Aβ peptide, or account for the improvement in AD model mice that occurs with a reduction in tau protein [34].

An alternative model, presented in Figs. 1.1–1.3, proposes that APP is indeed a dependence receptor, and that it functions normally as a molecular switch in *synaptic element interdependence* (Fig. 1.4): in this model, both the presynaptic element and the postsynaptic element are dependent on trophic support, including soluble factors such as netrin, substrate adherence molecules such as laminin, neurotransmitters, and neuronal activity, as well as other factors. In the presence of adequate trophic support, APP is cleaved at the α- and γ-secretase sites, generating three peptides – sAPPα, p3, and APP intracytoplasmic domain (AICD) – that support cell

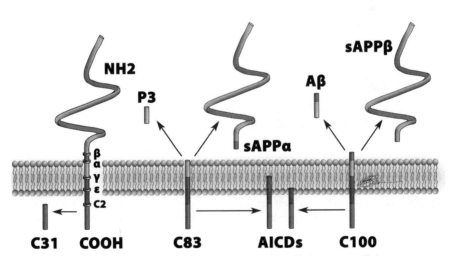

Figure 1.2   Alternative cleavage patterns of APP generate distinct extracellular, transmembrane, and intracytoplasmic fragments. (See color insert.)

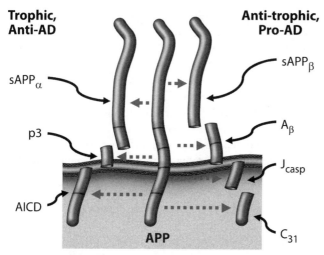

Figure 1.3   Alternative cleavage of APP to produce four peptides that mediate synaptic loss, neurite retraction, and ultimately, programmed cell death ("the four horsemen"); or three peptides that mediate synaptic maintenance and inhibit programmed cell death ("the wholly trinity"). Among the factors that mediate the decision between these two pathways are included trophic effects such as netrin-1 and anti-trophic effects such as Aβ peptide.

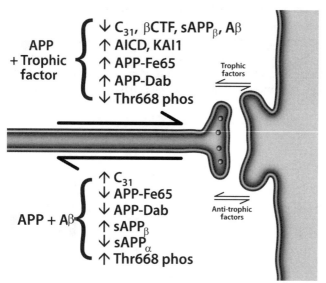

Figure 1.4   Synaptic element interdependence model of synaptic maintenance, reorganization, and Alzheimer's disease. The presynaptic and postsynaptic elements are interdependent, and provide both trophic influences (e.g., neurotrophins, netrin-1, laminin, collagen, and synaptic activity itself) and anti-trophic influences (e.g., amyloid-β peptide). Trophic support leads to the processing of APP into three peptides that support synaptic maintenance, whereas the withdrawal of trophic support leads to alternative processing, to four peptides that mediate synaptic inhibition, synaptic loss, neurite retraction and, ultimately, programmed cell death. In this model, the Aβ peptide functions as an anti-trophin and, since it leads to APP processing that produces additional Aβ peptide, it is "prionic," that is, Aβ begets additional Aβ.

survival and synaptic maintenance. However, a reduction in trophic support (e.g., due to head trauma) alters the processing of APP, thereby activating BACE cleavage of APP to alter the ratio of α/β cleavages, and leading to the production of four peptides – sAPPβ, Aβ, Jcasp, and C31 (Fig. 1.3) – that mediate a reduction in synaptic transmission, synaptic loss, neurite retraction and, ultimately, programmed cell death [1, 3, 4, 9, 35]. In this model, neuronal and synaptic injury in AD is suggested to result from an imbalance in physiological signaling pathways that mediate synaptic maintenance versus synaptic reorganization, mediated at least in part by APP, functioning in synaptic element interdependence (Fig. 1.4), as part of a plasticity module that includes other receptors such as the common neurotrophin receptor, p75[NTR] and the axon guidance receptor DCC, among others [40].

1.6 KEY MUTATIONS PROXIMAL OF APP PROCESSING TO Aβ

Mutations in APP that are associated with familial AD typically affect Aβ processing and lead to an increase in the ratio of Aβ1-42 to Aβ1-40. These mutations may be located in proximity to the β-cleavage site or the γ-cleavage site. Mutations near the α-secretase cleavage site affect the primary structure of the Aβ peptide, and are often associated with cerebral hemorrhagic syndromes, but in at least some cases, such as the Arctic mutation (see Table 1.1), also lead to AD.

TABLE 1.1 APP Mutations Around the Key Cleavage Sites Involved in APP Processing

Nearest cleavage site	Mutation	Type	References
Beta-site	Lys670 → Asn	Swedish	Mullan et al., 1992 [41]
	Met671 → Leu	Swedish	
Alpha-site	Ala692 → Gly	Flemish	Kumar-Singh et al., 2002 [42]
	Glu693 → Gln	Dutch	Van Broeckhoven et al., 1990 [43]
	Glu693 → Gly	Arctic	Nilsbeth et al., 2001 [44]
	Asp694 → Asn	Iowa	Grabowski et al., 2001 [45]
Gamma-site	Ala713 → Thr	Austrian	Carter et al. 1992 [46]
	Thr714 → Ile/Ala	Austrian/Iranian	Kumar-Singh et al., 2000 [47]; Pasalar et al., 2002 [48]
	Val715 → Met	French	Ancolio et al., 1999 [49]
	Ile716 → Val	Florida	Eckman et al., 1997 [50]
	Val717 → Phe/Gly/Ile	Indiana/ /London	Murell et al., 1991 [51]; Chartier-Harlin et al., 1991 [52]; Goate et al., 1991 [53]
Epsilon-site	Leu723 → Pro	Australian	Kwok et al., 2000 [54]
	Lys724 → Asn	Belgium	Theuns et al., 2006 [55]

1.7 FINAL REMARKS

BACE processing of APP represents an important therapeutic target in AD. However, such processing may be part of a larger set of pathogenetic events in this disease, featuring imbalanced signal transduction mediated by APP and potentially other receptors.

ACKNOWLEDGMENTS

We thank Molly Susag and Loretta Sheridan for manuscript preparation, and members of the Bredesen laboratory for discussion and critical reading of the manuscript.

REFERENCES

1. Lu, D.C., Rabizadeh, S., Chandra, S., Shayya, R.F., Ellerby, L.M., Ye, X., Salvesen, G.S., Koo, E.H., and Bredesen, D.E. 2000. A second cytotoxic proteolytic peptide derived from amyloid β-protein precursor [see comments]. *Nat Med* **6**:397–404.
2. Madeira, A., Pommet, J.M., Prochiantz, A., and Allinquant, B. 2005. SET protein (TAF1beta, I2PP2A) is involved in neuronal apoptosis induced by an amyloid precursor protein cytoplasmic subdomain. *FASEB J* **9**:1905–1907.
3. Nikolaev, A., McLaughlin, T., O'Leary, D.D., and Tessier-Lavigne, M. 2009. APP binds DR6 to trigger axon pruning and neuron death via distinct caspases. *Nature* **457**:981–989.
4. Galvan, V., Gorostiza, O.F., Banwait, S., Ataie, M., Logvinova, A.V., Sitaraman, S., Carlson, E., Sagi, S.A., Chevallier, N., Jin, K., Greenberg, D.A., and Bredesen, D.E. 2006. Reversal of Alzheimer's-like pathology and behavior in human APP transgenic mice by mutation of Asp664. *Proc Natl Acad Sci U S A* **103**:7130–7135.
5. Graham, R.K., Deng, Y., Slow, E.J., Haigh, B., Bissada, N., Lu, G., Pearson, J., Shehadeh, J., Bertram, L., Murphy, Z., Warby, S.C., Doty, C.N., Roy, S., Wellington, C.L., Leavitt, B.R., Raymond, L.A., Nicholson, D.W., and Hayden, M.R. 2006. Cleavage at the caspase-6 site is required for neuronal dysfunction and degeneration due to mutant huntingtin. *Cell* **125**:1179–1191.
6. Saganich, M.J., Schroeder, B.E., Galvan, V., Bredesen, D.E., Koo, E.H., and Heinemann, S.F. 2006. Deficits in synaptic transmission and learning in amyloid precursor protein (APP) transgenic mice require C-terminal cleavage of APP. *J Neurosci* **26**:13428–13436.
7. Yang, F., Sun, X., Beech, W., Teter, B., Wu, S., Sigel, J., Vinters, H.V., Frautschy, S.A., and Cole, G.M. 1998. Antibody to caspase-cleaved actin detects apoptosis in differentiated neuroblastoma and plaque-associated neurons and microglia in Alzheimer's disease. *Am J Pathol* **152**:379–389.
8. Banwait, S., Galvan, V., Zhang, J., Gorostiza, O.F., Ataie, M., Huang, W., Crippen, D., Koo, E.H., and Bredesen, D.E. 2008. C-terminal cleavage of the amyloid-beta protein precursor at Asp664: a switch associated with Alzheimer's disease. *J Alzheimers Dis* **13**:1–16.
9. Lourenco, F.C., Galvan, V., Fombonne, J., Corset, V., Llambi, F., Muller, U., Bredesen, D.E., and Mehlen P. 2009. Netrin-1 interacts with amyloid precursor protein and regulates amyloid-beta production. *Cell Death Differ* **16**:655–663.
10. Zhao, M., Su, J., Head, E., and Cotman, C.W. 2003. Accumulation of caspase cleaved amyloid precursor protein represents an early neurodegenerative event in aging and in Alzheimer's disease. *Neurobiol Dis* **14**:391–403.
11. Bredesen, D.E., Ye, X., Tasinato, A., Sperandio, S., Wang, J.J., Assa-Munt, N., and Rabizadeh, S. 1998. p75NTR and the concept of cellular dependence: seeing how the other half die [see comments]. *Cell Death Differ* **5**:365–371.
12. Yao, R. and Cooper, G.M. 1995. Requirement for phosphatiylinositol-3 kinase in the prevention of apoptosis by nerve growth factor. *Science* **267**:2003–2006.

13. Bredesen, D.E., Mehlen, P., and Rabizadeh, S. 2004. Apoptosis and dependence receptors: a molecular basis for cellular addiction. *Physiol Rev* **84**:411–430.

14. Rabizadeh, S., Oh, J., Zhong, L.T., Yang, J., Bitler, C.M., Butcher, L.L., and Bredesen, D.E. 1993. Induction of apoptosis by the low-affinity NGF receptor. *Science* **261**:345–348.

15. Ellerby, L.M., Hackam, A.S., Propp, S.S., Ellerby, H.M., Rabizadeh, S., Cashman, N.R., Trifiro, M.A., Pinsky, L., Wellington, C.L., Salvesen, G.S., Hayden, M.R., and Bredesen, D.E. 1999. Kennedy's disease: caspase cleavage of the androgen receptor is a crucial event in cytotoxicity. *J Neurochem* **72**:185–195.

16. Barrett, G.L. and Bartlett, P.F. 1994. The p75 nerve growth factor receptor mediates survival or death depending on the stage of sensory neuron development. *Proc Natl Acad Sci U S A* **91**:6501–6505.

17. Barrett, G.L. and Georgiou, A. 1996. The low-affinity nerve growth factor receptor p75NGFR mediates death of PC12 cells after nerve growth factor withdrawal. *J Neurosci Res* **45**:117–128.

18. Bordeaux, M.C., Forcet, C., Granger, L., Corset, V., Bidaud, C., Billaud, M., Bredesen, D.E., Edery, P., and Mehlen, P. 2000. The RET proto-oncogene induces apoptosis: a novel mechanism for Hirschsprung disease. *EMBO J* **19**:4056–4063.

19. Bredesen, D.E. and Rabizadeh, S. 1997. p75NTR and apoptosis: Trk-dependent and Trk-independent effects. *Trends Neurosci* **20**:287–290.

20. Forcet, C., Ye, X., Granger, L., Corset, V., Shin, H., Bredesen, D.E., and Mehlen, P. 2001. The dependence receptor DCC (deleted in colorectal cancer) defines an alternative mechanism for caspase activation. *Proc Natl Acad Sci U S A* **98**:3416–3421.

21. Llambi, F., Causeret, F., Bloch-Gallego, E., and Mehlen, P. 2001. Netrin-1 acts as a survival factor via its receptors UNC5H and DCC. *EMBO J* **20**:2715–2722.

22. Mehlen, P., Rabizadeh, S., Snipas, S.J., Assa-Munt, N., Salvesen, G.S., and Bredesen, D.E. 1998. The DCC gene product induces apoptosis by a mechanism requiring receptor proteolysis. *Nature* **395**:801–804.

23. Rabizadeh, S. and Bredesen, D.E. 1994. Is p75NGFR involved in developmental neural cell death? *Dev Neurosci* **16**:207–211.

24. Stupack, D.G., Puente, X.S., Boutsaboualoy, S., Storgard, C.M., and Cheresh, D.A. 2001. Apoptosis of adherent cells by recruitment of caspase-8 to unligated integrins. *J Cell Biol* **155**:459–470.

25. Thibert, C., Teillet, M.A., Lapointe, F., Mazelin, L., Le Douarin, N.M., and Mehlen, P. 2003. Inhibition of neuroepithelial patched-induced apoptosis by sonic hedgehog. *Science* **301**:843–846.

26. Mah, S.P., Zhong, L.T., Liu, Y., Roghani, A., Edwards, R.H., and Bredesen, D.E. 1993. The proto-oncogene bcl-2 inhibits apoptosis in PC12 cells. *J Neurochem* **60**:1183–1186.

27. Bredesen, D.E. 1996. Keeping neurons alive: the molecular control of apoptosis (part I). *Neuroscientist* **2**:181–190.

28. Salvesen, G.S. and Dixit, V.M. 1997. Caspases: intracellular signaling by proteolysis. *Cell* **91**:443–446.

29. Gervais, F.G., Xu, D., Robertson, G.S., Vaillancourt, J.P., Zhu, Y., Huang, J., LeBlanc, A., Smith, D., Rigby, M., Shearman, M.S., Clarke, E.E., Zheng, H., Van Der Ploeg, L.H., Ruffolo, S.C., Thornberry, N.A., Xanthoudakis, S., Zamboni, R.J., Roy, S., and Nicholson, D.W. 1999. Involvement of caspases in proteolytic cleavage of Alzheimer's amyloid-beta precursor protein and amyloidogenic A beta peptide formation. *Cell* **97**:395–406.

30. Lu, D.C., Shaked, G.M., Masliah, E., Bredesen, D.E., and Koo, E.H. 2003. Amyloid beta protein toxicity mediated by the formation of amyloid-beta protein precursor complexes. *Ann Neurol* **54**:781–789.

31. Lu, D.C., Soriano, S., Bredesen, D.E., and Koo, E.H. 2003. Caspase cleavage of the amyloid precursor protein modulates amyloid beta-protein toxicity. *J Neurochem* **87**:733–741.

32. Butterfield, D.A. and Bush, A.I. 2004. Alzheimer's amyloid beta-peptide (1-42): involvement of methionine residue 35 in the oxidative stress and neurotoxicity properties of this peptide. *Neurobiol Aging* **25**:563–568.

33. Shaked, G.M., Kummer, M.P., Lu, D.C., Galvan, V., Bredesen, D.E., and Koo, E.H. 2006. Aβ induces cell death by direct interaction with its cognate extracellular domain on APP (APP 597-624). *FASEB J* **20**:1254–1256.

34. Roberson, E.D., Scearce-Levie, K., Palop, J.J., Yan, F., Cheng, I.H., Wu, T., Gerstein, H., Yu, G.Q., and Mucke, L. 2007. Reducing endogenous tau ameliorates amyloid beta-induced deficits in an Alzheimer's disease mouse model. *Science* **316**:750–754.

35. Nguyen, T.V., Galvan, V., Huang, W., Banwait, S., Tang, H., Zhang, J., and Bredesen, D.E. 2008. Signal transduction in Alzheimer disease: p21-activated kinase signaling requires C-terminal cleavage of APP at Asp664. *J Neurochem* **104**:1065–1080.

36. Beher, D., Hesse, L., Masters, C.L., and Multhaup, G. 1996. Regulation of amyloid protein precursor (APP) binding to collagen and mapping of the binding sites on APP and collagen type I. *J Biol Chem* **271**:1613–1620.

37. Caceres, J. and Brandan, E. 1997. Interaction between Alzheimer's disease beta A4 precursor protein (APP) and the extracellular matrix: evidence for the participation of heparan sulfate proteoglycans. *J Cell Biochem* **65**:145–158.

38. Williamson, T.L., Marszalek, J.R., Vechio, J.D., Bruijn, L.I., Lee, M.K., Xu, Z., Brown, R.H. Jr., and Cleveland, D.W. 1996. Neurofilaments, radial growth of axons, and mechanisms of motor neuron disease. *Cold Spring Harb Symp Quant Biol* **61**:709–723.

39. Nishimoto, I. 1998. A new paradigm for neurotoxicity by FAD mutants of betaAPP: a signaling abnormality. *Neurobiol Aging* **19**:S33–S38.

40. Fombonne, J., Rabizadeh, S., Banwait, S., Mehlen, P., and Bredesen, D.E. 2009. Selective vulnerability in Alzheimer's disease: amyloid precursor protein and p75(NTR) interaction. *Ann Neurol* **65**:294–303.

41. Mullan, M., Crawford, F., Axelman, K., Houlden, H., Lilius, L., Winblad, B., and Lannfelt, L. 1992. A pathogenic mutation for probable Alzheimer's disease in the APP gene at the N-terminus of beta-amyloid. *Nat Genet* **1**:345–347.

42. Kumar-Singh, S., Cras, P., Wang, R., Kros, J.M., van Swieten, J., Lubke, U., Ceuterick, C., Serneels, S., Vennekens, K., Timmermans, J.P., Van Marck, E., Martin, J.J., van Duijn, C.M., and Van Broeckhoven, C. 2002. Dense-core senile plaques in the Flemish variant of Alzheimer's disease are vasocentric. *Am J Pathol* **161**:507–520.

43. Van Broeckhoven, C., Haan, J., Bakker, E., Hardy, J.A., Van Hul, W., Wehnert, A., Vegter-Van der Vlis, M., and Roos, R.A. 1990. Amyloid beta protein precursor gene and hereditary cerebral hemorrhage with amyloidosis (in Dutch). *Science* **248**:1120–1122.

44. Nilsbeth, C., Westlind-Danielsson, A., Eckman, C.B., Condron, M.M., Axelman, K., Forsell, C., Stenh, C., Luthman, J., Teplow, D.B., Younkin, S.G., Naslund, J., and Lannfelt, L. 2001. The "Arctic" APP mutation (E693G) causes Alzheimer's disease by enhanced Abeta protofibril formation. *Nat Neurosci* **4**:887–893.

45. Grabowski, T.J., Cho, H.S., Vonsattel, J.P., Rebeck, G.W., and Greenberg, S.M. 2001. Novel amyloid precursor protein mutation in an Iowa family with dementia and severe cerebral amyloid angiopathy. *Ann Neurol* **49**:697–705.

46. Carter, D.A., Desmarais, E., Bellis, M., Campion, D., Clerget-Darpoux, F., Brice, A., Agid, Y., Jaillard-Serradt, A., and Mallet, J. 1992. More missense in amyloid gene. *Nat Genet* **2**:255–256.

47. Kumar-Singh, S., De Jonghe, C., Cruts, M., Kleinert, R., Wang, R., Mercken, M., De Strooper, B., Vanderstichele, H., Lofgren, A., Vanderhoeven, I., Backhovens, H., Vanmechelen, E., Kroisel, P.M., and Van Broeckhoven, C. 2000. Nonfibrillar diffuse amyloid deposition due to a gamma(42)-secretase site mutation points to an essential role for N-truncated A beta(42) in Alzheimer's disease. *Hum Mol Genet* **9**:2589–2598.

48. Pasalar, P., Najmabadi, H., Noorian, A.R., Moghimi, B., Jannati, A., Soltanzadeh, A., Krefft, T., Crook, R., and Hardy, J. 2002. An Iranian family with Alzheimer's disease caused by a novel APP mutation (Thr714Ala). *Neurology* **58**:1574–1575.

49. Ancolio, K., Dumanchin, C., Barelli, H., Warter, J.M., Brice, A., Campion, D., Frebourg, T., and Checler, F. 1999. Unusual phenotypic alteration of beta amyloid precursor protein (betaAPP) maturation by a new Val-715 → Met betaAPP-770 mutation responsible for probable early-onset Alzheimer's disease. *Proc Natl Acad Sci U S A* **96**:4119–4124.

50. Eckman, C.B., Mehta, N.D., Crook, R., Perez-tur, J., Prihar, G., Pfeiffer, E., Graff-Radford, N., Hinder, P., Yager, D., Zenk, B., Refolo, L.M., Prada, C.M., Younkin, S.G., Hutton, M., and Hardy, J. 1997. A new pathogenic mutation in the APP gene (I716V) increases the relative proportion of A beta 42(43). *Hum Mol Genet* **6**:2087–2089.

51. Murrell, J., Farlow, M., Ghetti, B., and Benson, M.D. 1991. A mutation in the amyloid precursor protein associated with hereditary Alzheimer's disease. *Science* **254**:97–99.

52. Chartier-Harlin, M.C., Crawford, F., Houlden, H., Warren, A., Hughes, D., Fidani, L., Goate, A., Rossor, M., Roques, P., Hardy, J. et al. 1991. Early-onset Alzheimer's disease caused by mutations at codon 717 of the beta-amyloid precursor protein gene. *Nature* **353**:844–846.

53. Goate, A., Chartier-Harlin, M.C., Mullan, M., Brown, J., Crawford, F., Fidani, L., Giuffra, L., Haynes, A., Irving, N., James, L. et al. 1991. Segregation of a missense mutation in the amyloid precursor protein gene with familial Alzheimer's disease. *Nature* **349**:704–706.

54. Kwok, J.B., Li, Q.X., Hallupp, M., Whyte, S., Ames, D., Beyreuther, K., Masters, C.L., and Schofield, P.R. 2000. Novel Leu723Pro amyloid precursor protein mutation increases amyloid beta42(43) peptide levels and induces apoptosis. *Ann Neurol* **47**:249–253.

55. Theuns, J., Marjaux, E., Vandenbulcke, M., Van Laere, K., Kumar-Singh, S., Bormans, G., Brouwers, N., Van den Broeck, M., Vennekens, K., Corsmit, E., Cruts, M., De Strooper, B., Van Broeckhoven, C., and Vandenberghe, R. 2006. Alzheimer dementia caused by a novel mutation located in the APP C-terminal intracytosolic fragment. *Hum Mutat* **27**:888–896.

CHAPTER 2

IDENTIFICATION OF BACE AS A TARGET IN ALZHEIMER'S DISEASE

Robert L. Heinrikson[1] and Sukanto Sinha[2]

[1]Proteos, Inc., Kalamazoo, MI and [2]Active Site Pharmaceuticals, Inc., Berkeley, CA

2.1 INTRODUCTION

Disease processes usually leave molecular clues as to the etiology, progression, or terminal events in the pathology. A major effort in contemporary research is focused on identifying causal relationships between these clues, or biomarkers, and disease that might translate into discovery and development of novel drugs to improve human health. For the most part, these biomarkers are protein in nature: peptides derived from parent proteins by aberrant processing, or proteins themselves that might be upregulated or downregulated in a particular pathology. Completion of the human genome project has, of course, set the stage for these searches by providing a vast database of protein sequences to facilitate identification of new biomarkers and enable connecting the dots linking them to disease.

This chapter concerns the discovery and characterization of a new target in the treatment of Alzheimer's disease (AD), a dreaded unmet and growing medical need. That target is β-site APP cleaving enzyme (BACE) or β-secretase, an enzyme that carries out the first and obligate step in liberation of the beta-amyloid peptide that is found in the brains of Alzheimer's patients. The sequence of events leading to the discovery of BACE parallels the process outlined in the paragraph above. In 1906, Alzheimer noted upon autopsy of the brain from a demented patient the existence of two structural abnormalities: neuritic plaques and neurofibrillary tangles. The neuritic plaques are spherical, multicellular lesions in limbic structures and association neocortices in the AD brain [1]. At that time, the technology for analysis of the plaque components did not exist, but some eight decades later, when protein sequencing had become a readily available method, Glenner and Wong [2] were able to establish the sequence of the 24 NH$_2$-terminal amino acids in a major peptide component of cerebral blood vessel-associated amyloid, now known as the amyloid (Aβ) peptide. Protein database searches led to the discovery that this Aβ peptide was, in all likelihood, generated proteolytically from a larger membrane-bound protein precursor, Aβ-precursor protein (APP). So, over the years the Aβ peptide

BACE: Lead Target for Orchestrated Therapy of Alzheimer's Disease, Edited by Varghese John
Copyright © 2010 John Wiley & Sons, Inc.

and APP have been identified as biomarkers that correlate with generation and deposition of neuritic plaque. These clues point, in turn, to the existence of at least two proteinases that carve out the Aβ peptide from APP and that constitute potentially important targets for inhibition in AD therapy.

2.1.1   APP

The amyloid precursor protein is a ubiquitously expressed Type I membrane protein that exists in three major forms created by alternative splicing and posttranslational modification (cf Reference 3). The smallest of the three is especially abundant in neurons and contains 695 amino acid residues. The larger 751- and 770-residue variants of APP are widely expressed in non-neuronal cells and contain a 56-residue extracellular domain homologous to the well-known Kunitz-type inhibitors of serine proteinases. In fact, from work going back to the late 1980s [4], these larger forms of APP were known as protease nexin-II because of their identification as inhibitors of this mechanistic set of proteolytic enzymes. The inference that the Aβ peptide was derived from an APP precursor was made by a comparative sequence analysis of the Glenner and Wong peptide [2] with protease nexin-II [5] and the deduced sequences of APP [6]. All the wild-type (Wt) APP forms are identical in the region of interest that encompasses Aβ, and this is the region of the protein extending from just outside the membrane on the extracellular domain, and back C-terminally into the membrane about 14 amino acids. This region of Aβ shows a great many mutations that influence the course of processing of Aβ and its toxicity.

2.1.2   Aβ

The amyloid peptide is generally considered to be 40 or 42 amino acids in length depending upon the site of C-terminal processing by the γ-secretase. Figure 2.1 provides a schematic overview of APP processing by the α, β, and γ-secretases [7]. For the purposes of this chapter, our focus will be on the β-site cleaving enzyme. In Fig. 2.1, numbering of sites is based upon the APP^{770} variant having the Kunitz protease inhibitor domain [8]. At the top of Fig. 2.1 is given the amino acid sequence of APP in the region of interest. BACE, or β-secretase, cleaves the Met-Asp^{672} bond and also the Tyr-Glu^{682} bond [9, 10]. This latter processing site is predominant in rat primary neuronal cultures [11]. When the Lys-Met residues at P2 and P1 are mutated to Asn-Leu, such as happens in a cohort of individuals having the so-called Swedish (Sw) mutation [11], processing at Leu-Asp^{672} is enhanced about 10-fold, and the result invariably leads to the early onset of AD. Processing at the C-terminus of Aβ occurs in the membrane usually either at Val-Ile to give $Aβ_{40}$, or at Ala-Thr to give the more highly amyloidogenic $Aβ_{42}$. Also shown in Fig. 2.1 is the site of processing by the α-secretase, a predominant activity that yields fragments of Aβ that are non-amyloidogenic (Panel A). In Panel B is shown the amyloidogenic pathway in which the action of the β- and γ-secretases give rise to $Aβ_{1-40}$ or $Aβ_{1-42}$, the major peptidic components of neuritic plaque.

   Much research has gone into understanding the amyloidogenicity of the Aβ peptides, their physical properties, and ways to prevent their formation that might

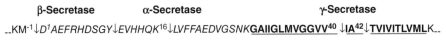

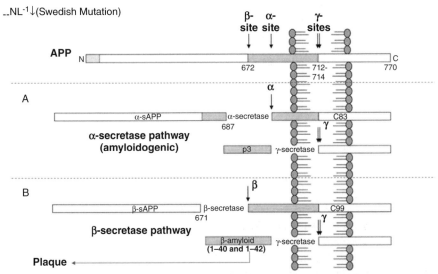

Figure 2.1   Schematic overview of APP processing by the α-, β-, and γ-secretases. The top panel shows the amino acid sequence of APP upstream of the transmembrane segment (underlined, boldface), and encompassing the sequences of $A\beta_{1-40}$ and $A\beta_{1-42}$ (D^1-V^{40} and D^1-A^{42}, respectively). The extracellular portion of Aβ is indicated in italics. β-secretase cleaves at D^1 and Y^{10}; the α-secretase at K^{16}, and the γ-secretase at V^{40} and/or A^{42}. Below the sequence is a representation of APP_{770} emphasizing its membrane localization and the residue numbers of interest in β- and γ-secretase processing. Panel A represents the non-amyloidogenic α-secretase pathway in which sAPPα and C83 (CTF83) are generated. Subsequent hydrolysis by the γ-secretase produces a p3 peptide that does not form amyloid deposits. Panel B represents the amyloidogenic pathway in which cleavage of APP by the β-secretase to liberate sAPPβ and C99 (CTF99) is followed by γ-secretase processing to release the β-amyloid peptides ($A\beta_{1-40}$ and $A\beta_{1-42}$) found in neuritic plaque. (Adapted from Reference 7.)

provide new drugs for AD therapy. Such drugs might induce dissolution of the amyloid aggregates in plaque, or prevent formation of Aβ by compounds that would inhibit the action of the β- or γ-secretases. Clearly, the work of Glenner and Wong [2] and the recognition of APP as the precursor of the Aβ peptides [5, 6] set the stage for an intense search to identify the β- and γ-secretases responsible for production of these amyloid peptides.

2.2   THE SEARCH FOR β-SECRETASE

Knowledge of the features of Aβ, its N- and C-termini, and surrounding amino acids in APP immediately focused attention on what kind of proteolytic enzymes might have been responsible for generating the amyloid peptides [12]. The β-cleavage clearly occurred in the extracellular portion of APP, a process that could have taken place outside the cell thus shedding the major portion of APP, or at some time during transit of APP through the secretory apparatus. The γ-secretase cleavage sites occur at positions predicted to be directly in the middle of the membrane (Fig. 2.1), a most unusual circumstance, given common understanding of proteolytic processing at the time. Now, it is believed that these γ-site cleavages might be mediated by an unusual protease activity that results from juxtaposition of two aspartyl residues in the transmembrane region of proteins called presenilins [13].

In the following narrative, efforts from five independent laboratories that led to the identification of the β-secretase will be described. One approach used expression cloning to identify genes that modulate Aβ production [14]; another involved isolation of the native enzyme from human brain [15]. Three other laboratories followed a notion that the β-secretase might be a new aspartyl protease [16–18], an inference supported by the fact that cathepsin D, a member of the aspartyl protease mechanistic set, was known to mediate both β- and γ-site cleavages in peptide substrates [19]. All of these individual approaches identified the same β-secretase, now commonly known as BACE or BACE1 (which is the isoform of the enzyme that is predominantly expressed in the brain).

Before discussing the discovery of BACE, it might be useful to give an overview of the protein. The amino acid sequence of BACE is shown in Fig. 2.2; the numbering system used here is based upon proBACE, beginning at Thr^1. The pre-proprotein has 501 amino acids comprising a signal peptide of 21 residues, a 432-residue catalytic proBACE unit, a 27-residue transmembrane region, and a 21-residue cytoplasmic domain. BACE is a new member of the mechanistic set of proteinases known as aspartyl proteinases, and it is unusual in being a Type I transmembrane protein. BACE co-localizes with APP in the trans-Golgi/endoplasmic reticulum compartment [14, 17]. Aspartyl proteases cleave peptide bonds by water activated through its association with two aspartyl residues in the catalytic site [20, 21]. The hallmark consensus sequence for the catalytic aspartyl residues is **Asp-Thr/Ser-Gly**, and these signatures are seen at positions 72–74 and 268–270 in proBACE. The existence of these sequences in the two halves of aspartyl enzymes and the internal homology between the halves suggest that aspartyl proteases arose by gene duplication of an ancestral message, followed by divergence [22]. Indeed, one finds in nature the retroviral proteases such as the HIV-protease [23] that correspond to only one-half of a typical member of the class, and must dimerize to yield an active entity. Comparison of the proBACE sequence with other zymogens of the aspartyl proteinase family suggests that the catalytic domain ought to begin somewhere around Gly^{37} to Val^{40}, but BACE isolated from human brain shows a single N-terminal sequence beginning at Glu^{25} [15]. Moreover, preproBACE expressed in mammalian cells is present as a near-equimolar mixture of proBACE beginning at Thr^1 and protein beginning at Glu^{25} [24]. Precursor BACE forms are peculiar compared with the other aspartyl proteinase zymogens in that removal of a prosegment has little effect on activity [24] and forms beginning at Thr^1, Glu^{25}, or Val^{40} all have nearly the same specific catalytic activity. Although the $Arg-Arg^{36}$ sequence suggests a reasonable site for removal of the prosegment based upon processing of related aspartyl prote-

M⁻²¹ AQALPWLLLWMGAGVLPAHG T¹ QHGIRLPLRSGLGGAPLGLRLPR↓E²⁵TDEEP³⁰

EEPGRR³⁶GSF ↓V⁴⁰ EMVDNLRGKSGQGYYVEMTV⁶⁰ GSPPQTLNILV DTG SSNFAV⁸⁰

GAAPHPFLHRYYQRQLSSTY¹⁰⁰ RDLRKGVYVPYTQGKWEGEL¹²⁰ GTDLVSIPHGP *N*V

TVRANLA¹⁴⁰ AITESDKFFI*N* GSNWEGILG¹⁶⁰ LAYAEIARPDDSLEPF FDSL¹⁸⁰ VKQTHVP

NLFSLQLCGAGFP²⁰⁰ L*N* QSEVLASVGGSMIIGGID²²⁰ HSLYTGSLWYTPIRREWYYE²⁴⁰

VIIVRVEINGQDLKMDCKEY²⁶⁰ NYDKSIVDSG TTNLRLPKKV²⁸⁰ FEAAVKSIKAASSTE

KFPDG³⁰⁰ FWLGEQLV C WQAGTTPWNIF³²⁰ PVISLYLMGEVT*N* QSFRITI³⁴⁰ LPQQYLRP

VEDV ATSQDD CY³⁶⁰ KFAISQSSTGTVMGAVIMEG³⁸⁰ FYVVFDRARKRIGFAVSA CH⁴⁰⁰

VHDEFRTAAVEGPFVTLDME⁴²⁰DC GYNIPQTDES⁴³² TLMTIAYV⁴⁴⁰ MAAICALFMLP ·

LCLMVCQWR⁴⁶⁰ CLRCLRQQHDDFADDIS⁴⁷⁷ LLK⁴⁸⁰

Figure 2.2   The complete amino acid sequence of human preproBACE. The 21 amino acid residue leader sequence is in italics, and the 24-aa prosegment is in bold. R↓E²⁵and F↓V⁴⁰ indicate furin and HIV-1 protease [20] cleavage sites, respectively. The two catalytic aspartyl residues are indicated by the **D⁷²TG** and **D²⁶⁸SG** consensus sequences. Four glycosylated asparagines 132, 151, 202, and 333 are in bold-italics, and the predicted O-linked glycosylation site at Thr⁵⁹ is depicted in bold. The 27-residue transmembrane domain is underlined and the cytoplasmic domain extends from K⁴⁶⁰ to the C-terminal K⁴⁸⁰. Six half-cystine residues are paired by disulfide bridges as indicated: (Cys¹⁹⁵ – Cys³⁹⁹, •; Cys²⁵⁷ – Cys⁴²², ♣; Cys³⁰⁹ – Cys³⁵⁹, ♦). A phosphorylation site is at Ser⁴⁷⁷. Most studies done with BACE have been with the catalytic, extracellular domain, terminating at or near S⁴³². Chain-terminating histidine tags to facilitate purification may be incorporated following Ser⁴³² without affecting catalytic activity. (Adapted from Reference 24).

ases, BACE initiating at Gly³⁷ has not been observed from recombinant or natural systems. Interestingly, the HIV protease cleaves proBACE very efficiently and specifically at the Phe-↓-Val⁴⁰ bond to give fully active enzyme [24]. To summarize, the prosegment of BACE is generally referred to as residues Thr¹ to Arg²⁴, and BACE is thought to begin at Glu²⁵. Nevertheless, the concept of the prosegment as a modulator of catalytic activity is not well understood in BACE and may come into play as it functions in its natural biological setting in the secretory pathway.

BACE contains consensus sequences for N-linked glycosylation at asparagines 132, 151, 202, and 333, and an O-linked sugar is predicted at Thr⁵⁹. Glycosylation is not required for catalytic activity, and in fact, the highest resolution X-ray structures [25] have been derived for the non-glycosylated BACE catalytic domain produced in bacteria (cf Chapter 6). The enzyme has been expressed in mammalian, insect, and bacterial host cells, both as the catalytic domain and as precursor forms. Constructs of the catalytic domain generally terminate at or near Ser⁴³². This assures that all three disulfide bonds are included in the structure. More will be said about production of recombinant BACE forms, crystallization, and modeling approaches for inhibitor design in Chapter 6 of this book, and the recent papers of Emmons et al. [24] and Tomasselli et al. [25] provide sources of further discussion and references. With this overall view of BACE and its precursor forms, we turn to the story of how this unique membrane-bound aspartyl protease was discovered independently by five laboratories at the close of the last century.

2.2.1 Amgen Approach: Expression Cloning [14]

A classic expression cloning approach was utilized by scientists at Amgen to identify the enzyme that cleaves at the N-terminus of the Aβ sequence. Human embryonic kidney (HEK293) cells had been widely used from 1988 onward to study all aspects of APP expression and metabolism in cells [26], and Aβ and β-sAPP formation from both Wt [27] and Sw APP [28] had already been previously described in these cells. Therefore, the Amgen group reasoned that the enzymes that generate Aβ must, by definition, also reside in such cells, and an expression library constructed from HEK293 cell cDNA would be expected to encode the cDNA for both β- and γ-secretases. As described in Vassar et al. [14], the primary screening strategy for identifying such enzymes was (1) to transiently transfect the cDNA library, in pools of ~100 clones, into HEK293 cells stably transfected with Sw APP, and (2) to simultaneously monitor the conditioned medium from such transfections using two separate sandwich enzyme linked immunosorbant assay (ELISA)-based assays for Aβ, one that measured all forms of Aβ (cf Fig. 2.1) starting at position 1 ($A\beta_{1-x}$) and another that measured all forms of Aβ ending at position 42 ($A\beta_{x-42}$). Analysis of sequences from cDNA pools that, when transfected, resulted in relative increases in one or the other of these two measures of Aβ production led to the identification of a 2256 bp cDNA that encoded a novel protein sequence exhibiting significant homology to the pepsin family of aspartyl proteases. Again, the novelty here was a C-terminal extension with a predicted transmembrane domain. Transfection of this cDNA into HEK293 cells overexpressing Wt APP led to increases in Aβ, as measured by either $A\beta_{1-x}$ or $A\beta_{x-42}$ assays, and also led to a decrease in sAPPα, as might be expected upon overexpression of a β-secretase enzyme. Transfection into HEK293 cells overexpressing Sw APP led to an increase in sAPPβ and a decrease in sAPPα, but no additional increase was detected in Aβ forms being secreted into the conditioned medium of the doubly transfected cells. Analysis of cellular forms of APP with antibodies directed to the C-terminal region of APP revealed that overexpression of the new cDNA along with Sw APP also greatly increased the C-99 fragment that would result upon cleavage of APP by β-secretase, as well as a second C-terminal fragment that started at position 11 of the Aβ sequence, that has come to be known as C-89. A portion of naturally occurring Aβ is known to start at Glu-11, and the C-89 fragment would be the likely precursor of Glu[11] Aβ. Since the overexpression of the novel aspartyl protease resulted in increased levels of metabolites (Aβ, sAPPβ, C-99, C-83) that would be predicted to be generated by β-secretase activity from both Wt and Sw APP (Fig. 2.1), these results indicated that the newly identified enzyme possessed the properties of β-secretase, rather than a γ-secretase. These investigators went on to name this novel protein BACE, a name that has since been widely adopted.

2.2.2   Elan Approch: BACE Isolation from Human Brain [15]

An entirely different, biochemical approach was used by scientists at Elan Pharmaceuticals to identify β-secretase. Knowing that primary neuronal cultures generate larger amounts of Aβ from endogenous APP than do HEK293 cells transfected with Wt APP, and that this is owing to larger amounts of β-secretase cleavage as the APP transits through its maturation pathway, this group reasoned that higher levels of enzyme activity are probably to be found in cells of neuronal origin than in cells of peripheral origin (such as HEK293). The lack of Aβ production in cell culture observed upon transfection of truncated forms of APP that lack the full transmembrane domain of full-length (FL) APP [29] suggested that either stable membrane association, or the entire transmembrane domain, may be required for effective recognition of the APP substrate by β-secretase.

The Elan group therefore devised fusion protein substrates, consisting of the *Escherichia coli* maltose-binding protein (MBP) fused N-terminally to the C-terminal 125 amino acids of APP (MBP-C125) with which to probe for β-secretase enzymatic activity in cells and tissues. Cleavage of this substrate at the β-secretase site generates a novel N-terminal fragment (MBP-C26) and C-99. Using neoepitope antibodies specific to the C-terminal end of MBP-C26, ELISA assays were constructed that could sensitively and specifically detect β-secretase cleavage of this substrate. Although incubation of the fusion protein substrate in *soluble* extracts of either HEK293 cells or primary neuronal cultures at pH 4–8 did not result in detectable cleavage at the β-secretase site, a β-secretase-like enzymatic activity was detected when the *membrane pellets* from these cells were extracted with Triton X-100, and the incubation was carried out in the presence of the detergent. This crude enzyme preparation cleaved the Sw C125 substrate much more efficiently than the corresponding Wt peptide, consistent with the much larger amounts of Aβ generated from Sw APP than Wt APP in cell culture. The crude enzyme activity appeared most robustly upon incubation at pH 4.5–6, and was significantly attenuated at pH >7, indicating a preference for acidic pH. This was consistent with cellular studies of Aβ formation and β-secretase cleavage that suggested that they occurred within intracellular acidic compartments, such as endosomes. Higher levels of enzymatic activity were found in neuronal cultures than in the peripheral cells, and a survey of various mouse organs indicated that the highest levels of enzymatic activity were detected in the brain, with very little, if any, detected in peripheral organs. Strikingly, the enzymatic activity was not inhibited by classical inhibitors of the four major classes of proteases (serine, cysteine, metallo, and aspartyl). Although partial purification of the enzyme activity from postmortem human brain was quickly achieved using lectin affinity chromatography, purification to homogeneity had to await the understanding of the substrate preference of the enzyme, and the subsequent design of a specific inhibitor affinity ligand, as described below.

Characterization of the substrate preference of the partially purified enzyme activity revealed a greatly increased preference for Leu at P1 over Met at that position, in accordance with the *in vivo* preference for the Sw over Wt APP substrate (Fig. 2.1). The P1′ residue could be altered without significant consequence to cleavage efficiency, and substitution of Val for the native Asp at P1′ resulted in a peptide substrate that competed for cleavage of the MBPC125 substrate with an $IC_{50} \sim 3\,\mu M$. Replacement of the P1 Leu with statine (Sta) resulted in a noncleavable peptide (P10-P4' Stat-Val) that inhibited the activity of the enzyme with an $IC_{50} \sim 0.03\,\mu M$. The enzyme activity was subsequently purified 300,000-fold using a sequential four-step procedure, incorporating an affinity purification step involving binding and elution from an immobilized P10-P4' Stat-Val inhibitor.

The purified enzyme gave a single band migrating on sodium dodecyl sulfate polyacrylamide gel electrophoresis (SDS-PAGE) as a ~70 kDa, single chain protein. N-terminal sequence analysis of the human brain enzyme revealed a single new peptide sequence beginning at Glu[25] (Fig. 2.2), which was utilized to obtain an FL cDNA clone, encoding a polypeptide comprising 501 amino acids. Co-expression of the new cDNA along with either Wt or Sw APP into HEK293 cells resulted in increased β-secretase cleavage of both substrates, as well as increases in total Aβ ($A\beta_{1-x}$ and $A\beta_{1-42}$). Co-expression with the Sw APP resulted in almost complete attenuation of α-secretase cleavage, indicating that a combination of the better Sw APP substrate with overexpressed enzyme activity can direct almost all APP into the β-secretase pathway. *In vitro*, the purified enzyme cleaved FL, Wt, or Sw APP at a single site each, generating the corresponding sAPPβ and C-99 fragments.

2.2.3 Pharmacia Approach: Hypothesis and Genome Searches [16]

In 1997, CNS scientists and protein chemists at Pharmacia brainstormed the question as to what kind of protease might be responsible for processing at the β-site(s) in APP. The company had a long tradition of experience with aspartyl protease targets, including renin in the late 1980s [30, 31] and the HIV-protease in the early 1990s [23, 32]. The question of specificity in this class of proteolytic enzymes is not as easily understood as with the serine proteases, and they can hydrolyze peptide bonds over an extended range of pH from pepsin at pH 2 to renin at pH 7–8. Moreover, they vary widely in specificity. The aspartyl protease renin is among the most specific of proteases in having a single known substrate, angiotensinogen. In contrast, the HIV and retroviral enzymes can, in principle, cleave almost any peptide bond, given an appropriate array of amino acids at surrounding sites. Considerable effort was spent at Pharmacia to define the specificity of the HIV protease [33, 34] to aid in design of inhibitors for AIDS therapy [32].

The focus of attention was on regions encompassing the β-site cleavages that take place in the following stretches of sequence as designated by arrows: ...Ile-Ser-Glu-Val-Lys-**Met**-↓-**Asp**[1]-Ala-Glu-Phe-Arg-His[5]..., and again a few residues downstream, thus: ...Arg-His[5]-Asp-Ser-Gly-**Tyr**[10]-↓-**Glu**-Val-His-His-Gln.... The hydrophobic Met and Tyr residues in P1 positions might signal a chymotrypsin-type specificity; Glu or Asp at P1' are rarely, if ever, seen as signals for N-terminal cleavage. Analysis of the specificity of the HIV protease showed that negatively charged Asp and especially Glu residues in the vicinity of the substrate cleavage site were favorable for hydrolysis, whereas a Lys in any position from P2 to P2' prevented cleavage [32, 33]. It was of interest, therefore, to note the presence of Asp and Glu residues in the region encompassing the Asp[1] and Glu[11] processing sites, and also to know that replacement of the Lys residue by Asn in the Sw KM→NL mutation (Fig. 2.1), was part of an alteration in APP sequence that favored cleavage at Asp^1 by 10-fold.

These observations led to the hypothesis that the β-secretase might be an aspartyl protease, an inference supported by the fact that another prominent member of this mechanistic set, cathepsin D, is able to process at both β- and γ-sites [19] *in vitro*. But it appeared that cathepsin D was not the β-secretase, since it had been shown that APP processing to Aβ peptides occurs normally in cathepsin-D-null mice [35]. The most likely possibility was that if BACE was, in fact, an aspartyl protease, it was one yet to be discovered.

Two things were needed to begin the effort to identify a new aspartyl protease: a search algorithm and an appropriate genomic database. Given what has been said above, it was clear that a generalized representation of a modern preproaspartyl protease would be a chain of about 400 amino acids in which the consensus active site sequences, **Asp-Thr/Ser-Gly** (DTG or DSG), would appear twice, once about 80 residues from the N-terminus, and again about 150–200 residues downstream in the second half of the double-domain molecule. The database for the primary search was that of the nematode, *Caenorhabditis elegans*, a small multicellular eukaryote whose genomic sequence was near completion at that time. This nematode has about 19,000 genes, and it offered a resource for enumerating a complete set of aspartyl proteases that could then be used as a bridge to human sequence databases. The aspartyl protease search algorithm was used to interrogate the WormPep database of predicted *C. elegans* proteins and 10 candidate aspartyl proteases were thus identified, together with their chromosomal locations [16]. A secondary search of human expressed sequence tag (EST) databases with the 10 putative aspartyl proteases identified 7 known and 4 new candidate enzymes that were numbered Asps1–4 based upon their order of discovery. Although two of the nematode genes corresponded to human cathepsin D, most of them had no clear vertebrate orthologues. One (T18H9.2), however, bridged to two unusual sequences, Asp1 and Asp2, that showed a DTG sequence in the N-terminal half and DSG in the C-terminal domain [16]. The other two new candidates (Asp3 and Asp4) had been reported in the literature as napsins A and B [36].

Complete sequences for Asp1 and Asp2 identified by the nematode T18H9.2 locus were generated by a combination of EST sequencing, 5′ rapid amplification of cDNA ends by polymerase chain reaction (PCR), and library screening. Both had a feature previously unseen in known aspartyl proteases in that they contained a C-terminal extension with a predicted transmembrane domain [16]. Asp1 mapped to human chromosome 21q22 within the Down's syndrome critical region, and Asp2 to chromosome 11q23-24. Both proteins were shown by Northern hybridization to human tissue blots to be widely expressed, but at highest levels in pancreas. Asp2 also showed high expression in brain, somewhat higher than Asp1. Two Asp2 ESTs were identified in a human astrocyte cDNA library, indicating that Asp2 may be expressed in both neurons and glial cells.

With four new potential candidates for the β- (or γ-) secretase, a panel of antisense oligomers was used to test their possible involvement in APP processing using a stable clone of HEK293 cells engineered to process APP to Aβ peptides at high levels [16]. Transfection of this HEK293 clone, as well as IMR-32 (Institute for Medical Research, Camden, NJ) neuroblastoma cells (expressing neuronal nicotinic acetylcholine receptors) and an engineered mouse Neuro-2A cell line, both of which release $A\beta_{1-40}$ and $A\beta_{1-42}$ in easily measureable concentrations, with a panel of 16 antisense oligomers (four each targeting Asps1–4) showed that only those directed toward Asp2 had a major effect on release of $A\beta$ peptides into the medium. Reversed-sequence oligomers had no effect. The magnitude of these effects ranged from 40% to 80% reduction of both $A\beta_{1-40}$ and $A\beta_{1-42}$ in roughly equal amounts. These findings in three different cell lines provided good support for the idea that Asp2 is involved, directly or indirectly, in $A\beta$ processing in cells of both somatic and neuronal origin.

Because of the intramembrane locale of the γ-site cleavages (Fig. 2.1), it was unlikely that Asp2 could have both β- and γ-secretase activity. In fact, identification of Asp2 as the β-secretase was verified by analysis of the fragments of APP produced in the various cell lines mentioned above. This study was made possible by the availability of monoclonal antibodies to various discrete regions of APP. Residues 1–16 of $A\beta$ (Asp^1–Lys^{16}) contain the epitope to mAb 6E10 and that portion of APP that is amino terminal to Asp^1 is recognized by mAb 22C11. In the antisense experiments, knockdown of the Asp2 gene led to an increase of a soluble form of APP (sAPPα) generated by the α-secretase that was recognized by both of these monoclonal antibodies. In cells not treated with the antisense oligonucleotide, there was a relative increase in sAPPβ that was recognized only by 22C11. With respect to the C-terminal parts of APP remaining after β- or α-secretase cleavage, these would be expected to contain 99 and 83 amino acids (C-Terminal Fragments, CTF99 and CTF83), respectively (Fig. 2.1). As would be expected, the amount of CTF99 was reduced in cells treated with Asp2 antisense oligomers, and was increased in cells transfected with Asp2. These and other cell biological experiments supported the idea that Asp2 specifically facilitates β-site cleavage of APP, an effect that is enhanced in APP with the KM→NL Sw mutation. Asp2 is, therefore, the β-secretase or BACE, and will be henceforth referred to by this generally accepted designation. The amino acid sequence is shown in Fig. 2.2.

Asp1 was also recognized as a unique member of the aspartyl proteinase family by virtue of the fact that it also contains predicted C-terminal transmembrane and cytoplasmic domains [16]. Studies of the purified recombinant Asp1 (now commonly referred to as BACE2) indicate that this enzyme can also process APP, but at a site just downstream of the α-secretase processing site at Lys^{16}-↓-Leu^{17} (Fig. 2.1). The BACE2 cleavage sites [37, 38] are at the Phe^{19}-↓-Phe^{20}, and Phe^{20}-↓-Ala^{21} bonds in the sequence: ... Leu^{17}-Val-Phe-Phe-Ala-Glu-Asp ... (Fig. 2.1). The existence of Glu and Asp residues in P′ sites adjacent to the BACE2 cleavages is another interesting example of the enhancing effect of negatively charged residues adjacent to bonds hydrolyzed by BACE and the HIV protease [34]. BACE2 processing, therefore, would lead to non-amyloidogenic peptide products, similar to those produced via the activity of the α-secretase, and thus limit production of pathogenic forms of $A\beta$. This highlights the concern that inhibitors of BACE developed for treatment of AD not show inhibitory activity toward this very similar relative, BACE2.

2.2.4   SmithKlein Beecham (SKB): Hypothesis and Genome Searches [17]

Scientists at SKB, like those at Pharmacia, also had extensive experience with aspartyl protease targets, and many of the seminal publications on renin and the HIV protease came from these laboratories. Not surprisingly, therefore, workers at SKB were among the earliest to consider the possibility that the β-secretase might be an aspartyl protease. They reported identification of a novel transmembrane aspartyl protease designated, coincidentally with the term used by Pharmacia, Asp2, with high levels of expression in the brain (European Patent Application EPO855444), and later published evidence that Asp2 is the β-secretase [17]. Much of the narrative presented above concerning the Pharmacia discovery pertains to this work as well and need not be repeated here.

The SKB group identified Asp2 using a proprietary EST database screened against a hallmark aspartyl protease structure and subsequently cloned the FL cDNA from a melanoma Marathon-Ready cDNA preparation from Clontech Laboratories, Inc. The cDNA sequence encoded a sequence for their Asp2 that is identical to that shown in Fig. 2.2 above so again, the SKB Asp2 is BACE. Hussain et al. [17] validated this conclusion by a number of cell biological studies similar to those noted above in the other discovery laboratories. Transient transfection of SH-SY5Y APP$_{695}$ cells with BACE gave a significant increase in secretion of sAPPβ, consistent with β-site cleavage (Fig. 2.1). As a control for these studies, cells were transfected with mutant Asp2 in which the catalytic Asp residues were changed to Asn; in these studies there was no increase in sAPPβ. Because of the known β-site activity of cathepsin D [19], this enzyme was transfected into the SH-SY5Y APP$_{695}$ cells and, in contrast to the result with Asp2, there was no increase in sAPPβ. To look at production of C-terminal fragments expected from β- and α-secretase, Asp2 was transfected into COS-7 APP$_{751}$ cells and into the same cells stably transfected with APP bearing the Sw mutation (KM^{652}→NL), and the cells were probed with an antibody that recognizes both CTF83 and CTF99, and one that recognizes only CTF99. Cells transfected with Asp2 showed significant increases of CTF99 compared with control cells not transfected with Asp2, and cells transfected with cathepsin D where both CTF83 and CTF99 were identified. Controls were also performed using the active site mutants of Asp2 mentioned above, where there was no increase in CTF99.

The SKB group also examined distribution of Asp2 in AD hippocampus using a polyclonal antiserum raised against a peptide segment of Asp2. Clear staining of neuronal tissue was observed, but no staining associated with astrocytes, microglia, or oligodendrocytes. These same anti-peptide sera allowed detection of Asp2 in the recombinant cell lines expressing APP$_{695}$ and APP$_{751}$ mentioned above. As reported by others [39, 40], APP localizes to the Golgi/endoplasmic reticulum of the secretory apparatus, and based upon confocal analysis of *myc*-tagged Asp2 and APP in COS-7 APP$_{751}$ cells, these workers were able to show a similar localization for Asp2. These results suggest that APP and BACE may segregate as they are processed and transported within the cell. Hydrolysis of APP by BACE at the β-site appears to be a process of heterogeneous catalysis where the susceptible β-cleavage in membrane anchored APP is oriented in a favorable position for processing by the membrane-bound BACE.

2.2.5   Oklahoma Medical Research Foundation (OMRF): Hypothesis and Genome Searches [18]

Scientists at the OMRF have spearheaded advances in the field of aspartyl proteases, from their pioneering work on the sequence analysis of pepsin, the prototype aspartyl enzyme [41], identification of one of the two active site Asp residues [42], inference of an internal duplication of structure in the two halves of these enzymes [22], and extensions of these findings to a broad category of representatives of this mechanistic set of proteases. Using human aspartyl protease motifs, their search of human EST libraries for new human aspartyl proteases led to the identification of two unique membrane anchored enzymes, named memapsin 2 and memapsin 1, corresponding respectively, to BACE and BACE2. Again, much of the background for this effort was already presented above for the discoveries at Pharmacia and SKB.

The sequence for memapsin 2 is identical to that shown in Fig. 2.2 for the β-secretase. The cDNA sequence was derived from EST AA136368, EST AA207232, and EST R55398 from the National Center for Biotechnology Information (NCBI) EST database. Completed sequences from corresponding bacterial clones 947471, 214526, and 392689 assembled into ~80% of the preproBACE cDNA, and standard methods of 5′-rapid amplification of cDNA ends and PCR were employed to give the FL cDNA sequence for memapsin 2 (BACE) shown in Fig. 2.2.

The OMRF group described expression of part of the memapsin 2 sequence in *E. coli*. Their construct, said to correspond to the catalytic domain, began eight residues upstream of Thr^1 (at Ala^{-8}; Fig. 2.2) and extended to Ala^{398}. This form of the protein would eliminate Cys^{399} and Cys^{422}, thereby preventing formation of two disulfide bridges, now known to link Cys^{399}-Cys^{195} and Cys^{422}-Cys^{257}. Although proteolytic activity was claimed in preparations of this protein following refolding from inclusion bodies and purification, BACE activity has been shown to require the presence of all three disulfide bridges [43], so it is not clear how this C-terminally truncated BACE could have shown proteolytic activity. Generally speaking, BACE catalytic domain constructs terminate at, or near Ser^{432} (Fig. 2.2). In fact, subsequent work from the OMRF laboratory, including the X-ray structural analysis [44], was done with a longer BACE form extending to Thr^{433} and including all three disulfide bridges.

As reported in the citations outlined above, tissue distribution of memapsin 2 showed high-level expression in pancreas and brain. The distance of the catalytic apparatus in the globular catalytic domain from the membrane surface was estimated to be about 20–30 amino acid residues. This fits well with the β-site in membrane-anchored APP of 28 amino acids, and confocal microscopy of both APP and memapsin 2 revealed their co-localization in lysosomal/endosomal compartments. This paper also provides data supporting memapsin 2 as the β-secretase, based upon cell biology experiments analyzing APP product proteins and peptides resulting from overexpression of the enzyme that confirm findings of the other discovery laboratories.

2.3 VALIDATION OF THE BACE TARGET

2.3.1 Summary of Evidence from Cell Biology

The five discovery efforts discussed above all arrived at essentially the same answers via diverse approaches. Several points may be emphasized.

1. All agree that the β-secretase is a new member of the pepsin family of aspartyl proteases with the same primary structure given in Fig. 2.2, and is unique in having predicted transmembrane and cytoplasmic domains in its C-terminal extension. Membrane association explains its intracellular localization in the secretory apparatus.

2. Evidence based upon cell biological experiments supports the conclusion that increased levels of BACE in a variety of cell systems are associated with increased processing at the APP β-site and vice versa, and these effects are BACE-specific.

3. The β-secretase is not involved with processing at the intramembrane γ-sites.

4. There is general agreement with the proposal of Sinha and Lieberberg [45] that β-site processing is rate limiting in Aβ production.

5. All groups also identified a second transmembrane protein, closely related to BACE that is now commonly known as BACE2. This enzyme can also process APP in the Aβ region but at sites that would produce non-amyloidogenic peptides.

An important landmark in validating the BACE target came from observations generated from BACE knockout mice.

2.3.2 Knockout Mice

The convergent identification by multiple independent research groups of the same polypeptide as β-secretase was dramatically and quickly validated, as mice deficient in the BACE gene became available and were analyzed for their APP-related phenotype [46–48]. The mouse BACE sequence is highly conserved to the human, and as in humans, a murine BACE2 was also documented. Mice deficient in BACE were found to be fertile, viable, and did not show any phenotypic differences from their Wt littermates in normal tissue morphology and brain histochemistry, as well as in blood and urine clinical chemistry measures. Primary neuronal cultures made from such mice showed *complete* loss of all Aβ forms generated from endogenous mouse APP, and primary cultures made from mice also expressing Sw APP did not show any generation of the human Aβ forms either. Both Aβ and sAPPβ were essentially undetectable in brain extracts of transgenic human Sw-APP mice deficient in BACE. The exact same conclusion was thus reached by the three different BACE knockout mice studies – this unique enzyme is *solely* responsible for Aβ generation from either endogenous or transgenic APP in mice, and no other enzyme (including BACE2) can compensate for its genetic deficiency.

Recently published studies [49] have revealed that PDAPP (PD-APP; platelet-derived growth factor promoter) transgenic mice, which express a human familial Alzheimer's Disease (FAD)-APP transgene and normally develop robust AD-like pathology with age, remained entirely free of amyloid deposits even at 13 months of age in a BACE-deficient background. When crossed with heterozygous BACE knockout animals, which exhibited ~50% of Wt BACE protein and enzymatic activity in their brain, the PDAPP transgenic mice showed greatly diminished amyloid plaques as well as dystrophic neurites at both 13 months and 18 months of age, and showed significant protection of the age-dependent loss of synaptophysin that is seen in these animals even at the 18 months of age time point. Thus, even a partial loss of BACE activity can afford significant protection against the development of plaque pathology and synaptic loss in a well-characterized transgenic model of AD pathology.

Although almost entirely normal by gross phenotypic measures, the BACE-deficient mice have shown some behavioral deficits. BACE-deficient mice display sensorimotor impairments and spatial memory deficits [50], both of which were more pronounced on the PDAPP background (overexpressing human FAD APP). These observations suggest that BACE-mediated processing of APP and perhaps other substrates play a role in "normal" learning, memory, and sensorimotor processes.

In addition, there does turn out to be a morphologically quantifiable developmental defect in BACE-deficient animals that appears to result from cleavage of a substrate other than APP. BACE-null mice have a reduced thickness of myelin sheaths around the axonal fibers [51, 52], which is maintained at the oldest ages examined. The hypomyelination is evident in both the central nervous system (CNS) (optic nerve) and the peripheral nervous system (PNS) (sciatic nerve), suggesting that it is owing to interference with a common mechanism of myelination, even though different cells mediate myelination in the CNS (oligodendrocytes) and the PNS (Schwann cells). Phenotypically, the reduced myelination results in a reduced nociception threshold in BACE-null animals. BACE appears to modulate developmental myelination via its cleavage of neuregulin-1, a protein that is known to affect myelination. Levels of neuregulin-1 are increased in BACE-deficient mice, and levels of a cleaved N-terminal fragment of the protein are decreased [51], in line with the expected loss of cleavage by BACE.

2.4 FINAL REMARKS

There was a good deal of excitement at the beginning of this century that a viable target was in hand for the development of drugs to fight AD. Given the assumption that Aβ in neuritic plaque from AD brain is causally linked to disease progression, it is obvious to focus on the β-secretase and the γ-secretase that generate this toxic β-amyloid peptide from APP precursors. Of the two, the β-secretase has many advantages as a target. Perhaps most importantly, BACE is a single molecular entity belonging to a large and well-characterized mechanistic set of proteolytic enzymes; its structure and mechanism are well established. This opens the door to structure-based drug design, an activity that has been underway for 20 years in the search for inhibitors of related enzymes like renin for hypertension and the HIV-protease for treatment of AIDS. The first renin inhibitor is now on the market [53], and protease inhibitors as co-therapies have been of great benefit in prolonging the lives of AIDS patients. Another argument in favor of the β-secretase target is that the γ-secretase cannot function without prior cleavage at the β-site [45] so that, in fact, a β-secretase inhibitor would also silence γ-secretase. Finally, results from the BACE knockout mice are most encouraging in that these mice show absence of Aβ in the circulation, and do not appear to show phenotypic liabilities of any kind. Knockouts of components of the γ-secretase complex are often lethal. Accordingly, the BACE target is clearly defined in molecular and mechanistic terms, and the biology says that its deletion is not only not lethal, but is also of no apparent consequence. In contrast, the mechanism and details as to how the components of the complex identified as the γ-secretase work in intramembrane catalysis remain open to question. Moreover, other important signaling systems require participation of similar type enzymes in intramembrane hydrolysis, and building specificity into a γ-secretase inhibitory drug is a challenge. Interestingly, however, screening for inhibitors of Aβ production turn up blockers of γ-secretase more often than of β-secretase, and it could be that a lead turned up by high-throughput screening will make it first to the finish line. Serendipity generally rules the day in drug discovery!

Having said all this, it is important to mention that aspartyl proteases also pose obstacles for development of inhibitors that will be effective drugs in clinical application. They have extended active site pockets, and effective, potent inhibitors are generally large, limiting oral uptake and greatly increasing cost of manufacture. A long-acting parenterally administered drug may be tolerable for AD because there exist few, if any, alternatives. But in producing a BACE inhibitor for AD, one must also deal with the blood–brain barrier, even with an injectable drug; this poses yet another challenge in the effort to produce an effective therapeutic [54]. Then there is the question of blocking BACE2, the closest relative to BACE, and an enzyme believed to have a beneficial effect in producing non-amyloid peptides from APP. It may be exceedingly difficult to design specificity into a BACE inhibitor such that it will have little, or no inhibitory activity toward BACE2.

Despite these challenges, β-secretase inhibitors are under vigorous investigation, although at the time of this writing none have demonstrated efficacy in lowering brain or cerebral spinal fluid (CSF) Aβ by the oral route in the absence of permeability glycoprotein (P-gp) or Cyp3A4 inhibition [55]. At least one compound, CTS-21166 (Comentis), has completed a small Phase I trial in healthy volunteers administered via the intravenous route, and has been shown to reduce plasma Aβ levels. Whether this or other compounds progress further into clinical development for the treatment of AD remains to be seen.

REFERENCES

1. Dickson, D.W. 1997. The pathogenesis of senile plaques. *J Neuropathol Exp Neurol* **56**:321–329.
2. Glenner, G.G. and Wong, C.W. 1984. Alzheimer's disease: initial report of the purification and characterization of a novel cerebrovascular amyloid protein. *Biochem Biophys Res Commun* **120**:885–890.
3. Selkoe, D.J. and Schenk, D. 2003. Alzheimer's disease: molecular understanding predicts amyloid-based therapeutics. *Annu Rev Pharmacol Toxicol* **43**:545–584.
4. Van Nostrand, W.E. and Cunningham, D.D. 1987. Purification of protease nexin II from human fibroblasts. *J Biol Chem* **262**:8508–8515.
5. Van Nostrand, W.E., Wagner, S.L., Suzuke, M., Choi, B.H., Farrow, J.S., Geddes, J.W., Cotman, C.W., and Cunningham, D.D. 1989. Protease nexin-II, a potent antichymotrypsin, shows identity to amyloid β-protein precursor. *Nature* **341**:546–549.
6. Kang, J., Lemaire, H.-G., Unterbeck, A., Alsboum, M., Masters, C.L., Grzeschik, K.H., Multhaup, G., Beyreuther, K., and Müller-Hill, B. 1987. The precursor of Alzheimer's disease amyloid A4 protein resembles a cell-surface receptor. *Nature (Lond)* **325**:733–736.
7. Heinrikson, R.L. 2004. Secretases. *Encycl of Biol Chem* **4**:7–10.
8. Ponte, P., Gonzalez-DeWhitt, P., Schilling, J., Miller, J., Hsu, D., Greenberg, B.D., Davis, K., Wallace, W., Lieberburg, I., Fuller, F., and Cordel, B. 1988. A new A4 amyloid mRNA contains a domain homologous to serine proteinase inhibitors. *Nature (Lond)* **331**:525–527.
9. Roher, A.E., Lowenson, J.D., Clarke, S., Wolkow, C., Wang, R., Cotter, R.J., Reardon, I.M., Zurcher-Neely, H.A., Heinrikson, R.L., Ball, M.J., and Greenberg, B.D. 1993. Structural alterations in the peptide backbone of β-amyloid core protein may account for its deposition and stability in Alzheimer's disease. *J Biol Chem* **268**:3072–3083.
10. Haass, C., Schlossmacher, M.G., Hung, A.Y., Vigo-Pelfrey, C., Mellon, A., Ostaszewski, B.L., Lieberburg, I., Koo, E.H., Schenk, D., Teplow, D.B., and Selkoe, D.J. 1992. Amyloid β-peptide is produced by cultured cells during normal metabolism. *Nature* **359**:322–325.
11. Gouras, G.K., Xu, H., Jovanovic, J.N., Buxbaum, J.D., Wang, R., Greengard, P., Relkin, N.R., and Gandy, S. 1998. Generation and regulation of β-amyloid peptide variants by neurons. *J Neurochem* **71**:1920–1925.
12. Mullan, M., Crawford, F., Axelman, K., Houlden, H., Lilius, L., Winblad, B., and Lannfelt, L. 1992. A pathogenic mutation for probably Alzheimer's disease in the APP gene at the N-terminus of beta amyloid. *Nat Genet* **1**:345–347.
13. Wolfe, M.S., Xia, W., Ostaszewski, B.L., Diehl, T.S., Kimberly, T.T., and Selkoe, D.J. 1999. *Nature* **398**:513–517.
14. Vassar, R., Bennett, B.D., Babu-Khan, S., Kahn, S., Mendiaz, E.A., Denis, P., Teplow, D.B., Ross, S., Amarante, P., Loeloff, R., Luo, Y., Fisher, S., Fuller, J., Edenson, S., Lile, J., Jarosinski, M.A., Biere, A.L., Curran, E., Burgess, T., Louis, J.C., Collins, F., Treanor, J., Rogers, G., and Citron, M. 1999. β-secretase cleavage of Alzheimer's amyloid precursor protein by the transmembrane aspartic protease BACE. *Science* **286**:735–741.
15. Sinha, S., Anderson, J.P., Barbour, R., Basi, G.S., Caccavello, R., Davis, D., Doan, M., Dovey, H.F., Frigon, N., Hong, J., Jacobson-Croak, K., Jewett, N., Keim, P., Knops, J., Lieberburg, I., Power, M., Tan, H., Tatsuno, G., Tung, J., Schenk, D., Seubert, P., Suomensaari, S.M., Wang, S., Walker, D., and John, V. 1999. Purification and cloning of amyloid precursor protein β-secretase from human brain. *Nature* **402**:537–540.
16. Yan, R., Bienkowski, M.J., Shuck, M.E., Miao, H., Tory, M.C., Pauley, A.M., Brashier, J.R., Stratman, N.C., Mathews, W.R., Buhl, A.E., Carter, D.B., Tomasselli, A.G., Parodi, L.A., Heinrikson, R.L., and Gurney, M.E. 1999. Membrane-anchored aspartyl protease with Alzheimer's disease β-secretase activity. *Nature* **402**:533–537.
17. Hussain, I., Powell, D., Howlett, D.R., Tew, D.G., Meek, T.D., Chapman, C., Gloger, I.S., Murphy, K.E., Southan, C.D., Ryan, D.M., Smith, T.S., Simmons, D.L., Walsh, F.S., Dingwall, C., and Christie, G. 1999. Identification of a novel aspartic protease (Asp2) as beta secretase. *Mol Cell Neurosci* **14**:419–427.

18. Lin, X., Koelsch, G., Wu, S., Downs, D., Dashti, A., and Tang, J. 2000. Human aspartic protease memapsin 2 cleaves the β-secretase site of β-amyloid precursor protein. *Proc Natl Acad Sci U S A* **97**:1456–1460.

19. Ladror, U.S., Snyder, S.W., Wang, G.T., Holzman, T.F., and Krafft, G.A. 1994. Cleavage at the amino and carboxyl termini of Alzheimer's amyloid-beta by cathepsin D. *J Biol Chem* **269**:18422–18428.

20. Tang, J., ed. 1976. *Acid Proteases, Structure, Function, and Biology.* New York: Plenum Press.

21. Tang, J. 1998. Pepsin A. In *Handbook of Proteolytic Enzymes* (A.J. Barrett, N.D. Rawlings, and J.F. Woessner, eds.). London: Academic Press, pp. 805–814.

22. Tang, J., James, M.N.G., Hsu, I.N., Jenkins, J.A., and Blundell, T.L. 1978. Structural evidence for gene duplication in the evolution of the acid proteases. *Nature* **315**:618–621.

23. Tomasselli, A.G., Howe, W.J., Sawyer, T.K., Wlodawer, A., and Heinrikson, R.L. 1991. The complexities of AIDS: an assessment of the HIV protease as a therapeutic target. *Chim Oggi* **9**:6–27.

24. Emmons, T.L., Shuck, M.E., Babcock, M.S., Holloway, J.S., Leone, J.W., Durbin, J.D., Paddock, D.J., Prince, D.B., Heinrikson, R.L., Fischer, H.D., Bienkowski, M.J., Benson, T.E., and Tomasselli, A.G. 2008. Large-scale purification of human BACE expressed in mammalian cells and removal of the prosegment with HIV-1 protease to improve crystal diffraction. *Protein Pept Lett* **15**:119–130.

25. Tomasselli, A.G., Paddock, D.J., Emmons, T.L., Mildner, A.M., Leone, J.W., Lull, J.M., Cialdella, J.I., Prince, D.B., Fischer, H.D., Heinrikson, R.L., and Benson, T.E. 2008. High yield expression of human BACE constructs in *Escherichia coli* for refolding, purification, and high resolution diffracting crystal forms. *Protein Pept Lett* **15**:131–143.

26. Oltersdorf, T., Fritz, L.C., Schenk, D.B., Lieberburg, I., Johnson-Wood, K.L., Beattie, E.C., Ward, P.J., Blacher, R.W., Dovey, H.F., and Sinha, S. 1989. The secreted form of the Alzheimer's amyloid precursor protein with the Kunitz domain is protease nexin-II. *Nature* **341**:144–147.

27. Seubert, T., Oltersdorf, T., Lee, M.G., Barbour, R., Blomquist, C., Davis, D.L., Bryant, K., Fritz, L.C., Galasko, D., Thal, L.J., Lieberburg, I., and Schenk, D.B. 1993. Secretion of beta-amyloid precursor protein cleaved at the amino terminus of the beta-amyloid peptide. *Nature* **361**:260–263.

28. Citron, M., Oltersdorf, T., Haass, C., McConlogue, L., Hung, A.Y., Seubert, P., Vigo-Pelfrey, C., Lieberburg, I., and Selkoe, D.J. 1992. Mutation of the beta-amyloid precursor protein in familial Alzheimer's disease increases beta-protein production. *Nature* **360**:672–674.

29. Citron, M., Teplow, D.B., and Selkoe, D.J. 1995. Generation of amyloid beta protein from its precursor is sequence specific. *Neuron* **14**(3):661–670.

30. Poorman, R.A., Palermo, D.P., Post, L.E., Murakami, K., Kinner, J.H., Smith, C.W., Reardon, I., and Heinrikson, R.L. 1986. Isolation and characterization of native human renin derived from Chinese hamster ovary cells. *Proteins: Struct, Funct Genet* **1**:139–145.

31. Heinrikson, R.L. and Poorman, R.A. 1990. The biochemistry and molecular biology of recombinant human renin and prorenin. In *Hypertension: Pathophysiology, Diagnosis, and Management*, Vol. I (J.H. Laragh and B.M. Brenner, eds.). New York: Raven Press, pp. 1179–1196.

32. Tomasselli, A.G., Thaisrivongs, S., and Heinrikson, R.L. 1996. Discovery and design of HIV protease inhibitors as drugs for treatment of AIDS. In *Advances in Antiviral Drug Design* (E. De Clercq, ed.). Greenwich, CT: JAI Press, pp. 173–228.

33. Poorman, R.A., Tomasselli, A.G., Heinrikson, R.L., and Kezdy, F.J. 1991. A cumulative specificity model for proteases from human immunodeficiency virus Types 1 and 2, inferred from statistical analysis of an extended substrate database. *J Biol Chem* **266**:14554–14561.

34. Tomasselli, A.G. and Heinrikson, R.L. 1994. Specificity of retroviral proteases: an analysis of viral and nonviral protein substrates. *Methods Enzymol* **241**:279–301.

35. Saftig, P., Peters, C., Figura, K. von, Craessaerts, K., Van Leuven, F., and De Strooper, B. 1996. Amyloidogenic processing of human amyloid precursor protein in hippocampal neurons devoid of cathepsin D. *J Biol Chem* **271**:27241–27244.

36. Tatnell, P.J. 1994. Napsins: new human aspartic proteinases. Distinction between two closely related genes. *FEBS Lett* **441**:43–48.

37. Emmons, T.L., Mildner, A.M., Lull, J.M., Leone, J.W., Fischer, H.D., Heinrikson, R.L., and Tomasselli, A.G. 2009. Large-scale refolding and purification of the catalytic domain of human BACE-2 produced in *E. coli*. *Protein Pept Lett* **16**: in press.

38. Yan, R., Munzner, J.B., Shuck, M.E., and Bienkowski, M.J. 2001. BACE2 functions as an alternative α-secretase in Cells. *J Biol Chem* **276**:34019-34027.
39. Kuentzel, S.L., Ali, S.M., Altman, R.A., Greenberg, B.D., and Raub, T.J. 1993. The Alzheimer β-amyloid protein precursor/protease nexin II is cleaved by the secretase in a trans-Golgi secretory compartment in human neuroglioma cells. *J Biochem* **295**:367-378.
40. Walter, J., Capell, A., Grunberg, J., Pesold, B., Schindzielorz, A., Prior, R., Podlisny, M.B., Fraser, P., Hyslop, P.S., Selkoe, D.J., and Haass, C. 1996. The Alzheimer's disease-associated presenilins are differentially phosphorylated proteins located predominantly within the endoplasmic reticulum. *Mol Med* **2**:673-691.
41. Tang, J., Sepulveda, P., Marciniszyn, J. Jr., Chen, K.C.S., Huang, W.-Y., Liu, D., and Lanier, J.P. 1973. Amino acid sequence of porcine pepsin. *Proc Nat Acad Sci U S A* **70**:3437-3439.
42. Chen, K.C.S. and Tang, J. 1972. Amino acid sequence around the epoxide-reactive residues in pepsin. *J Biol Chem* **247**:2566-2574.
43. Haniu, M., Denis, P., Young, Y., Mendiaz, E.A., Fuller, J., Hui, J.O., Bennett, B.D., Kahn, S., Ross, S., Burgess, T., Katta, V., Rogers, G., Vassar, R., and Citron, M. 2000. Characterization of Alzheimer's beta-secretase protein BACE. A pepsin family member with unusual properties. *J Biol Chem* **275**(28):21099-21106.
44. Hong, L., Koelsch, G., Lin, X., Wu, S., Terzyan, S., Ghosh, A.K., Zhang, X.C., and Tang, J. 2000. Structure of the protease domain of memapsin2 (β-secretase) complexed with inhibitor. *Science* **290**:150-153.
45. Sinha, S. and Lieberburg, I. 1999. Cellular mechanisms of beta-amyloid production and secretion. *Proc Natl Acad Sci U S A* **96**(20):11049-11053.
46. Cai, H., Wang, Y., McCarthy, D., Wen, H., Borchelt, D.R., Price, D.L., and Wong, P.C. 2001. BACE1 is the major beta-secretase for generation of Abeta peptides by neurons. *Nat Neurosci* **4**(3):233-234.
47. Luo, Y., Bolon, B., Kahn, S., Bennett, B.D., Babu-Khan, S., Denis, P., Fan, W., Kha, H., Zhang, J., Gong, Y., Martin, L., Louis, J.-C., Yan, Q., Richards, W.G., Citron, M., and Vassar, R.B. 2001. Mice deficient in BACE1, the Alzheimer's beta-secretase, have normal phenotype and abolished beta-amyloid generation. *Nat Neurosci* **4**(3):231-232.
48. Roberds, S.L., Anderson, J., Basi, G., Bienkowski, M.J., Branstetter, D.G., Chen, K.S., Freedman, S., Frigon, N.L., Games, D., Hu, K., Johnson-Wood, K., Kappenman, K.E., Kawabe, T.T., Kola, I., Kuehn, R., Lee, M., Liu, W., Motter, R., Nichols, N.F., Power, M., Robertson, D.W., Schenk, D., Schoor, M., Shopp, G.M., Shuck, M.E., Sinha, S., Svensson, K.A., Tatsuno, G., Tintrup, H., Wijsman, J., Wright, S., and McConlogue, L. 2001. BACE knockout mice are healthy despite lacking the primary beta-secretase activity in brain: implications for Alzheimer's disease therapeutics. *Hum Mol Genet* **10**(12):1317-1324.
49. McConlogue, L., Buttini, M., Anderson, J.P., Brigham, E.F., Chen, K.S., Freedman, S.B., Games, D., Johnson-Wood, K., Lee, M., Zeller, M., Liu, W., Motter, R., and Sinha, S. 2007. Partial reduction of BACE1 has dramatic effects on Alzheimer plaque and synaptic pathology in APP transgenic mice. *J Biol Chem* **282**(36):26326-26334.
50. Kobayashi, D., Zeller, M., Cole, T., Buttini, M., McConlogue, L., Sinha, S., Freedman, S., Morris, R.G., Chen, K.S. 2008. BACE1 gene deletion: impact on behavioral function in a model of Alzheimer's disease. *Neurobiol Aging* **29**(6):861-873.
51. Hu, X., Hicks, C.W., He, W., Wong, P., Macklin, W.B., Trapp, B.D., and Yan, R. 2006. BACE1 modulates myelination in the central and peripheral nervous system. *Nat Neurosci* **9**:1520-1525.
52. Willem, M., Garratt, A.N., Novak, B., Citron, M., Kaufmann, S., Rittger, A., DeStrooper, B., Saftig, P., Birchmeier, C., and Haass, C. 2006. Control of peripheral nerve myelination by the β-secretase BACE1. *Science* **314**:664-666.
53. Stanton, A. 2008. Now that we have a direct renin inhibitor, what should we do with it? *Curr Hypertens Rep* **10**(3):194-200.
54. Hussain, I., Hawkins, J., Harrison, D., Hille, C., Wayne, G., Cutler, L., Buck, T., Walter, D., Demont, E., Howes, C., Naylor, A., Jeffrey, P., Gonzalez, M.I., Dingwall, C., Michel, A., Redshaw, S., and Davis, J.B. 2007. Oral administration of a potent and selective non-peptidic BACE-1 inhibitor decreases beta-cleavage of amyloid precursor protein and amyloid-beta production in vivo. *J Neurochem* **100**(3):802-809.

55. Sankaranarayanan, S., Holahan, M.A., Colussi, D., Crouthamel, M.-C., Devanarayan, V., Ellis, J., Espeseth, A., Gates, A.T., Graham, S.L., Gregro, A.R., Hazuda, D., Hochman, J.H., Holloway, K., Jin, L., Kahana, J., Lai, M., Lineberger, J., McGaughey, G., Moore, K.P., Nantermet, P., Pietrak, B., Price, E.A., Rajapakse, H., Stauffer, S., Steinbeiser, M.A., Seabrook, G., Selnick, H.G., Shi, X.-P., Stanton, M.G., Swestock, J., Tugusheva, K., Tyler, K.X., Vacca, J.P., Wong, J., Wu, G., Xu, M., Cook, J.J., and Simon, A.J. 2009. First demonstration of cerebrospinal fluid and plasma A beta lowering with oral administration of a beta-site amyloid precursor protein-cleaving enzyme 1 inhibitor in nonhuman primates. *J Pharmacol Exp Ther* **328**(1):131–140.

CHAPTER 3

BACE BIOLOGICAL ASSAYS

Alfredo G. Tomasselli and Michael J. Bienkowski

Pfizer Inc., St. Louis, MO

3.1 INTRODUCTION

Each step of drug discovery and development is strictly dependent on reliable biochemical and biological assays. Assays are developed to identify compounds, referred to as leads, capable of modulating a select target and/or a biological process, and to allow optimization of these leads to drug candidates. Moreover, assays are used both to monitor the fate of the drug candidate *in vivo* with respect to its absorption, distribution, metabolism, excretion (ADME), and to track biomarkers as a means to assess or predict the course of the disease.

Striking advances over the past decade in genome and proteome research, in molecular biology technologies, and in the understanding of biological pathways, have brought about a myriad of opportunities to find and validate new targets to treat diseases. To exploit this wealth of opportunities, pharmaceutical companies have exponentially expanded their compound collections through efforts such as parallel syntheses, natural products acquisition, and alliances with various institutions all over the world. Yet, capitalization on the enormous investments in compound libraries and drug target mining rests on the ability to develop sensitive and accurate biochemical and/or biological assays capable of analyzing the millions of compounds from these libraries and correctly identifying molecules that modulate the selected target in the desired way. Correct identification of leads is a fundamental step that often sets the medicinal chemistry strategy for the drug discovery process.

This chapter will review β-site APP cleaving enzyme (BACE) biological assays set up both for high-throughput screening (HTS) and for screening of compounds from medicinal chemists. Development of protein and cell assays for the BACE discovery will be described. Basic enzyme kinetic terms and their relevance to BACE inhibitor screening will be discussed along with the various substrates that have been used in the development of BACE assays. This chapter will also briefly discuss the screening flow scheme for discovery and development of BACE inhibitors, including primary and secondary assays along with selectivity assays versus other aspartyl proteases such as cathepsin D.

BACE: Lead Target for Orchestrated Therapy of Alzheimer's Disease, Edited by Varghese John
Copyright © 2010 John Wiley & Sons, Inc.

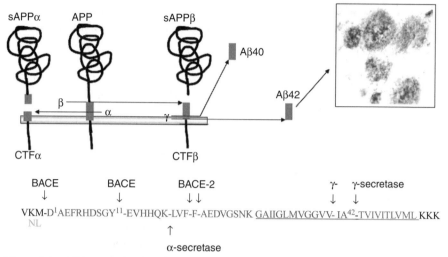

Figure 3.1 APP processing by secretases leading to the formation of APP fragments of which $A\beta_{1-42}$ and $A\beta_{11-42}$ are toxic forms. (See color insert.)

3.2 CLINICAL AND PHYSIOLOGICAL HALLMARKS OF ALZHEIMER'S DISEASE (AD)

AD, the most common form of senile dementia, is a progressive, devastating, neurodegenerative illness of the central nervous system that affects over 40 million people worldwide. Clinically, AD patients develop symptoms consisting in a gradual loss of memory which evolves into the more severe symptoms of mental confusion, language disturbances, personality and behavioral changes, and diminished abilities required for reasoning, orientation, and judgment. Physiologically, AD is characterized by the deposition of intracellular neurofibrillary tangles inside the neurons and extracellular amyloid plaques in the brain parenchyma. Tangles are formed from paired helical filaments containing hyperphosphorylated microtubule binding protein tau. Plaques found in the brains of AD patients typically contain peptides, referred to as the β-amyloid peptide ($A\beta$) that are generated from the amyloid precursor protein (APP) by two sequential proteolytic steps carried out by two enzymes referred to as β- and γ-secretases, respectively (Fig. 3.1) [1]. According to the widely accepted "amyloid hypothesis," increased production in the brain and/or decreased removal of $A\beta$ peptides from it are the triggers of the series of pathogenic events, including the tangle formation, leading to AD [2, 3].

3.3 APP PROCESSING

β-Secretase is the enzyme that catalyzes the first and prerequisite proteolytic step that yields the N-terminus of $A\beta$ by cleaving APP770 at two sites, at similar rates; specifically, between residues Met^{671} and Asp^{672}, and between Tyr^{682} and Glu^{683} [4,

5]. Asp^{672} will be referred to as Asp^1, and Glu^{682} as Glu^{11} to reflect their positions in the Aβ sequence (Fig. 3.1). BACE cleavages generate a soluble ectodomain sAPPβ, that is released into vesicle lumina and the extracellular space and leaves behind membrane-associated fragments of 99 and 89 amino acids, respectively. C99 and C89 are further cleaved by the action of the γ-secretase at various positions to generate Aβ peptides terminating after residues 37, 38, 39, 40, 42, and 43, that include the very toxic forms $Aβ_{1-42}$ and $Aβ_{11-42}$. The accumulation of these Aβ peptides is counteracted by the action of cellular enzymes referred to as α-secretases. Indeed, the most frequent cleavage of APP is an α-secretase cleavage occurring between Lys^{687} (K^{16}) and Leu^{688} (L^{17}) eliminating the region responsible for β-sheet formation. The resulting α-secretase-generated membrane associated fragments are then converted into non-amyloidogenic peptides by the γ-secretase, and the soluble ectodomain (sAPPα).

Blocking or modulating the action of β- and/or γ-secretase and/or potentiating the activity of the α-secretase represent important means of reducing the formation of Aβ below the threshold concentrations required to trigger the onset and/or sustain the progression of AD [6, 7]. Indeed, the inhibition of the two enzymes involved in the generation of Aβ, namely the β- and γ-secretase, is being pursued by numerous pharmaceutical companies [7] and clinical trials are underway, while α-secretase activity potentiation has received much less attention [6]. Various proteases have been proposed as potential α-secretases. They include neprilysin [8], insulin degrading enzyme [9], and at least three proteases of the ADAM (*a disintegrin and metalloprotease*) family: ADAM-9, ADAM-10, and ADAM-17 [6, 10]. γ-secretase has been identified by both biochemical and genetic studies to be formed by a complex of at least four membrane-bound proteins: presenilin, nicastrin, Aph1, and Pen2 [11, 12]), with presenilin being the catalytic core of the complex [13–15]. β-secretase was discovered as a membrane-anchored aspartyl protease by the independent efforts of four groups and was also called BACE and Asp2 [16–19]. Soon after its discovery, the BACE role as the β-secretase was definitively validated by studies of BACE (–/–) mice [20, 21]. BACE highly homologous enzyme, BACE-2, was discovered along with BACE [16–19]. BACE-2 was shown to be able to process APP at Met^{671} and Asp^{672} in cell culture under physiological conditions [22], but BACE-2 (–/–) animal models showed that this was not the case *in vivo* and was excluded as being a potential β-secretase [21]. BACE-2 predominant activity toward APP resides in the cleavages between Phe^{19} and Phe^{20}, and between Phe^{20} and Ala^{21} [23] to produce, like in the case of the α-secretase, non-amyloidogenic peptides. In fact, because of this potential beneficial role, and other yet unknown functions, inhibitors directed to BACE need to spare BACE-2. Additional molecular targets to be mindful of are other members of the aspartyl protease family, including cathepsin D/E and renin.

3.4 ASPARTYL PROTEASE CLASSIFICATION

Aspartyl proteases have been classified in two clans, AA and AD [24]. The AA clan contains two families (A1 and A2). Both families are referred to as classical aspartic proteases because they harbor the sequence $D^{32}S/TG \ldots D^{228}S/TG$ (Fig. 3.2). Family

M^{-21L}*AQALPWLLLWMGAGVLPAHG*T^{1P}**QHGIRLPLRSG**
LGGAPLGLRLPR^{24P}↓E^{25P}TDEEP^{30P}EEPGRRGSFV^{40P}E¹
MVDNLRGKSGQGYYVEMTV²⁰GSPPQTLNILV**DTG**SS
NFAV⁴⁰GAAPHPFLHRYYQRQLSSTY⁶⁰RDLRKGVYVP
YTQGKWEGEL⁸⁰GTDLVSIPHGP*N*VTVRANIA¹⁰⁰AITES
DKFFI*N*GSNWEGILG¹²⁰LAYAEIARPDDSLEPFFDSL¹⁴⁰
VKQTHVPCNLFSLQLC̲GAGFP¹⁶⁰L*N*QSEVLASVGGSM
IIGGID¹⁸⁰H̲SLYTGSLWYTPIRREWYYE²⁰⁰VIIVRVEING
QDLKMDC̲KEY²²⁰NYDKSIV**DSG**TTNLRLPKKV²⁴⁰FEA
AVKSIKAASSTEKFPDG²⁶⁰FWLGEQLVC̲WQAGTTPW
NIF²⁸⁰PVISLYLMGEVT*N*QSFRITI³⁰⁰LPQQYLRPVEDVA
TSQDDC̲Y³²⁰KFAISQSSTGTVMGAVIMEG³⁴⁰FYVVFDR
ARKRIGFAVSAC̲H³⁶⁰VHDEFRTAAVEGPFVTLDME³⁸⁰
DC̲GYNIPQTDEST̲LMTIAYV⁴⁰⁰MAAICALFMLPLCLM
VCQWR⁴²⁰CLRCLRQQHDDFADDISLLK⁴⁴⁰

Figure 3.2 The primary structure of BACE with features relevant to the enzyme cellular trafficking and functions. (See color insert.)

A1 comprises Pepsin-A/-C, cathepsin D/E, renin, napsin A, BACE, and BACE-2. Family A2 comprises retroviral proteases, which the virus integrates in the human genome, for example, HIV-1/HIV-2. On the other hand, intramembrane cleaving aspartic proteases such as presenilin, (PS-1 and PS-2), signal peptide peptidase (SPP), and SPP-like proteases (SPPL-2, -3, and -4), all of them harboring the signature YD²⁵⁷ and GxGD³⁸⁵ (PS-1 numbering), comprise yet a third functional family.

3.5 BACE STRUCTURE

BACE is a complex enzyme that undergoes proteolytic processing to yield the mature form; the primary structure of the protein as synthesized in the endoplasmatic reticulum is given in Fig. 3.2. It is composed of a 21-aa leader sequence (M⁻²¹ … G⁻¹) and a 24-aa prosegment (T^{1P} … R^{24P}), which are both removed in the Golgi apparatus [18, 25, 26] to yield what appears to be the mature enzyme (E^{25P} … K⁴⁴⁰) isolated from brain [17]. Though the prosegment ends at R^{24P}, the suffix P is used next to the amino acid number for the segment T^{1P} … V^{40P}, after which we adopt the numbering E¹ MVD … to follow the numbering of the majority of the reports on BACE 3D structure and kinetics. The stretch of 408 aa E^{25P} … S³⁹² harbors the classic catalytic triad D³²TG … D²²⁸SG, six cysteine residues paired to form three disulfide bridges: Cys¹⁵⁵–Cys³⁵⁹, Cys²¹⁷–Cys³⁸², and Cys²⁶⁹–Cys³¹⁹ [27] critical for activity, and four glycosylated asparagines, 92, 111, 162, 293 [27]. Residue S³⁹² precedes the BACE transmembrane domain of 27-aa (T³⁹³ … R⁴²⁰) that targets this protein to the Golgi and anchors it to the membrane. The primary structure is completed by a cytoplasmic tail of 21 residues (R⁴²⁰ … K⁴⁴⁰) containing posttranslational modifications involved in BACE trafficking and localization; these are palmitoylation at three cysteine residues and phosphorylation at Ser^{437} [14, 26]. The protein lacking C-terminal transmembrane and cytosolic domains folds in a bilobed structure reminiscent of other aspartyl proteases such as cathepsin D, pepsin A, and renin [28]. The two catalytic aspartyl residues, Asp^{32} and Asp^{228}, are in proximity and directly interact with the hydroxyl group of the statine moiety in the complex of BACE with OM99-2 [28]. The catalytic site is protected from the solvent by a hairpin loop, referred to as "the flap region." Of relevance to both substrate and inhibitor design is the nature of the active site pockets showing hydrophobic character at S3, S1, S2′, and S3, while the S4, S2, and S3′ are more hydrophilic. While the truncated enzyme is a monomer in both the 3D structure and in aqueous solution, Westmeyer et al. [29] reported that endogenous and overexpressed full-length BACE is a homodimer under native conditions and showed both higher affinity and turnover rate for substrates than monomeric-soluble BACE. In addition, they showed that even the BACE ectodomain dimerized when attached to the membrane [29]. Yet, Kopcho et al. [30] have reported that full-length BACE has catalytic activity similar to its non-glycosylated, soluble catalytic domain. Most of the kinetic and all the crystallographic studies have been done with the BACE-soluble catalytic domain.

3.6 MECHANISM, KINETICS, INHIBITION, AND SPECIFICITY

3.6.1 Catalytic Mechanism

Understanding the mechanism of reaction by which a protease catalyzes the irreversible cleavage of a substrate is very valuable, especially if one is able to catch catalytic events that can be exploited in inhibitor design. Indeed, the design of a huge number of aspartyl proteases inhibitors has used insights into these enzymes' catalytic mechanism. BACE, like other aspartyl proteases, performs catalysis by a general acid–general base mechanism where the enzyme brings two aspartic acids in close proximity to one another, one of which is protonated and the other is not (Fig. 3.3) [31]. By this mechanism, the substrate is positioned between the two catalytic Asp residues, and the protonated Asp uses its proton to form a hydrogen bond with the carbonyl oxygen of the cleavage bond. The non-protonated Asp interacts with the lytic water and, by extracting a proton from it, produces a hydroxide ion and an electrophilic acidic proton, which coordinately attacks the peptide bond via the formation of a tetrahedral transition state. Collapse of the tetrahedral intermediate results in the release of two peptide products and restores the enzyme for another round of catalysis. The formation of catalytic hydroxyl and tetrahedral intermediate has been an important finding in aspartyl proteases catalysis, which has been extensively used to design inhibitors. In these inhibitors, the scissile P_1-$P_1′$ peptide bond of the substrate has been replaced by a non-hydrolyzable isostere with tetrahedral geometry (Figs. 3.4 and 3.5); several inhibitors based on non-hydrolyzable isosteres are approved drugs to treat AIDS, and also in development to treat AD.

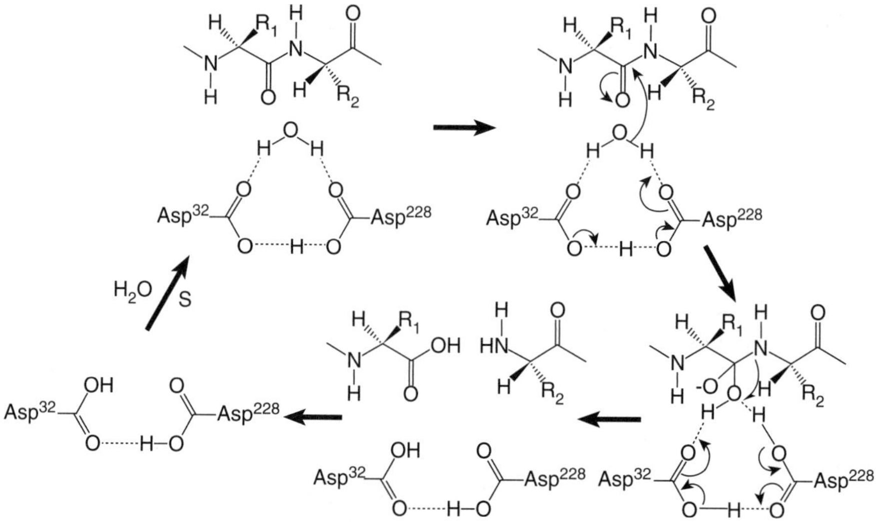

Figure 3.3   Highlights of a proposed mechanism of action for BACE. There is no solid proof on which catalytic Asp residue is protonated in free BACE. Therefore, Asp^{228} protonation indicated in this reaction is speculative.

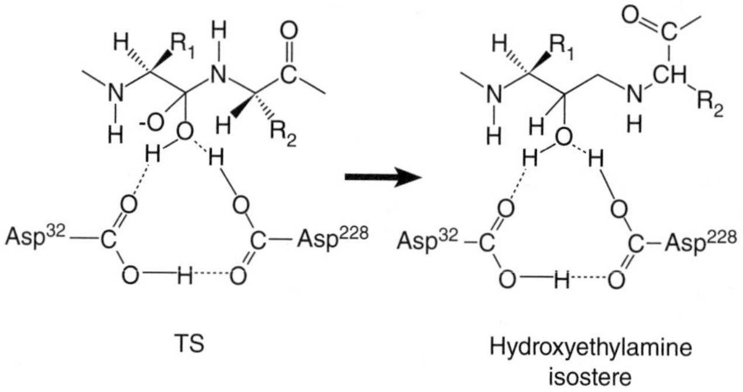

Figure 3.4   Application of the transition-state concept to design inhibitor.

3.6.2   Kinetic Analysis

Details of all the important concepts of enzyme kinetics and inhibition have been extensively reported in enzymology textbooks. The Michaelis–Menten model is described where an enzyme E and a single substrate S form the enzyme–substrate (ES) complex that is subsequently converted to product(s), P, with release of the enzyme:

$$E + S \underset{k_{-1}}{\overset{k_1}{\rightleftharpoons}} ES \overset{k_2}{\rightarrow} E + P \tag{Eq. 3.1}$$

Under the conditions in which BACE is assayed, [S] $\gg$ [E], a kinetic situation is reached when the rate of formation of ES is balanced by the rate of its conversion

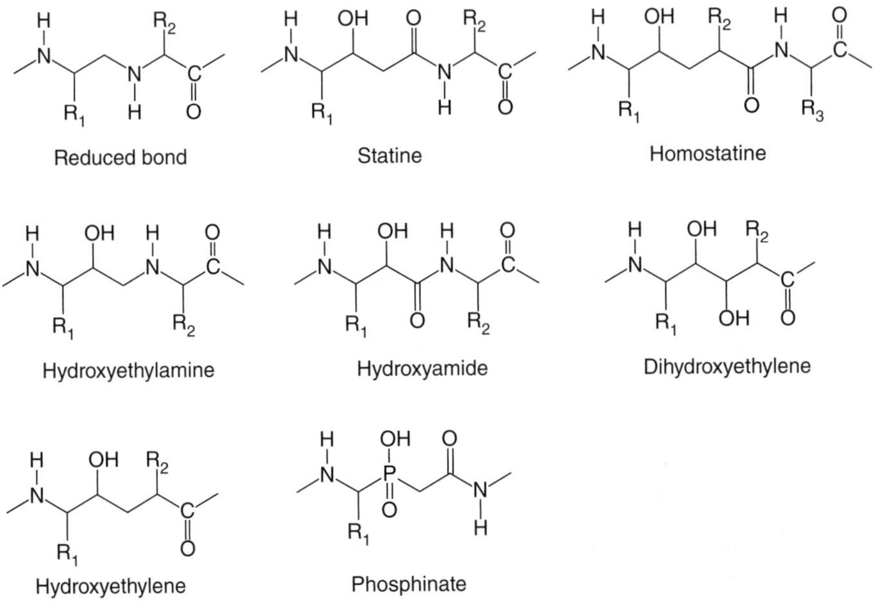

Reduced bond   Statine   Homostatine

Hydroxyethylamine   Hydroxyamide   Dihydroxyethylene

Hydroxyethylene   Phosphinate

Figure 3.5   Transition-state template commonly employed to design aspartyl proteases inhibitors.

to E and P, leaving the concentration of ES constant. During this phase, the Michaelis–Menten equation (Eq. 3.2 can be derived from Eq. 3.1). Equation 3.2 allows calculating the initial velocity of reaction (V) as a function of the substrate concentration ([S]). V_{max} is the maximal velocity, attainable at substrate saturation, and $K_M = (k_{-1} + k_2)/k_1$ is the substrate concentration at which $V = V_{max}/2$, where k_1 is the second-order rate constant of association, k_{-1} is the first-order rate constant of dissociation, and $k_2 = k_{cat}$ is the first-order rate constant representing the enzymatic catalysis per second or turnover number:

$$V_{max} = k_{cat} \times [E]$$

$$V = \frac{V_{max}[S]}{K_M + [S]} \qquad \text{(Eq. 3.2)}$$

3.6.3 Inhibition

With regard to enzyme inhibition, the equations relating kinetic and inhibition parameters are given below for competitive (Eq. 3.3), uncompetitive (Eq. 3.4), and noncompetitive/mixed (Eq. 3.5) inhibition.

Competitive inhibition is characterized by an inhibitor competing with the substrate for the active site. Inhibition can be completely overcome by substrate escalation. As [S] increases, V_{max} does not change while the effective K_M increases. [I] is the inhibitor concentration, V_i is the initial velocity of reaction in the presence of inhibitor, and K_i is the inhibition constant:

$$V_i = \frac{V_{max}[S]}{[S] + K_M(1 + [I]/K_i)} \qquad \text{(Eq. 3.3)}$$

Uncompetitive inhibition occurs when the inhibitor binds to the ES complex, but not the free enzyme. As a consequence, the inhibitor decreases both the effective V_{max} and the effective K_M in the same proportions:

$$V_i = \frac{V_{max}[S]}{[S](1+[I]/\alpha K_i)+K_M} \quad \text{(Eq. 3.4)}$$

In noncompetitive/mixed inhibition, the inhibitor binds to both the ES complex and free enzyme. In noncompetitive inhibition, the inhibitor displays equal affinity for both the free enzyme and the ES complex species ($\alpha = 1$), while in mixed inhibition, the affinity for the two species is different ($\alpha \neq 1$). When $\alpha = 1$, V_{max} changes, while K_M does not. When $\alpha \neq 1$, both V_{max} and K_M change, but not in equal proportions, as is seen for uncompetitive inhibition:

$$V_i = \frac{V_{max}[S]}{[S](1+[I]/\alpha K_i)+K_M(1+[I]/K_i)} \quad \text{(Eq. 3.5)}$$

Very important to compound library screening is the determination of IC_{50}, which represents the concentration of inhibitor needed to accomplish 50% inhibition:

$$V_i/V = \frac{1}{1+[I]/IC_{50}} \quad \text{(Eq. 3.6)}$$

For competitive (Eq. 3.7), uncompetitive (Eq. 3.8), and noncompetitive/mixed (Eq. 3.9) inhibition, Cheng and Prusoff [32] have derived the following relationships between and IC_{50} and K_i:

$$IC_{50} = K_i(1+[S]/K_M) \quad \text{(Eq. 3.7)}$$
$$IC_{50} = \alpha K_i(1+K_M/[S]) \quad \text{(Eq. 3.8)}$$
$$IC_{50} = \frac{[S]+K_M}{K_M/K_i+[S]/\alpha K_i} \quad \text{(Eq. 3.9)}$$

Thus, in competitive inhibition, an increase in [S] increases IC_{50}, while in uncompetitive inhibition an increase in [S] decreases IC_{50}. In noncompetitive/mixed inhibition, an increase in [S] either leaves IC_{50} unchanged ($\alpha = 1$), or causes less drastic changes as seen in competitive or uncompetitive inhibitions ($\alpha \neq 1$).

3.6.4   Substrate Specificity

The coordinated action of two catalytic Asp residues and a nucleophilic H_2O molecule to cleave a peptide bond is only the last of a series of steps in BACE catalysis. In fact, this process starts with the recognition and binding of selected substrates containing sequences several amino acids long. An in depth understanding of the substrate specificity is very important for several reasons. First of all, it allows designing a peptide that can be used to develop a sensitive and reliable assay. Second, it can guide the designing of enzyme inhibitors. Third, it might help in the identification of potential physiological substrates. Soon after its discovery, it became evident that BACE was not specific for cleavage of a single peptide bond.

BACE was able to cleave wild-type (Wt) APP at the ...Lys-Met↓Asp-Ala ... and ... Gly-Tyr↓Glu-Val ... bonds at very low rate. Moreover, an increase of about 50-fold in the rate of cleavage of Swedish (Sw) mutant APP was observed. In spite of the latter finding, it was initially estimated that even a substrate based on the Sw mutant APP would require concentrations of enzyme so high that it would compromise the potency determination of subnanomolar inhibitors and underscored once more the need to find superior substrates. Yet, it turned out that a combination of very sensitive fluorophores and detection equipment made the Sw mutant substrate widely used as described in this narrative.

The 3D structure of BACE complexed to a peptide-derived inhibitor with the hydroxyethylene transition-state isostere revealed that the substrate binding site accommodates eight side chains [28]. Several groups have examined the P_4-P_4' residue preferences in the BACE subsites S_4-S_4' with the goal of identifying best substrates for assay and/or inhibitor development [33–35].

Turner et al. [33] assigned the amino acids preferences summarized in Table 3.1 based on a combinatorial library study. They concluded that the P_1 subsite is the most stringent and P subsites are in general more specific than the P' subsites. They assembled the eight most favored residues to design a substrate, E-I-D-L↓M-V-L-D (Table 3.1, row 2), whose $k_{cat}/K_M = 20.8 \, \mu M^{-1} min^{-1}$ ($0.35 \, \mu M^{-1} s^{-1}$) was 14-fold better than that of a peptide harboring the Sw mutation at its cleavage site E-V-N-L↓D-A-E-F. With respect to peptidomimetic inhibitor design, these investigators selected the peptidomimetic inhibitor EVNL*AAEF (Table 3.1, row 8, where the asterisk represents the hydroxyethylene tansition-state isostere) and substituted the P_3, P_2, P_2', and P_3' with random amino acids (less Cys) while they kept the L*A constant. They found the amino acid preference specified in Table 3.1 and designed the inhibitor, OM-003, E-L-D-L*A-V-E-F, with K_i of 0.31 nM. This is a good example of

TABLE 3.1 BACE Amino Acid Preferences at P_4-P_4' Positions for Substrate (Rows 1–6) and Inhibitor (Rows 8–11) According to Turner et al. [33]

1	P_4	P_3	P_2	P_1	P_1'	P_2'	P_3'	P_4'
2	Glu	Ile	Asp	Leu	Met	Val	Leu	Asp
3	Gln	Val	Asn	Phe	Glu	Ile	Trp	Glu
4	Asp	Leu	Met	Met	Gln	Ala	Val	Trp
5				Tyr				
6	**Glu**	**Ile**	**Asp**	**Leu**	**Met**	**Val**	**Leu**	**Asp**
7								
8	*Glu*	*Val*	*Asn*	*Leu**	*Ala*	*Ala*	*Glu*	*Phe*
9		Leu	Asp			Val	Glu	
10		Ile	Glu				Gln	
11	**Glu**	**Leu**	**Asp**	**Leu***	**Ala**	**Val**	**Glu**	**Phe**

Note: Amino acids preference decreases from top to bottom of the Table, and was deduced from studying peptide libraries. Optimal substrate from these studies is shown in bold in row 6. Inhibitor has been generated starting from the inhibitor indicated in row 8 by changing amino acids in positions P_3-P_2 and P_2'-P_3' with every amino acid except Cys. The asterisk represents the hydroxyethylene transition-state isostere.

studies of the specificity of an enzyme that have generated a good substrate for assay development and a powerful inhibitor.

Knowledge of substrate specificity is further expanded by discussing two additional studies. The first study is based on combinatorial libraries [35], while the other [34] is based on combining data obtained by protein cleavage such as oxidized insulin B-chain, ubiquitin, and APP, and on cleavage of a series of peptides designed starting from kinetic information gleaned from cleavage of these proteins.

The combinatorial library study of Grüninger-Leitch et al. reported Glu > Asp as the preferred amino acid (aa) for the P_4 site [35]. Surprisingly, substitution of Glu with Gln, a preferred amino acid at P_4 according to Turner et al. [33] resulted in a significant loss of activity, while Glu to Lys almost extinguished activity [35]. A possible explanation is that those substitutions bring loss of a negative charge between the P_4 side chain and two neighboring Arg residues [33]. However, we found that replacement of P_4 Glu with Gly was essentially without loss of activity [34]. With respect to the P_3 position, Tomasselli et al. [34] and others [33] have shown that Ile is superior to Val in P_3. Grüninger-Leitch et al. [35] studied a library in which Leu was kept constant at P_1, and reported that Asn, Glu, and Asp were the three amino acids with maximal occurrence at P_2, while Ser and Thr were found at position P_2 only in combination with Ser at P_1'. This finding was extended in our studies that showed that Ser in P_2 in combination with Tyr or Leu in position P_1 is a well-accepted amino acid when Glu or Asp are in position P_1' [34]. At the most stringent position, P_1, the most abundant amino acids are Leu, Tyr, Phe, Nle, and Met [(33–35]. The P' side is less rigorous than the P side in its tolerance for amino acids, but some combinations are better than others. For example, the triplets EVE, or AVE, or DVE, or EVD are excellent motifs at the P_1'-P_3', but a relatively mild change to introduce Asp at both P_1' and P_3' dramatically reduces enzymatic activity [34].

Our studies led to the design of the substrate GLTNIKTEEISEISY↓ EVEFRWKK and its shorter version SEISY↓EVEFRWKK. As explained later, these peptides were employed as such in high-pressure liquid chromatography (HPLC) assays to determine IC_{50} and K_i and were equipped with fluorescence-quencher tags to screen compound libraries. Moreover, the ISY↓EV was inserted in the APP sequence and was employed in cell assays [34].

3.6.5 Natural Proteins as BACE Substrates

The poor activity displayed by BACE with regard to APP cleavage and the broad specificity displayed in studies of peptides cleavage would point to the existence of BACE substrates other than APP. Cole and Vassar have discussed putative non-APP BACE substrates reported in the literature, pointing out that all the substrates discovered thus far are membrane proteins [36]. Identification of proteins of physiological significance is important in designing strategies to inhibit BACE. Some of the substrates are, like APP, cleaved by both BACE and γ-secretase. They include the APP homologous, amyloid precursor-like proteins, APLP1 and APLP2 of undefined functions, the voltage-gated sodium channels (VGSC) responsible for the initiation and propagation of action potentials, and the lipoprotein receptor-related protein (LRP) which is a multifunctional endocytic receptor which has signaling roles in neurons. BACE cleaves neuregulin 1 (NRG1), a protein that influences the myelination of central and peripheral axons. BACE (–/–) mice, but not BACE (–/+), show some impairment in normal learning and memory processes, and it has been suggested they are related to lack of NRG1 cleavage. Other BACE substrates are also of interest because they involve inflammatory responses. They include the modulator of leukocyte adhesion molecule P-selectin glycoprotein ligand 1 (PSGL-1), α2, 6-sialyltransferase (ST6Gal1), and the interleukin-1 receptor II (IL-R2). Interestingly, NRG1 VGSC, LRP, PSGL-1, and ST6Gal1 seem to be cleaved by BACE *in vivo* [36].

3.7 ASSAY STRATEGIES FOR INHIBITOR FINDING AND DEVELOPMENT

Pharmaceutical companies routinely screen libraries composed of several hundred thousands to several million compounds to come up with a small percentage of compounds that produce the desired effect. These latter compounds are usually weak modulators referred to as "hits" and they need to be validated as to whether they are worth further optimization. Consequently, the assays need to be highly sensitive, low in cost, amenable to HTS, and preferentially homogeneous with no wash steps required. Animal testing is the ultimate assay which verifies that prerequisites such as potency, specificity, bioavailability, lack of toxicity, and good pharmacokinetics are met in order to proceed to clinical trials. A potential flow scheme for discovery and development of BACE inhibitors is given (Scheme 3.1).

A cellular assay capable of determining the amount of Aβ produced in the absence and in the presence of an inhibitor is, of course, of primary importance as a prerequisite to animal model testing. However, using it as the sole assay for screening millions of compounds would not be satisfactory for at least two reasons. First of all, those compounds that do not penetrate the cell or are metabolized inside the cell would show up as negatives and therefore would be lost. It could be argued, however, that such compounds might not be desirable leads for optimization. Second, the positively identified leads would not be necessarily targeting BACE, as other mechanisms of inhibition of Aβ production could be operative. In the latter case, the subsequent lead optimization would necessitate a difficult trial and error approach because the targets of those leads would not be known. The process of lead finding is exemplified when the molecular target is known and can be obtained in relatively large quantities such as BACE. Two approaches can be taken here. One is to express and purify the target and/or its relevant domains, for example, catalytic domain, and perform HTS. Hopefully, some leads can be identified and tested directly in cell assays and/or subjected to the optimization process. In fact, if the enzyme can be co-crystallized with the lead compounds, as is the case for BACE, crystallography can be employed to provide important information to drive the medicinal chemistry optimization process. Yet, while X-ray crystallography and its associated discipline,

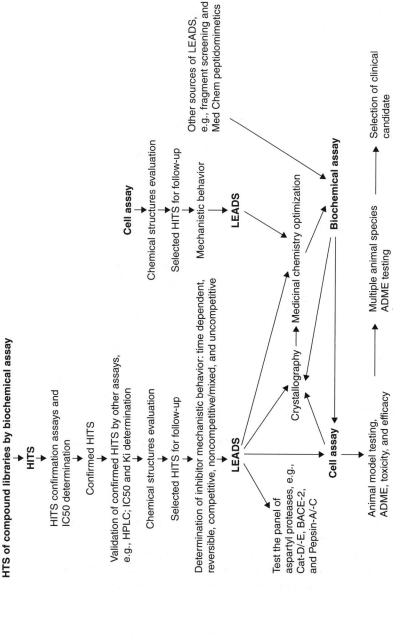

Scheme 3.1 Possible pathways from HTS to clinical candidates.

HTS of compound libraries by biochemical assay

HITS

HITS confirmation assays and
IC50 determination

Confirmed HITS

Validation of confirmed HITS by other assays,
e.g., HPLC; IC50 and Ki determination

Chemical structures evaluation

Selected HITS for follow-up

Determination of inhibitor mechanistic behavior: time dependent,
reversible, competitive, noncompetitive/mixed, and uncompetitive

LEADS

Test the panel of
aspartyl proteases, e.g.,
Cat-D/-E, BACE-2,
and Pepsin-A/-C

Crystallography — Medicinal chemistry optimization

Cell assay

Cell assay

Chemical structures evaluation

Selected HITS for follow-up

Mechanistic behavior

LEADS

Biochemical assay

Other sources of LEADS,
e.g., fragment screening and
Med Chem peptidomimetics

Animal model testing,
ADME, toxicity, and efficacy

Multiple animal species
ADME testing

Selection of clinical
candidate

computational chemistry, are of great value in helping optimizing a lead [37], they cannot tell whether optimization has occurred. In order to verify if optimization is successful, there is a need for both a biochemical and a cell assay that determine IC_{50} and/or K_i for the purified target and the IC_{50} for the target in its intracellular environment. Another approach is to first start with a cell assay devised for HTS wherein the target is overexpressed and/or its substrate is optimized and made specific for it to unambiguously generate a product that can be easily monitored. The advantage here is that one screens against the target protein in a cellular environment that is close to its natural environment. The disadvantage is that the cell assay would not reveal the mechanistic behavior of the inhibitor; getting this information requires a biochemical assay, but in this instance, the latter will be used as an assay for optimization of selected leads. Irrespective of the approach, the optimization process can take many cycles of compound crystallization, modeling, and chemical synthesis. Biochemical and biological assays are both needed and ultimately determine the compounds' suitability for animal testing. In addition, because of the huge effort involved in lead identification and optimization leading to animal tests, it is very important to adapt a biochemical assay to a cell assay, and to establish consistency between the two.

A common strategy is to start screening with a biochemical assay; fixed concentrations of target protein, substrate, inhibitor, and assay medium are selected in order to identify "hits." Hit validation is carried out by testing at various concentrations in so-called secondary assays. Secondary assays can be performed with the same assay that was used to find the hits and/or with different assays. In the secondary assays, several questions are answered: for example, is a compound that shows up positive in a fluorescence-based assay an inhibitor, or is it the result of an artifact due to interference of the absorbance of the compound with the fluorescence of the substrate? What are the values of its IC_{50} and K_i and its mechanistic behavior (time dependent, reversible, competitive, uncompetitive, and noncompetitive/mixed)? An HPLC assay that directly determines the initial and final amounts of the substrate and products can be employed to overcome the issues of interference with fluorescence determinations. Moreover, an indication of inhibitor behavior can be simply attained by the effect of substrate concentration on IC_{50}; for example, competitive inhibition would show an increase in IC_{50} upon substrate escalation.

While the K_i is independent of substrate and enzyme concentration and thus constitutes a solid criterion for inhibitor selection, the IC_{50} can be influenced by these factors and does not necessarily reflect true inhibitor affinity. However, the IC_{50} is still an important determination of the inhibitor functional strength. It is often the case that in cell assays, we do not know parameters such as substrate and enzyme concentration, as well as the composition and conditions of the intracellular medium where the reaction takes place. Under these circumstances, determining the IC_{50} as a criterion for inhibitor selection is very valuable. In fact, an agreement between the IC_{50} of the cell assay and the IC_{50} determined in the biochemical assay (biochemical efficiency) is an indication that most of the inhibitor has reached its target, while a disagreement will point to possible problems such as the inhibitor's inability to cross the membrane and/or being metabolized to ineffective forms.

Various biochemical and cell assays and their application in BACE inhibitor discovery are described.

3.8   COMMON ASSAYS USED TO IDENTIFY AND STUDY INHIBITORS

3.8.1   Capture Assay (CA)

This assay is noncontinuous and nonhomogeneous. In the CA, a substrate carrying a biotin molecule at one terminus and a fluorescent tag at the opposite terminus is incubated with BACE in the absence (control) and in the presence of an inhibitor. The enzyme is either preincubated with an inhibitor or added to the solution containing an inhibitor and allowed to incubate for a determined amount of time; the reaction is stopped by the addition of buffer at pH 8.0 or higher. An aliquot of the mixture is then transferred to a streptavidin (SA)-coated plate and washed in order to remove unbound material. The plates are read to assess the extent of inhibition by comparison with the control assay reaction without the inhibitor. The washing step has an advantage because it removes light absorbing and fluorescent compounds present in the reaction mixture, and a disadvantage because it introduces an extra step.

3.8.2   Fluorescence Polarization (FP) Assay

Because small fluorescent molecules (fluorophores) rotate and tumble quickly, they have low emission polarization values when they are excited by plane-polarized light. If, however, they are bound to large molecules, the resulting complexes rotate slowly and have high emission polarization values. When excited by vertically polarized light, the intensity of the emitted light can be monitored in vertical (V) and horizontal (H) planes and the equation:

$$P = (V - H)/(V + H) \qquad \text{(Eq. 3.10)}$$

relates the polarization (P), to both the vertical (V) and horizontal (H) components of the emitted light. P has no dimensions and is not dependent on the intensity of the emitted light or on the concentration of the fluorophore. The term "mP" (milliP) is used in calculations, where $1\,mP$ = one thousandth of a P. In the FP assay, like in the CA, BACE is incubated with a substrate carrying a biotin molecule at one terminus and a fluorescent tag at the opposite terminus. Enzyme reaction and inhibition are also carried out as in the CA. Upon reaction termination, the substrate is captured with SA in solution. The inhibited reaction would show higher emission polarization values than the non-inhibited reaction and the extent of inhibition is assessed by comparison with the non-inhibited control. The FP assay is amenable to HTS formats and, contrary to the CA, is a homogeneous assay that does not require washing steps. In both CA and FP assays, enzyme inhibition at various inhibitor concentrations allows determining K_i and IC_{50} values. The drawback of FP is poor sensitivity with P usually reaching values of 150–200 mP compared with a background level of 50 mP, a fact that makes it difficult to distinguish signal from noise.

3.8.3   Fluorescence Resonance Transfer (FRET) and Time Resolved (TR)-FRET Assay

Both FRET and TR-FRET assays are based on the energy transfer between a fluorescent donor and acceptor provided that the emission spectrum of the donor has a good overlap with the absorption spectrum of the acceptor, and they are positioned within the Förster radius of each other (this is about 3–6 nm and defined as the distance at which half the excitation energy of the donor is transferred to the acceptor). In one application of this concept, the light emitted by the donor is absorbed by the acceptor (quencher), but is not reemitted. For example, a BACE substrate carrying a fluorescent tag, such as 5-[(2-aminoethyl)amino]naphthalene-1-sulfonic acid (EDANS) or Lucifer Yellow at one terminus, and a fluorescent quencher, such as 4-(4-dimethylaminophenylazo) benzoic acid (DABCYL) or 2,4-dinitrophenyl (DNP) is located at the opposite C-terminus to foster fluorescence quenching. The fluorophore emission occurs upon BACE cleavage as a consequence of FRET interruption. FRET is a homogeneous and continuous assay, highly sensitive, and easily adaptable to HTS. However, FRET assays have traditionally used pairs of donor : acceptor, such as those indicated above, with small Stokes shifts and excitation and emission in the wavelength ranges overlapping those of many compounds contained in HTS libraries, and might produce large numbers of false results in HTS. These negative aspects of FRET are overcome by the use of the TR-FRET technology, which exploits the properties of caged lanthanides such as Eu^{3+}cryptate, Eu^{3+}chelates, or terbium chelates. These lanthanides have a relatively large Stokes shifts and emission lifetime much longer than those of compounds contained in HTS libraries. For example, Eu^{3+}cryptate/chelate in the examples given below have excitation maximum at ~337 nm, main emission at ~620 nm, and lifetime in the range of 320–2,200 µs. Introducing a time delay of 50–200 µs between the excitation and fluorescence measurement allows avoiding overlap with the short-lived signals of a variety of compounds used in the HTS. TR-FRET is, like FRET, a homogeneous and continuous assay where a fluorophore like Eu^{3+}cryptate/chelate is placed at one extremity of the substrate and an energy acceptor at the other extremity. In TR-FRET, the donor (fluorophore) is excited at one wavelength and emits fluorescence at a longer wavelength. The emitted light is absorbed by an acceptor (another fluorophore) and is reemitted at longer wavelength; alternatively, the emitted light is absorbed by an acceptor (a quencher) and not reemitted.

3.8.4   Chemiluminescence (CL) and Electrochemiluminescence (ECL) Assays

In CL, light is emitted as a consequence of a chemical reaction. The enzyme alkaline phosphatase (AP) cleaves phosphate moieties from a variety of different molecules. Various substrates have been reported that allow direct measurement of the product formed by CL and fluorescent methods. A classical and widely used chemiluminescent substrate is *p*-nitrophenyl phosphate (PNPP) whose hydrolysis results in the formation of a colored compound with maximal absorbance at 405 nm. The Great EscAPe SEAP System from Clontech (Mountain View, CA), for example, offers the fluorescent substrate 4-methylumbelliferyl phosphate (MUP), which allows monitoring of SEAP expression through excitation at 360 nm and fluorescence emission at 449 nm, and the chemiluminescent substrate CSPD (Invitrogen Corp., Carlsbad, CA) whose hydrolysis can be monitored by a luminometer or X-ray film.

ECL is a phenomenon by which molecules such as $Ru(bpy)_3^{2+}$ (bpy is 2,2'-bipyridine) emit light through a process consisting of oxidation–reduction cycles fostered by application of a voltage from an electrode. In biochemical/biological assays, ECL molecules are incorporated in an antibody and are used to monitor a specific process. This technology offers the advantage of low background, and the reaction can be controlled because it depends on electricity as a means to start the reaction. Quantitatively, the emission intensity, I_L, is related to the rate of reaction under observation, dC/dt (molecules reacting per second), according to the equation:

$$I_L = \Phi L(dC/dt)$$ (Eq. 3.11)

The proportionality constant ΦL is the CL or ECL quantum yield or efficiency, in photons emitted per molecule reacting.

3.8.5 HPLC Assay

HPLC is widely used for hits validation, to evaluate and/or confirm the mechanistic mode of inhibition, and to determine and/or confirm kinetic parameters such as K_i and IC_{50} determined by other assays. The advantage of an HPLC assay is that of being a technique that uses column chromatography to separate unreacted substrate from formed products during an enzymatic reaction. It thus accounts for substrate disappearance and product formation, and fluorescent or absorbing inhibitors do not interfere with the background signal observed with other fluorogenic and chromogenic assays. The disadvantage of the technique is that it has low throughput affording about 200–250 samples/day and cannot be used for HTS of large libraries.

3.9 BACE ASSAYS

3.9.1 Inhibitor Screening Assays for BACE Activity In Vitro and In Vivo

The substrate GLTNIKTEEISEISY↓EVEFRWKK and its shorter version SEISY↓EVEFRWKK developed as a result of our efforts to study BACE specificity, were employed as such in 96- and 384-well format HPLC assays to determine IC_{50} and K_i. The assay is simple as it consists of incubating BACE substrate with and without inhibitor for a specific amount of time. The products of the reaction are separated by a reverse phase column, and the formation of a tryptophan-containing product is followed by fluorimetry consisting of excitation at 280 nm and monitoring emission at 348 nm. These studies allowed to determine a $k_{cat}/K_M = 70.4\,\mu M^{-1}s^{-1}$, and $= 4.5\,\mu M^{-1}s^{-1}$ for the former and latter substrates, respectively [34].

The peptides Biotin-KVEANY↓EVEGERC[cys-oregongreen]KK and Biotin-GLTNIKTEEISEISY↓EVEFR [cys-oregon green]KK were used in our laboratory for the CA and the FP assay, respectively. The progress of the reaction was monitored at a determined time by reading on an LJL Analyst (Ex 485 nm/Em 530 nm), and on an LJL Acquest (Ex 485 nm/Em 530 nm) for the CA and FP, respectively (LJL Biosystems, Inc., Sunnyvale, CA).

Moreover, the sequence ISY↓EV was inserted in the APP at β-site (Asp1) or β′-site (Glu11) and proved that it is a cellular substrate superior to APP_{Sw}. The APP_{ISYEV} substrate was very specific for measuring BACE activity in cells; in fact, BACE-2 poorly cleaved APP_{ISYEV}. This optimized APP substrate is useful to elucidate the cellular enzymatic actions of BACE and to monitor the cellular efficacy of inhibitors that might be of therapeutic benefit in AD.

Pietrak et al. [38] screened a peptide library against recombinant BACE and identified the octapeptide sequence EVNF↓EVEF as a lead substrate for assay development. They converted that substrate into the coumarin-labeled 10-mer peptide for adaptation to an HPLC assay in a 96-well format requiring 5 min per sample. The Coumarin-REVNF↓EVEFR had a $k_{cat}/K_M = 34\,\mu M^{-1}s^{-1}$ that they estimated to be 1000 times better than a Wt APP-based substrate. This assay afforded them using concentrations of BACE as low as 100 pM thus permitting the determination of K_i in the nanomolar and subnanomolar range. They tested several inhibitors; one of these inhibitors, referred to as Compound 2, gave an $IC_{50} \sim 15$ nM. These investigators also found that this substrate was cleaved by BACE-2 ($k_{cat}/K_M = 0.017\,\mu M^{-1}s^{-1}$ at pH 4.5) and cathepsin D ($k_{cat}/K_M = 0.043\,\mu M^{-1}s^{-1}$ at pH 3.3), and used it to find $IC_{50} \sim 230$ nM and 7620 nM for BACE-2 and cathepsin D, respectively.

Compound 2 was tested in a homogeneous cell assay based on ECL [37]. The investigators stably transfected HEK293T cells with APP_{NFEV} and 1 day after plating treated the cells with a medium containing a compound or 1% dimethylsulfoxide (DMSO) (v/v) for 20–24 h. They derivatized the antibodies to EV40 residues 5–11 (6E10) and residues 34–40 (G2-10) with biotin and ruthenium molecules, respectively, and used them to treat the conditioned medium from the HEK293T cells. After overnight incubation, they treated the solution with SA-coated magnetic beads and subjected it to ECL analysis, and $IC_{50} \sim 33.0$ nM was found.

Oh et al. [39] used AP to develop a cell assay to monitor site-specific proteolysis of BACE in *Drosophila*. They fused AP lacking its own signal sequence to the truncated luminal domain of a *Drosophila* Golgi integral membrane protein, GMII, via dodecameric β-sites peptides. They expressed the resulting constructs, GMII-β-sites-AP, in *Drosophila* S2 cells under the control of the *Drosophila* hsp70 or metallothionein promoter. These constructs contain a Golgi membrane protein, which allow their retention inside this organelle. BACE cleavage of the β-sites fosters the release of AP into the culture medium where its activity was determined by the reaction with PNPP and measurement of absorbance at 405 nm with a microplate reader (Molecular Devices). Among the constructs selected, cleavage was observed only in the one containing the Sw mutation. Three peptidomimetic compounds identified as LB83190, LB83192, and LB83202, and whose IC_{50}'s in a biochemical assay were $0.715\,\mu M$, $0.714\,\mu M$, and $0.127\,\mu M$, respectively, were tested in the *Drosophila* cell assay. While LB83202 was not cell penetrable, IC_{50} values of $12.5\,\mu M$ and $7.8\,\mu M$ were found for LB83190, LB83192, respectively, also pointing to the poor penetration of these two peptidomimetic inhibitors. This is a simple method that allows to determine compound inhibition, cell penetrability, and toxicity; it is easier to use and less expensive than other techniques measuring $A\beta$ secretion into the media.

More recently, Coppola et al. [40] applied the same principle of fusing a Golgi retention signal to a peptide containing BACE cleavage followed by AP. Secretion of AP upon BACE cleavage was monitored by the SEAP activity using the Great EscAPe SEAP chemiluminescent detection kit. They used this assay to test non-steroidal anti-inflammatory drugs (NSAIDs) as inhibitors of BACE and concluded that aspirin and sulindac sulfide directly inhibit BACE activity.

There are various applications of the FRET assay for BACE. Grüninger-Leitch et al. reported the BACE substrate Lys(DABCYL)-SEV*XX*↓DAEFR-Glu(Gly-PEGA)-Lucifer Yellow (*XX* variable aa) with fluorescence excitation at 430 nm and emission at 520 nm [35], and Ermolieff et al. [41] reported the substrate Arg-Glu(EDANS)-Glu-Val-Asn-Leu↓Asp-Ala-Glu-Phe-Lys(DABCYL)-Arg and (7-methoxycoumarin-4-yl) acetyl (MCA))-Ser-Glu-Val-Asn-Leu↓Asp-Ala-Glu-Phe-Lys(DNP) [41] in the study of enzyme specificity and inhibitor profiling; kinetic and inhibition parameters have been mentioned earlier in this chapter.

Porcari et al. [42] reported an application of the TR-FRET assay to identify BACE inhibitors and described both kinetic and end-point measurements. Porcari et al. [42] used Eu^{3+}chelate coupled to the N-terminus and a quenching organic fluorophore (QSY 7) to the C-terminus of the peptide CEVNL↓DAEFK. When the peptide is uncleaved, fluorescence is quenched but is interrupted when the peptide is cleaved. They followed BACE enzymatic activity by excitation at 330 nm and fluorescence emission monitoring at 615 nm by continuous TR-FRET measurements and determined a $K_m = 290\,nM$ that was useful to select a substrate concentration of 200 nM to identify both competitive and noncompetitive inhibitors. Moreover, the assay was validated by reproducing the IC_{50} values of various literature inhibitors, including two Stat-Val peptides for one of which further inhibition studies allow to determine a noncompetitive mode of action and a $K_i = 40\,nM$.

Kennedy et al. [43] compared the activity of autoprocessed mature BACE to the activity of pro-BACE and their inhibition profiles toward selected inhibitors. They used the TR-FRET technology in which the light emitted by the donor is absorbed by the acceptor and reemitted at a higher wavelength. Specifically, the substrate Eu^{3+}cryptate-KTEEISEVNL↓DAEFRHDC-Biotin-(SA-XL665) where the energy acceptor cross-linked allophycocyanin protein (SA-XL665) complexed to SA was used. The Eu^{3+}cryptate-XL665 pair allows the simultaneous monitoring of 620 nm (Eu^{3+}chelate emission maximum) and 665 nm (XL665 emission maximum). The FRET occurs between the Eu^{3+}chelate and the SA-XL665 moieties, leading to quenching of the 620 nm emission and increase of the 665 nm emission. The technology allows monitoring the cleavage reaction progress by simultaneously monitoring the reaction at 620 nm, or at 665 nm, or the 665/620 ratio. These investigators [43] evaluated IC_{50} for the non-hydrolyzable statine inhibitor KTEEISEVN-(Statine)-VAEF, and the homostatine EVNL(ψHET)AAEF and ELDL(ψHET)AVEF for both pro-BACE and auto-cleaved BACE to conclude that these two enzymatic species behave very similarly toward these inhibitors.

Hussain et al. [44] used the fluorescent substrate FAM-[SEVNLDAEFK]-TAMRA for a FRET assay to identify inhibitors from a rational drug design approach. Also, this assay was suitable to monitor the activity of BACE, BACE-2, and cathepsin D. Quantification of substrate cleavage was assessed using an LJL analyst spectrophotometer (485 nm excitation, 535 nm emission). They identified a competitive inhibitor, GSK188909, for which they determined an $IC_{50} \sim 5$ nM, 170 nM, 2600 nM, and 1490 nM for BACE, BACE-2, cathepsin D, and renin (assayed with Dabcyl-γ-Abu-IHPFHLVIHT-Edans), respectively. Testing GSK188909 in human neuroblastoma cells, expressing APP_{Wt} or APP_{Sw} was carried out. Inhibition was quantitated by assaying cell lysates for $A\beta_{40}$ or $A\beta_{42}$ using a BioVeris (BV)™ immunoassay employing Aβ-specific antibodies. They used antibodies to $A\beta_{40}$ residues 5–11 (6E10) and residues 34–40 (G2-10) derivatized with biotin and BV Ruthenium NHS ester tag, respectively, and antibodies to $A\beta_{42}$ residues 5–11 (6E10) and C-terminal residues MVGGVVIA derivatized with biotin and BV Ruthenium NHS ester tag, respectively. After incubation, antibody–Aβ complexes were captured with SA-coated Dynabeads® and were subjected to ECL analysis in a BV M384 analyzer. They observed an inhibitor concentration-dependent decrease in $A\beta_{40}$ and $A\beta_{42}$ secretion into the media with an approximately IC_{50} of 5 nM in SHSY5Y-APP_{Wt} cells and 30 nM in SHSY5Y-APP_{Sw} cells.

The Ruthenium-based assay was also employed to investigate the Aβ lowering activity of GSK188909 *in vivo* by using TASTPM mice that express both human $APP_{Sw}^{K595N/M596L}$ and PS-1^{M146V} transgenes in the brain and exhibit age-associated Aβ accumulation and deposition. Though they observed bioavailability in mice, this inhibitor's brain penetration was low and required permeability glycoprotein (P-gp) inhibitor GF120918 that they administered at 250 mg/kg orally (po) 5 h prior to the administration of GSK188909 po also at 250 mg/kg. They achieved a brain exposure of 5.43 ± 3.504 μM (median 6.25 μM) GSK188909, which fostered a decrease in both guanidine soluble $A\beta_{40}$ (68%, $p < 0.0001$, $n = 18$) and guanidine soluble $A\beta_{42}$ (55%, $p < 0.0001$, $n = 18$) in the brain 9 h post dose.

3.9.2   BACE Assays Used in Expression and Purification of the Enzyme

An accurate determination of the purified enzyme specific activity is regarded, together with its purity and authenticity, as its certificate of quality. Sensitive substrates to monitor recombinant expression and purification of BACE from insect, mammalian, and *Escherichia coli* cell lines have been described [45–48]. In many instances, the recombinant enzyme is refolded from inclusion bodies and the extent of refolding is not known [47, 48]. In these situations, a tight binding competitive inhibitor is designed, when possible, to mimic the substrate, and is used to titrate the enzyme to assess which percentage is properly refolded. It is also common to hook this inhibitor to a resin to separate the refolded and active enzyme from the inactive form; this practice has been reported for both native and recombinant enzyme [17, 46, 47].

3.9.3 Assays for BACE Protein Levels and Activity in AD Patients

In order to test the idea that BACE protein and activity are increased in regions of the brain of AD patients that develop amyloid plaques, Fukumoto et al. [49] developed an antibody CA capable of measuring BACE protein level and BACE-specific activity in frontal, temporal, and cerebellar brain homogenates from 61 brains with AD and 33 control brains. The BACE protein assay consists of a sandwich enzyme-linked immunosorbent assay (ELISA) employing the antibody MAB5308 (mouse monoclonal anti-BACE, C-terminus), which captures BACE from brain homogenates. BACE detection is carried out by the anti-BACE N-terminal antibody PA1-756 followed by horseradish peroxidase (HRP)-linked anti-rabbit IgG (HRP-α-rb) and activation of the QuantaBlu fluorescent substrate. Fluorimetric measurements of the HRP chemiluminescent reaction were carried out at 320 nm excitation and 400 nm emission. For the BACE-specific activity assay, BACE is also captured by MAB5308, and the quenched fluorescent substrate (7-methoxycoumarin-4-yl)acetyl[MOCA]-Ser-Glu-Val-Asn-Leu$\downarrow$Asp-Ala-Glu-Phe-Arg-N-(2,4-dinitrophenyl)[DNP]-Lys-Arg-Arg-NH2 or Arg-Glu(5-[aminoethyl] aminonaphthalene sulfonate[EDANS])-Glu-Val-Asn-Leu$\downarrow$ Asp-Ala-Glu-Phe-Lys(4'-dimethylaminoazo-benzene-4-carboxylate[DABCYL])-Arg is added. BACE cleavage of the substrate removes the quenching and allows quantitation of the fluorescence as indicated earlier. These investigators found that enzymatic activity increased by 63% in the temporal neocortex and 13% in the frontal neocortex in brains with AD, but not in the cerebellar cortex. BACE protein level in the brains with AD increased by 14% in the frontal cortex and by 15% in the temporal cortex, but no difference in the cerebellar cortex.

Zetterberg et al. [50] developed an assay based on the BACE-specific substrate biotin-KTEEISEVNFEVEFR whose shorter version was used earlier by Pietrak et al. [38] to determine BACE activity in the cerebrospinal fluid (CSF) of AD patients. The product generated by BACE cleavage was measured with rabbit polyclonal NF neoepitope-specific antibody in combination with AP-conjugated goat anti-rabbit IgG. This turned out to be a very sensitive assay as it was able to detect 1.0 pM of recombinant BACE as assessed versus recombinant BACE standards.

They concluded that patients affected by AD had higher CSF BACE activity (median, 30 pM [range, 11–96 pM]) than controls (median, 23 pM [range, 8–43 pM]) ($p = 0.02$). Patients with mild cognitive impairment (MCI) who subsequently progressed to AD had higher baseline BACE activity (median, 35 pM [range, 18–71 pM]) than patients with MCI who remained stable (median, 29 pM [range, 14–83 pM]) ($p < 0.001$) and subjects with MCI who developed other forms of dementia (median, 20 pM [range, 10–56 pM]) ($p < 0.001$). They also found positive BACE activity correlation with CSF levels of secreted APP isoforms and Aβ_{40} in the AD and control groups and in all MCI subgroups ($p < 0.05$) except the MCI subgroup that developed AD.

3.10 FINAL REMARKS

This chapter reviews biochemical and cell assays regarding β-secretase, also referred to as β-site converting enzyme (BACE), an appealing target for developing drugs to treat AD. A brief introduction is presented regarding the clinical and physiological hallmarks of AD along with the role of β- and γ-secretase in generating Aβ peptides, which are believed to be critical to the onset and progression of AD. The importance of the biochemical and biological assays as primary assays for HTS to identify modulators from large collections of compounds is discussed along with the role of these assays in secondary screenings to confirm which compounds are worthy of medicinal chemistry optimization and to monitor the optimization process. The cell assay is described as a tool verifying that optimized inhibitors are effective in the cellular environment as a prerequisite to animal model testing. The development of sensitive and reliable BACE assays stems from an understanding of the specificity of this enzyme for substrates; the latter is discussed along with some key aspects of the catalytic mechanism of aspartyl proteases. Indeed, the catalytic mechanism and enzyme specificity are highlighted as important to both assay development and to inhibitor design. In addition, basic enzyme kinetic concepts such as k_{cat} and K_m are examined. The importance of accurately determining the inhibition parameters IC_{50} and K_i for BACE and related aspartyl proteases from both the screening and optimization processes is discussed along with the concepts of mechanism of inhibition, for example, competitive, uncompetitive, and noncompetitive/mixed. Finally, a flow scheme from library screening to drug candidate selection is given to emphasize points of go/no-go decisions for compound advancement in the inhibitor development process.

ACKNOWLEDGMENT

We would like to thank Huey Shieh, Thomas L. Emmons, and Arthur Wittwer (Pfizer Inc.) for valuable discussions.

REFERENCES

1. Selkoe, D.J. 2001. Alzheimer's disease: genes, proteins, and therapy. *Physiol Rev* **81**:741–766.
2. Hardy, J.A. and Selkoe, D.J. 2002. The amyloid hypothesis of Alzheimer's disease: progress and problems on the road to therapeutics. *Science* **297**:353–356.
3. Golde, T.E., Dickson, D., and Hutton, M. 2006. Filling the gaps in the abeta cascade hypothesis of Alzheimer's disease. *Curr Alzheimer Res* **3**:421–430.
4. Vassar, R. 2004. BACE1: the beta-secretase enzyme in Alzheimer's disease. *J Mol Neurosci* **23**:105–114.
5. Liu, K., Doms, R.W., and Lee, V.M. 2002. Glu[11] site cleavage and N-terminally truncated Aβ production upon BACE overexpression. *Biochemistry* **41**:3128–3136.
6. Fahrenholz, F. and Postina, R. 2006. α-Secretase activation – an approach to Alzheimer's disease therapy. *Neurodegen Dis* **3**:255–261.
7. Christensen, D.D. 2007. Changing the course of Alzheimer's disease: anti-amyloid disease-modifying treatments on the horizon. *Prim Care Companion J Clin Psychiatry* **9**:32–41.
8. Iwata, N., Tsubuki, S., Takaki, Y., Shirotani, K., Lu, B., Gerard, N.P., Gerard, C., Hama, E., Lee, H.-J., and Saido, T.C. 2001. Metabolic regulation of brain Aβ by neprilysin. *Science* **292**:1550–1552.
9. Kuroshkin, I.V. and Goto, S. 1994. Alzheimer's β-amyloid peptide specifically interacts with and is degraded by insulin degrading enzyme. *FEBS Lett* **345**:33–37.

10. Allinson, T.M., Parkin, E.T., Turner, A.J., and Hooper, N.M. 2003. ADAMs family members as amyloid precursor protein α-secretases. *J Neurosci Res* **74**:342–352.

11. Yu, G., Nishimura, M., Arawaka, S., Levitan, D., Zhang, L., Tandon, A., Song, Y.Q., Rogaeva, E., Chen, F., Kawarai, T., Supala, A., Levesque, L., Yu, H., Yang, D.S., Holmes, E., Milman, P., Liang, Y., Zhang, D.M., Xu, D.H., Sato, C., Rogaev, E., Smith, M., Janus, C., Zhang, Y., Aebersold, R., Farrer, L.S., Sorbi, S., Bruni, A., Fraser, P., and George-Hyslop, P. 2000. Nicastrin modulates presenilin-mediated notch/glp-1 signal transduction and betaAPP processing. *Nature* **407**:48–54.

12. Francis, R., McGrath, G., Zhang, J., Ruddy, D.A., Sym, M., Apfeld, J., Nicoll, M., Maxwell, M., Hai, B., Ellis, M.C., Parks, A.L., Xu, W., Li, J., Gurney, M., Myers, R.L., Himes, C.S., Hiebsch, R., Ruble, C., Nye, J.S., and Curtis, D. 2002. Aph-1 and pen-2 are required for Notch pathway signaling, gamma-secretase cleavage of betaAPP, and presenilin protein accumulation. *Dev Cell* **3**:85–97.

13. De Strooper, B., Saftig, P., Craessaerts, K., Vanderstichele, H., Guhde, G., Annaert, W., Von Figura, K., and Van Leuven, F. 1998. Deficiency of presenilin-1 inhibits the normal cleavage of amyloid precursor protein. *Nature* **391**:387–390.

14. Li, Y.M., Xu, M., Lai, M.T., Huang, Q., Castro, J.L., DiMuzio-Mower, J., Harrison, T., Lellis, C., Nadin, A., Neduvelil, J.G., Register, R.B., Sardana, M.K., Shearman, M.S., Smith, A.L., Shi, X.P., Yin, K.C., Shafer, J.A., and Gardell, S.J. 2000. Photoactivated gamma-secretase inhibitors directed to the active site covalently label presenilin 1. *Nature* **405**:689–694.

15. Esler, W.P., Kimberly, W.T., Ostaszewski, B.L., Diehl, T.S., Moore, C.L., Tsai, J.Y., Rahmati, T., Xia, W., Selkoe, D.J., and Wolfe, M.S. 2000. Transition-state analogue inhibitors of gamma-secretase bind directly to presenilin-1. *Nat Cell Biol* **2**:428–434.

16. Yan, R., Bienkowski, M.J., Shuck, M.E., Miao, H., Tory, M.C., Pauley, A.M., Brashler, J.R., Stratman, N.C., Mathews, W.R., Buhl, A.E., Carter, D.B., Tomasselli, A.G., Parodi, L.A., Heinrikson, R.L., and Gurney, M.E. 1999. Membrane anchored aspartyl protease with Alzheimer's disease β-secretase activity. *Nature* **402**:533–537.

17. Sinha, S., Anderson, J.P., Barbour, R., Basi, G.S., Caccavello, R., Davis, D., Doan, M., Dovey, H.F., Frigon, N., Hong, J., Jacobson-Croak, K., Jewett, N., Keim, P., Knops, J., Lieberburg, I., Power, M., Tan, H., Tatsuno, G., Tung, J., Schenk, D., Seubert, P., Suomensaari, S.M., Wang, S., Walker, D., Zhao, J., McConlogue, L., and John, V. 1999. Purification and cloning of amyloid precursor protein β-secretase from human brain. *Nature* **402**:537–540.

18. Vassar, R., Bennett, B.D., Babu-Khan, S., Kahn, S., Mendiaz, E.A., Denis, P., Teplow, D.B., Ross, S., Amarante, P., Loeloff, R., Luo, Y., Fisher, S., Fuller, J., Edenson, S., Lile, J., Jarosinski, M.A., Biere, A.L., Curran, E., Burgess, T., Louis, J.C., Collins, F., Treanor, J., Rogers, G., and Citron, M. 1999. Beta-secretase cleavage of Alzheimer's amyloid precursor protein by the transmembrane aspartic protease BACE. *Science* **286**:735–741.

19. Hussain, I., Powell, D., Howlett, D.R., Tew, D.G., Meek, T.D., Chapman, C., Gloger, I.S., Murphy, K.E., Southan, C.D., Ryan, D.M., Smith, T.S., Simmons, D.L., Walsh, F.S., Dingwall, C., and Christie, G. 1999. Identification of a novel aspartic protease (Asp 2) as β-secretase. *Mol Cell Neurosci* **14**:419–427.

20. Roberds, S.L., Anderson, J., Basi, G., Bienkowski, M.J., Branstetter, D.G., Chen, K.S., Freedman, S.B., Frigon, N.L., Games, D., Hu, K., Johnson-Wood, K., Kappenman, K.E., Kawabe, T.T., Kola, I., Kuehn, R., Lee, M., Liu, W., Motter, R., Nichols, N.F., Power, M., Robertson, D.W., Schenk, D., Schoor, M., Shopp, G.M., Shuck, M.E., Sinha, S., Svensson, K.A., Tatsuno, G., Tintrup, H., Wijsman, J., Wright, S., and McConlogue, L. 2001. BACE knockout mice are healthy despite lacking the primary β-secretase activity in brain: implications for Alzheimer's disease therapeutics. *Hum Mol Genet* **10**:1317–1324.

21. Cai, H., Wang, Y., McCarthy, D., Wen, H., Borchelt, D.R., Price, D.L., and Wong, P.C. 2001. BACE1 is the major β-secretase for generation of Aβ peptides by neurons. *Nature Neurosci* **4**:233–234.

22. Hussain, I., Powell, D.J., Howlett, D.R., Chapman, G.A., Gilmour, L., Murdock, P.R., Tew, D.G., Meek, T.D., Chapman, C., Schneider, K., Ratcliffe, S.J., Tattersall, D., Testa, T.T., Southan, C., Ryan, D.M., Simmons, D.L., Walsh, F.S., Dingwall, C., and Christie, G. 2000. ASP1 (BACE2) cleaves the amyloid precursor protein at the b-secretase site. *Mol Cell Neurosci* **16**:609–619.

23. Yan, R., Munzner, J.B., Shuck, M.E., and Bienkowski, M.J. 2001. BACE2 functions as an alternative α-secretase in cells. *J Biol Chem* **276**:34019–34027.

24. Clans of peptidases. Available at http://merops.sanger.ac.uk/.

25. Capell, A., Steiner, H., Willem, M., Kaiser, H., Meyer, C., Walter, J., Lammich, S., Multhaup, G., and Haass, C. 2000. Maturation and pro-peptide cleavage of beta-secretase. *J Biol Chem* **275**:30849–30854.

26. Benjannet, S., Elagoz, A., Wickham, L., Mamarbachi, M., Munzer, J.S., Basak, A., Lazure, C., Cromlish, J.A., Sisodia, S., Checler, F., Chretien, M., and Seidah, N.G. 2001. Post-translational processing of beta-secretase (beta-amyloid-converting enzyme) and its ectodomain shedding. The pro- and transmembrane/cytosolic domains affect its cellular activity and amyloid-beta production. *J Biol Chem* **276**:10879–10887.

27. Haniu, M., Denis, P., Young, Y., Mendiaz, E.A., Fuller, J., Hui, J.O., Bennett, B.D., Kahn, S., Ross, S., Burgess, T., Katta, V., Rogers, G., Vassar, R., and Citron, M. 2000. Characterization of Alzheimer's beta-secretase protein BACE. A pepsin family member with unusual properties. *J Biol Chem* **275**:21099–21106.

28. Hong, L., Koelsch, G., Lin, X., Wu, S., Terzyan, S., Ghosh, A.K., Zhang, X.C., and Tang, J. 2000. Structure of the protease domain of memapsin 2 (β-secretase) complexed with inhibitor. *Science* **290**:150–153.

29. Westmeyer, G.G., Willem, M., Lichtenthaler, S.F., Lurman, G., Multhaup, G., Assfalg-Machleidt, I., Reiss, K., Saftig, P., and Haass, C. 2004. Dimerization of beta-site beta-amyloid precursor protein-cleaving enzyme. *J Biol Chem* **279**:53205–53212.

30. Kopcho, L.M., Ma, J., Marcinkeviciene, J., Lai, Z., Witmer, M.R., Cheng, J., Yanchunas, J., Tredup, J., Corbett, M., Calambur, D., Wittekind, M., Paruchuri, M., Kothari, D., Lee, G., Ganguly, S., Ramamurthy, V., Morin, P.E., Camac, D.M., King, R.W., Lasut, A.L., Ross, O.H., Hillman, M.C., Fish, B., Shen, K., Dowling, R.L., Kim, Y.B., Graciani, N.R., Collins, D., Combs, A.P., George, H., Thompson, L.A., and Copeland, R.A. 2003. Comparative studies of active site-ligand interactions among various recombinant constructs of human beta-amyloid precursor protein cleaving enzyme. *Archives Biochem Biophys* **410**:307–316.

31. Toulokhonova, L., Metzler, W.J., Witmer, M.R., Copeland, R.A., and Marcinkeviciene, J. 2003. Kinetic studies on beta-site amyloid precursor protein-cleaving enzyme (BACE). *J Biol Chem* **278**:4582–4589.

32. Cheng, Y. and Prusoff, W.H. 1973. Relationship between the inhibition constant (K1) and the concentration of inhibitor which causes 50 per cent inhibition (I50) of an enzymatic reaction. *Biochem Pharmacol* **1**;22(23):3099–3108.

33. Turner, R.T. III, Koelsch, G., Hong, L., Castanheira, P., Ghosh, A. and Tang, J. 2001. Subsite specificity of memapsin 2 (β-secretase): implications for inhibitor design. *Biochemistry* **40**:10001–10006.

34. Tomaselli, A.G., Qahwash, I., Emmons, T.L., Lu, Y., Leone, J.W., Lull, J.M., Fok, K.M., Bannow, C.A., Smith, C.W., Bienkowski, M.J., Heinrikson, R.L., and Yan, R. 2003. Employing a superior BACE1 cleavage sequence to probe cellular APP processing. *J Neurochemistry* **84**:1006–1017.

35. Grüninger-Leitch, F., Schlatter, D., Küng, E., Nelböck, P., and Döbeli, H. 2002. Substrate and inhibitor profile of BACE (β-secretase) and comparison with other mammalian aspartic proteases. *J Biol Chem* **277**:4687–4693.

36. Cole, S.L. and Vassar, R. 2007. The Alzheimer's disease β-secretase enzyme, BACE1. *Molecul Neurodegen* **2**:22–47.

37. See Chapter 6 of this book.

38. Pietrak, B.L., Crouthamel, M.-C., Tugusheva, K., Lineberger, J.E., Xu, M., DiMuzio, J.M., Steele, T., Espeseth, A.S., Stachel, S.J., Coburn, C.A., Graham, S.L., Vacca, J.P., Shi, X.-P., Simon, A.J., Hazuda, D.J., and Lai, M.-T. 2005. Biochemical and cell-based assays for characterization of BACE-1 inhibitors. *Anal Biochem* **342**:144–151.

39. Oh, M., Kim, S.Y., Oh, Y.S., Choi, D.Y., Sin, H.J., Jung, I.M., and Park, W.J. 2003. Cell-based assay for β-secretase activity. *Anal Biochem* **323**:7–11.

40. Coppola, J.M., Hamilton, C.A., Bhojani, M.S., Larsen, M.J., Ross, B.D., and Rehemtulla, A. 2007. Identification of inhibitors using a cell-based assay for monitoring Golgi-resident protease activity. *Anal Biochem* **364**:19–29.

41. Ermolieff, J., Loy, J.A., Koelsch, G., and Tang, J. 2000. Proteolytic activation of recombinant pro-memapsin 2 (pro-β-secretase) studied with new fluorogenic substrates. *Biochemistry* **39**:12450–12456.

42. Porcari, V., Magnoni, L., Terstappen, G.C., and Fecke, W. 2005. A continuous time-resolved fluorescence assay for identification of BACE1 inhibitors. *Assay Drug Dev Technol* **3**:287–297.

43. Kennedy, M.E., Wang, W., Song, L., Lee, J., Zhang, L., Wong, G., Wang, L., and Parker, E. 2003. Measuring human β-secretase (BACE1) activity using homogeneous time-resolved fluorescence. *Anal Biochem* **319**:49–55.

44. Hussain, I., Hawkins, J., Harrison, D., Hille, C., Wayne, G., Cutler, L., Buck, T., Walter, D., Demont, E., Howes, C., Naylor, A., Jeffrey, P., Gonzalez, M.I., Dingwall, C., Michel, A., Redshaw, S., and Davis, J.B. 2007. Oral administration of a potent and selective non-peptidic BACE-1 inhibitor decreases β-cleavage of amyloid precursor protein and amyloid-β production *in vivo*. *J Neurochem* **100**:822–840.

45. Bruinzeel, W., Yon, J., Giovannelli, S., and Masure, S. 2002. Recombinant insect cell expression and purification of human β-secretase (BACE-1) for X-ray crystallography. *Protein Expr Purif* **26**:139–148.

46. Emmons, T.L., Shuck, M.E., Babcock, M.S., Holloway, J.S., Leone, J.W., Durbin, J.D., Paddock, D.J., Prince, B.D., Fischer, H.D., Bienkowski, M.J., Heinrikson, R.L., Benson, T.E., and Tomasselli, A.G. 2008. Large-scale purification of human BACE expressed in mammalian cells and removal of the prosegment with HIV-1 protease to improve crystal diffraction. *Protein Pept Lett* **15**:119–130.

47. Tomasselli, A.G., Paddock, D.J., Emmons, T.L., Mildner, A.M., Leone, J.W., Lull, J.M., Cialdella, J.I., Prince, B.D., Fischer, H.D., Heinrikson, R.L., and Benson, T.E. 2008. High yield expression of human BACE constructs in *E. coli* for refolding, purification, and high resolution 3D structures. *Protein Pept Lett* **15**:131–143.

48. Sardana, V., Xu, B., Zugay-Murphy, J., Chen, Z., Sardana, M., Darke, P.L., Munshi, S., and Kuo, L.C. 2004. A general procedure for the purification of human β-secretase expressed in *Escherichia coli*. *Protein Expr Purif* **34**:190–196.

49. Fukumoto, H., Cheung, B.S., Hyman, B.T., and Irizarry, M.C. 2002. β-secretase protein and activity are increased in the neocortex in Alzheimer disease. *Ach Neurol* **59**:1381–1390.

50. Zetterberg, H., Andreasson, U., Hansson, O., Wu, G., Sankaranarayanan, S., Andersson, M.E., Buchhave, P., Londos, E., Umek, R.M., Minthon, L., Simon, A.J., and Blennow, K. 2008. Elevated cerebrospinal fluid BACE1 activity in incipient Alzheimer disease. *Arch Neuro* **65**:1102–1107.

CHAPTER 4

PEPTIDIC, PEPTIDOMIMETIC, AND HTS-DERIVED BACE INHIBITORS

James P. Beck and Dustin J. Mergott

Lilly Research Laboratories, Eli Lilly and Company, Indianapolis, IN

4.1 INTRODUCTION

Substantial effort has been expended on attempts to develop peptidic and peptido-mimetic BACE-1 inhibitors via mostly traditional substrate-based design or occasionally high-throughput screening (HTS)-based medicinal chemistry approaches. Several exceptional reviews have been published that treat various aspects of these drug discovery efforts spanning nearly the last decade [1]. Most reviews have been organized by inhibitor class of the transition-state isostere (TSI) mimic. In contrast, the examples presented in this chapter are organized first by company, research institution, or collaboration, and then further by TST. The goal of this compilation is to review and summarize the most impactful contributions from key organizations contributing to BACE-1 inhibitor design.

4.2 ELAN/PHARMACIA (PFIZER)

Peptidic and peptidomimetic substrate-based inhibitors of BACE were designed using the knowledge of the specificity and kinetics of BACE-1. The Elan team published on the development of the first statine-based [2] cell-permeable [3] BACE-1 inhibitors that demonstrated dose-dependent and mechanism-specific reduction of $A\beta$ in human embryonic kidney (HEK) cells (Fig. 4.1, **1–3**). The evolution of the Elan BACE-1 inhibitors began with the definition of the P_1 and P_1' in a BACE substrate spanning P_{16}-P_5' with replacement of the P_1 residue with a noncleavable statine residue and replacement of the P_1' Asp with valine. The conversion of peptidic inhibitors into cell-permeable peptidomimetic inhibitors was done in a sequence of steps, initiating with a conceptual division of the peptide into three regions: an N-terminal portion (non-prime side), a central statine-containing isostere, and a C-terminal portion (prime side). Individually targeted for modification, the amino

BACE: Lead Target for Orchestrated Therapy of Alzheimer's Disease, Edited by Varghese John
Copyright © 2010 John Wiley & Sons, Inc.

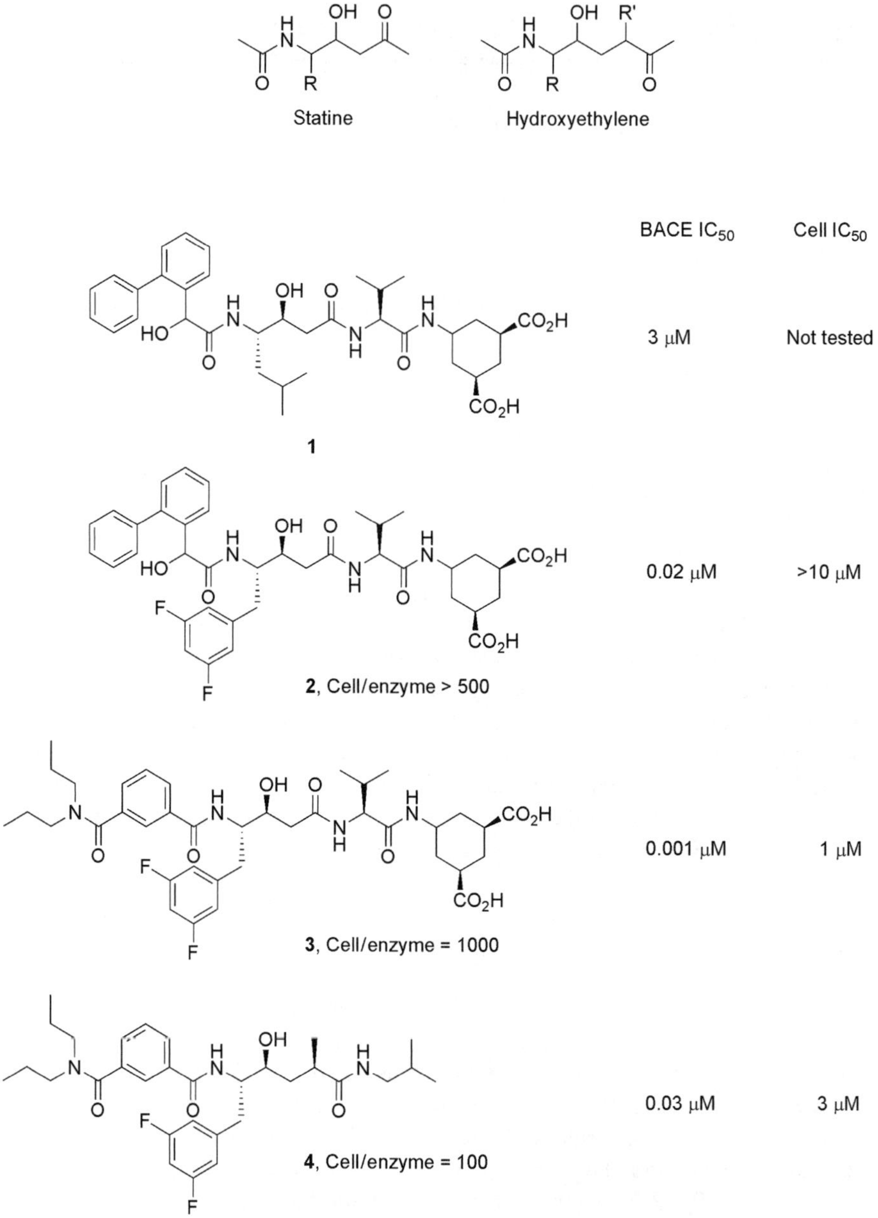

Figure 4.1   Elan BACE inhibitors.

acid residues of these sections were replaced with functionalities exhibiting less peptide character, while retaining BACE-1 enzyme activity. The most potent N-terminal replacements were α-hydroxyarylacetic acids while the C-terminal "AEF" region was transformed into cyclohexyl dicarboxylate derivative which served as an effectively constrained surrogate. The resultant inhibitor (**1**, BACE-1

$IC_{50} = 3\,\mu M$) was further modified at the central P_1 by replacing leucine with 3,5-difluorophenylalanine – a feature that would continue in all future Elan (and later Elan/Pharmacia) structure-activity relationships (SAR) on BACE-1 inhibitors (*vide infra*) [4]. The combination of these optimal features led to the potent inhibitor **2**; the corresponding dimethylester (not shown) was found to also be cell permeable (BACE-1 $IC_{50} = 0.12\,\mu M$, Cell $IC_{50} = 4\,\mu M$) and inhibited β-sAPP (amyloid precursor protein) formation upon immunoprecipitation analysis, confirming the mechanism-specific BACE-1 inhibition. Another key SAR discovery came when Elan researchers incorporated the known isophthalamide asparagine replacement [5] bridging P_2-P_3 in the inhibitor, therein affording statine **3** with a cell/enzyme ratio of 1000. An order of magnitude improvement in the cell/enzyme ratio was obtained when the statine TSI was replaced with hydroxyethylene [6] (Fig. 4.1, **4**) and with a further truncation of the C-terminal substitution. Although excellent enzyme activity could be obtained through further SAR in the hydroxyethylene series [7], the cell/enzyme ratio could not be improved upon, and therefore, attention turned to the hydroxyethylamine (HEA) isostere where the perceived advantage of the more basic amine was anticipated to facilitate cell transport and improve overall blood–brain barrier penetration of these peptidomimetic inhibitors.

In August of 2000, Elan and Pharmacia announced they had entered into a research and development partnership to discover and commercialize BACE-1 inhibitors. Shortly thereafter, this team published a series of patents on HEA BACE-1 peptidomimetic inhibitors (Fig. 4.2) [8]. These HEA inhibitors exhibited a strong preference for the *(R)* stereochemistry at the transition state secondary hydroxyl compared with statine and HE inhibitors, which preferred the *(S)* stereochemistry. Comparing hydroxyethylene inhibitor **4** with HEA inhibitor **5** (Fig. 4.2), the cell to enzyme ratio was improved from 100-fold to 1.8-fold. Another order of magnitude improvement to both the enzyme and cell activity was then achieved by (1) adding a methyl group to the isophthalamide phenyl to better fill S_2; (2) replacing the P_1'-P_2' substitution with benzyl; and then (3) adding the substitution at the meta-position of the benzyl to better occupy S_2'; the result of these combinations afforded HEA inhibitor **8** (Fig. 4.2) [9, 10]. Closely related to this work, Petukhov and colleagues at the University of Illinois at Chicago have very recently published on P_2 biaryl and fused-ring HEAs building off the isopthalamide (not shown) [11]. The 1st generation of HEA inhibitors to come from Elan/Pharmacia team also includes acyclic substitution (non-isophthalamide) at P_2 (Fig. 4.3, **9–13**) with either phenylalanine [12] or 3,5-difluorophenylalanine [13] occupying the S_1 pocket. One hypothesis in the design of these analogs was that selectivity over cathepsin D (Cat-D) would be improved relative to the isophthalamides occupying S_2. This hypothesis was based on the presence of the two methionine residues in Cat-D (Met307 and Met 309) that helps to form the S_2 pocket in contrast to Arg235 found in BACE-1. This data supported the hypothesis – whereas HEA inhibitor **8** afforded a Cat-D/BACE-1 selectivity of 13-fold, the corresponding selectivities for acyclic HEAs **9–11** were 250-, 186-, and 235-fold, respectively [13]. *In vivo* effects for these acyclic HEAs were not disclosed [14]. The macrocyclic inhibitors **14** and **15** (Fig. 4.3) further contribute to the 1st-generation HEAs from Elan/Pharmacia [15]. Although no enzyme data was disclosed for these inhibitors, the conserved optimal substitution from earlier

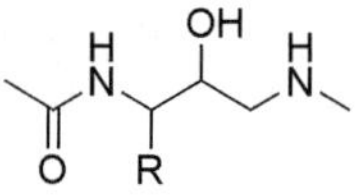

Hydroxyethylamine
(1st generation)

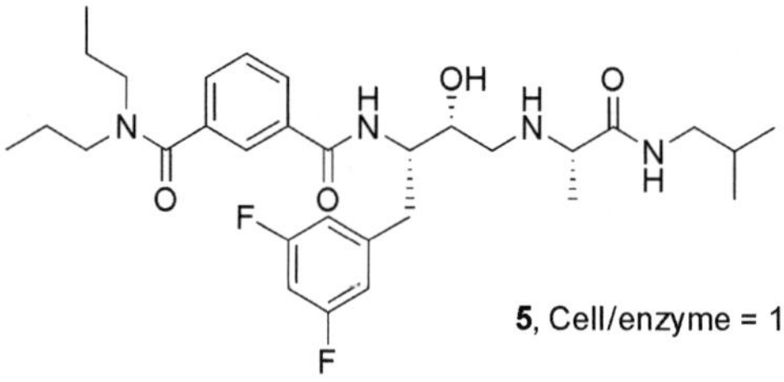

	BACE IC$_{50}$	Cell IC$_{50}$

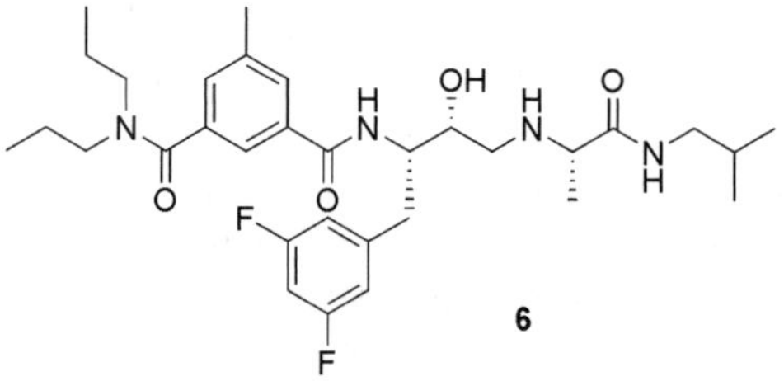

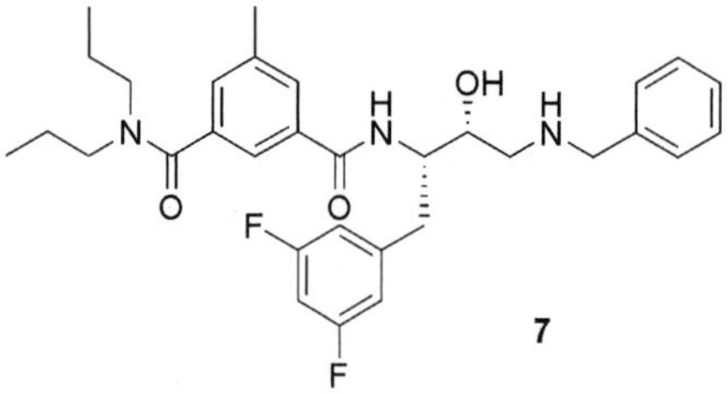

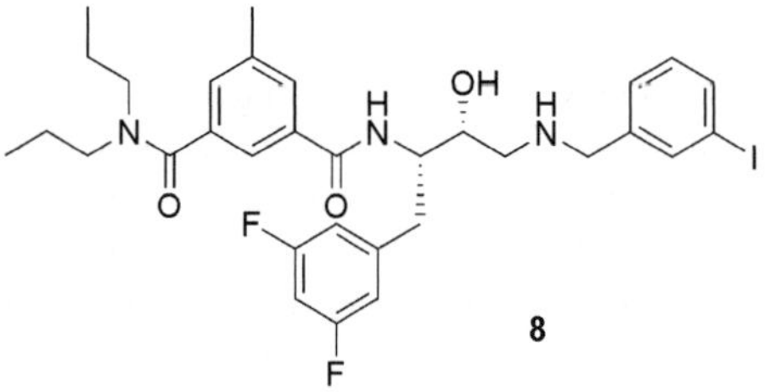

5, Cell/enzyme = 1.8

130 nM · 230 nM

6

70 nM · 80 nM

7

130 nM · 40 nM

8

5 nM · 3 nM

Figure 4.2   Elan/Pharmacia BACE inhibitors.

HEAs in the 1st-generation SAR almost certainly lends a substantial degree of activity to these macrocycles.

Prodrugs of HEA BACE inhibitors have been reported in two patent applications from the Elan/Pharmacia team. First described were ester and carbamate derivatives of the central secondary hydroxyl group [16]. The second, and more

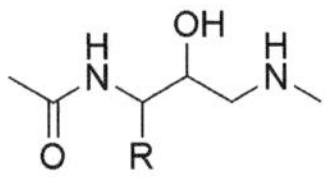

Hydroxyethylamine
(1st generation, cont.)

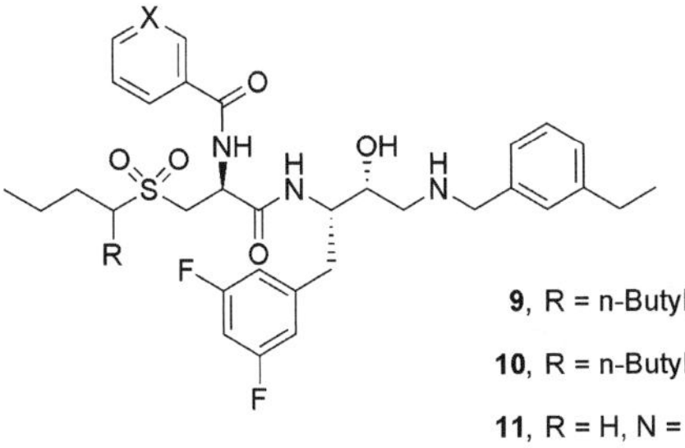

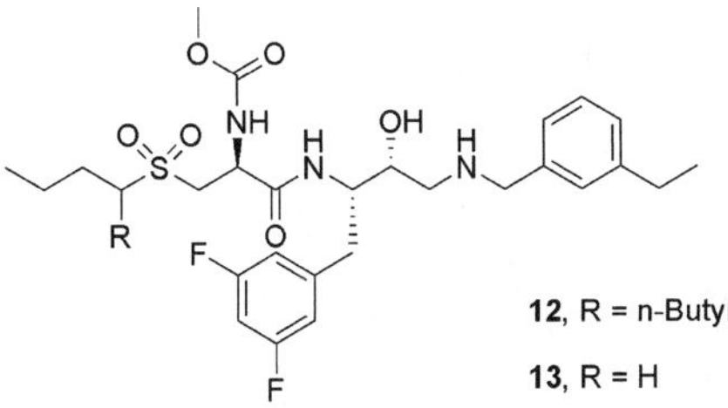

	BACE IC_{50}	Cell IC_{50}
9, R = n-Butyl, X = CH	2 nM	14 nM
10, R = n-Butyl, X = N	1 nM	1 nM
11, R = H, N = H	2 nM	1 nM
12, R = n-Butyl	3 nM	2 nM
13, R = H	4 nM	2 nM

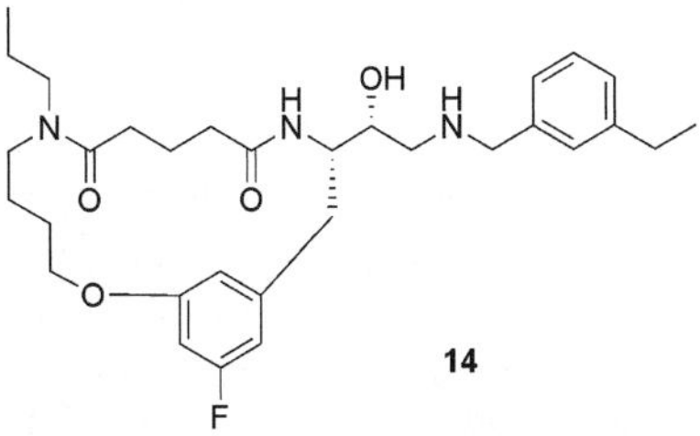

14

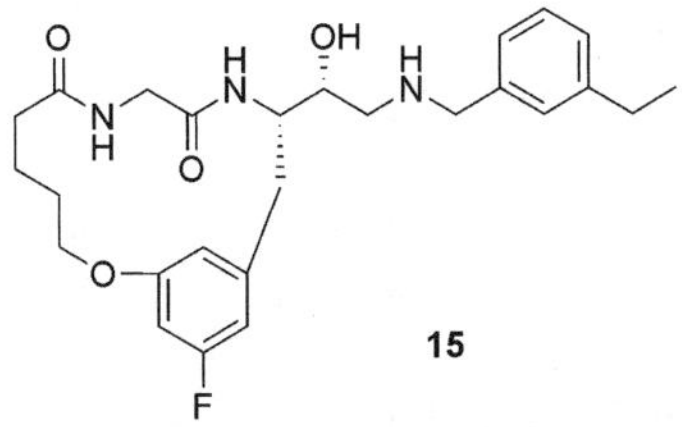

15

Figure 4.3   Elan/Pharmacia BACE inhibitors.

detailed, prodrug disclosure was based on the proven concept of O- to N-acyl migration [17], a strategy for improving delivery described previously for renin [18] and HIV aspartyl proteases [19]. The facile O- to N-acyl migration that is shown (Fig. 4.4, **16,17**) to occur results in part from the high aqueous solubility of the amines (**16**). In fact, depending on the nature of the substitution, prodrug **16** (R_1 = cyclopropyl, R_2 = ethyl or acetylene) rearranges to BACE-1 inhibitor **17** in as short as 1.0–1.5 h in pH 7.0 at 40°C (^{19}F-NMR used to follow the progress of the reactions).

In 2003, a "2nd generation" of Elan/Pharmacia HEAs began appearing in the patent literature. Focused exclusively on the P_1-P_3 SAR of the HEA peptidomimet-

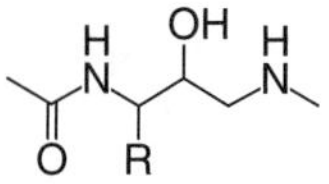

Hydroxyethylamine prodrug (acyl migration)
(1st generation)

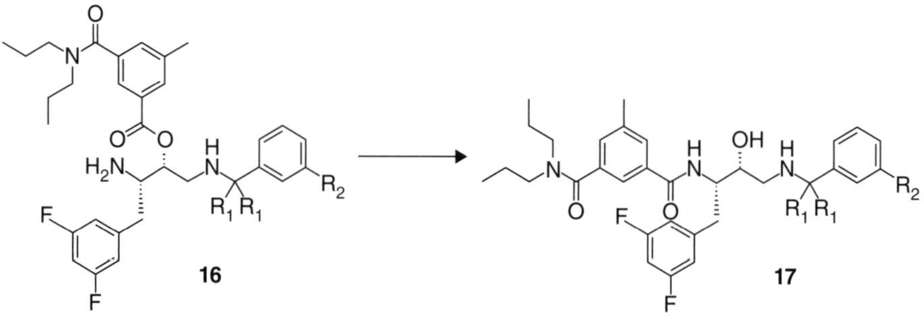

	40°C, pH 7		40°C, pH 4	
	HEA product	N-acyl product	HEA product	N-acyl product
R_1 = H, H R_2 = CF_3	24 h, 57%	24 h, 43%	30 h, 79%	30 h, 21%
R_1 = H, H R_2 = ethyl	24 h, 62%	24 h, 38%	24 h, 88%	24 h, 12%
R_1 = cylcopropyl R_2 = ethyl	1.5 h, 97%	—	24 h, 100%	—
R_1 = cylopropyl R_2 = acetylene	1 h, 100%	—	48 h, 86%	—

Figure 4.4   Elan/Pharmacia BACE inhibitors.

ics, the goal of this work was to attenuate the significant P-glycoprotein (P-gp) efflux observed in the 1st-generation HEAs. A diverse range of non-prime side functionality was explored in these inhibitors (Fig. 4.5, **18–25**) as evidenced by the reported aminopyridyl (**18**) [20], dihydrobenzoxazine and dihydrobenzothiazine (**19,21**) [20], indole (**20**) [20], phenyl- and oxazolesulfonamide (**22,23**) [20], keto-piperazine (**24**) [21], phenacyl (**25**) [20], and ureas and carbamates [22].

In 2004, Maillard et al. published a key significant breakthrough in BACE-1 aspartyl protease inhibitor design with a series of N-acetyl-2-hydroxy-1,3-diaminoalkanes (Fig. 4.6, **26–28**), termed the "3rd-generation HEAs" [23]. Key to this accomplishment was the designed removal of the P_2 and P_3 inhibitor groups (N-terminal truncated) with focus paid on optimizing the P_2' and P_3' substituents. The result of these efforts were to identify BACE-1 inhibitors with dramatically lowered molecular weight, lowered lipophilicity, lowered atomic polar surface area, and improved solubility. For example, inhibitor **8** contains 41 heavy atoms with a molecular weight of 678 compared with inhibitor **27** with just 30 heavy atoms and a molecular weight of 417; despite the weaker BACE-1 activity, inhibitor **27** actually has the better ligand efficiency [24] when compared to inhibitor **8**. In support of the improved druggability profile of these 3rd-generation HEA BACE-1 inhibitors,

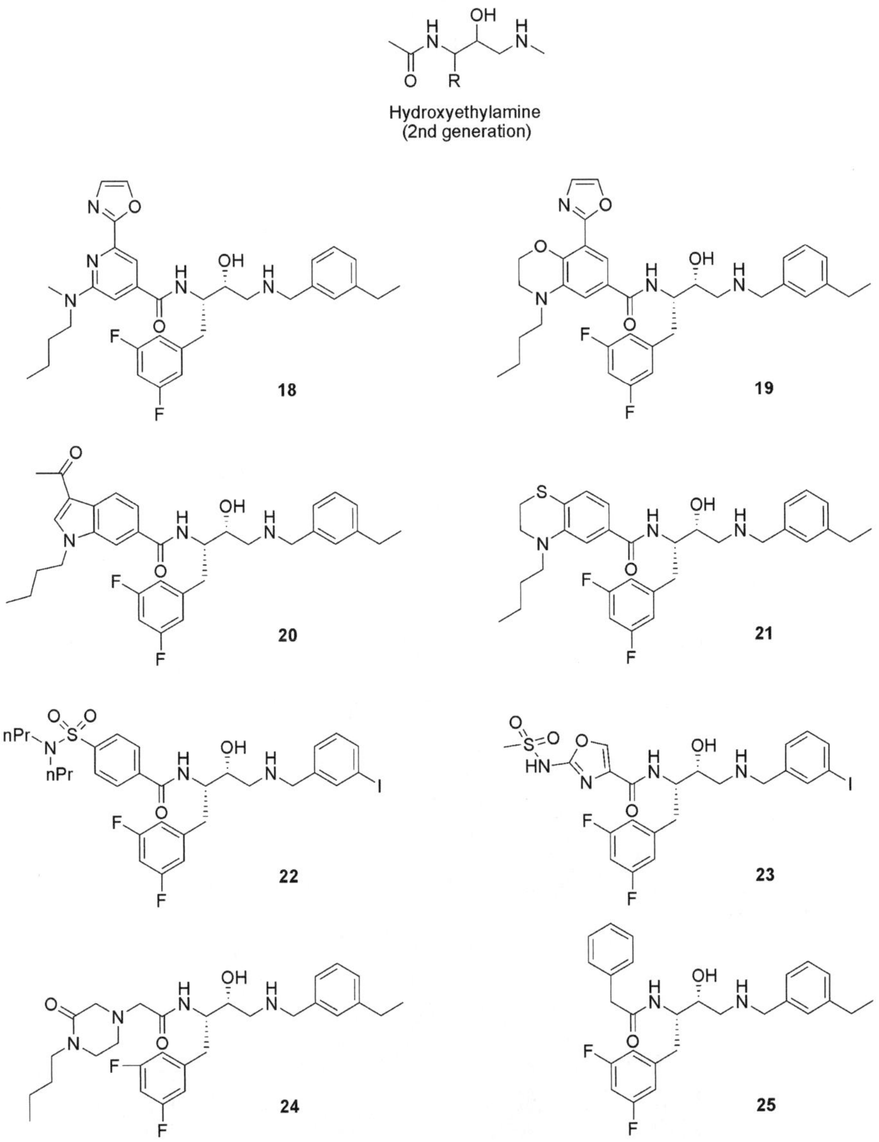
Hydroxyethylamine
(2nd generation)
18
19
20
21
22
23
24
25

Figure 4.5 Elan/Pharmacia BACE inhibitors.

Elan/Pharmacia disclosed [25] efficacy and oral bioavailability on a number of inhibitors. For example, inhibitor **27** afforded a 35% significant reduction of brain Aβ in the cortex of PDAPP mice when dosed orally at 100 mg/kg. Through extensive SAR [26], it was found that the P_2' group was very tolerant of diverse substitution and functionality, including heteroaryl (Fig. 4.6, **29**), oximes (Fig. 4.6, **30**), P_1 spirocycles with a P_2 benzyl (**26**) or amide linker (Fig. 4.6, **31**), and a pyrrolidine (Fig. 4.6, **32**). Furthermore, SAR (Fig. 4.7) in this genre of HEAs yielded N-acetyl

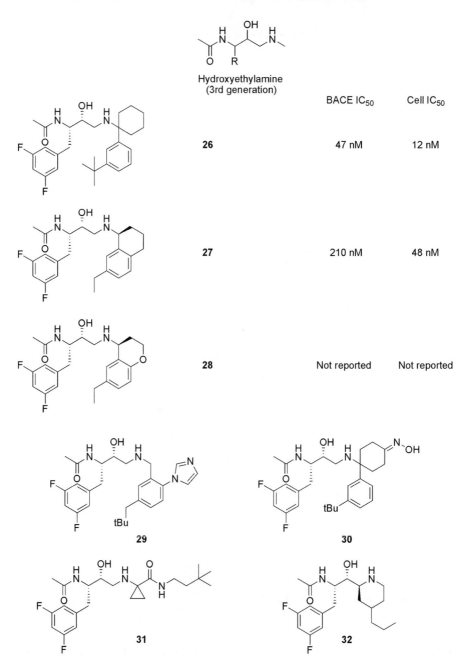

Figure 4.6   Elan/Pharmacia BACE inhibitors.

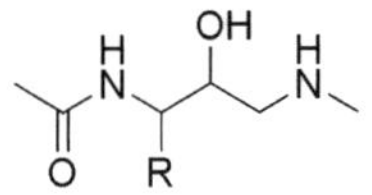

Hydroxyethylamine
(3rd generation, continued)

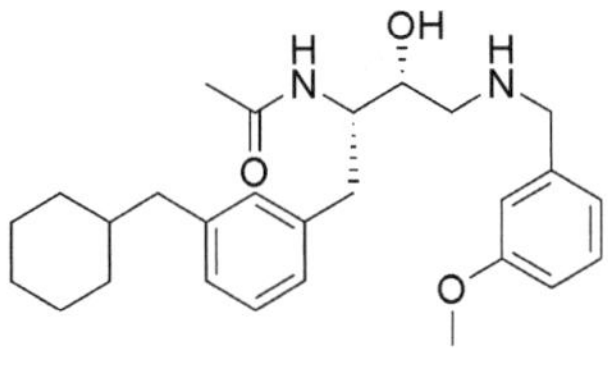

33

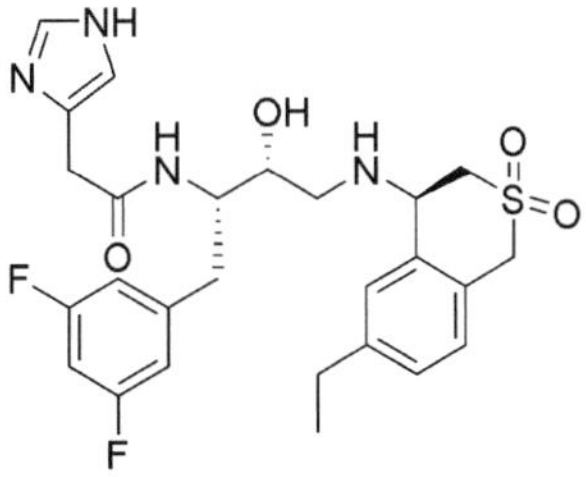

34

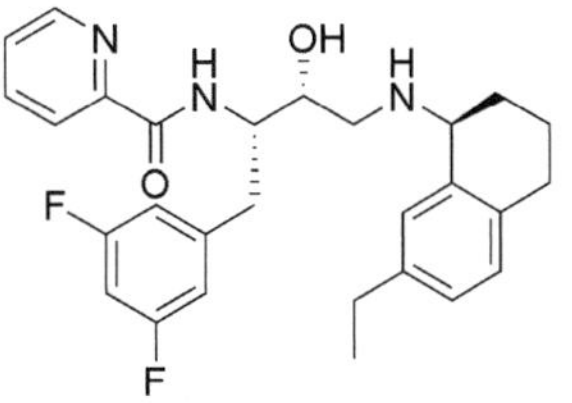

35

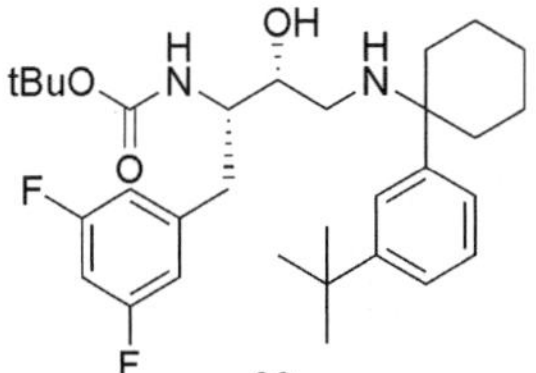

36

Figure 4.7 Elan/Pharmacia BACE inhibitors.

(N-terminal truncated) P_1-P_3 bridging HEAs [27] (Fig. 4.7, **33**), and with optimized P_2' functionality from the 3rd generation, a reexploration of P_2 with aryl and alkyl aryl/heteroaryl [28] (Fig. 4.7, **34,35**) and with ureas and carbamates (Fig. 4.7, **36**) [29]. Evidence of the impact of this work from Elan/Pharmacia's 3rd-generation HEA BACE-1 inhibitors is the influence on inhibitor design in subsequent disclosures from the field (*vide infra*).

Retaining the P_1-P_3 isophthalamide or thiazolesulfonamide groups, aza-hydroxyethylamines (Fig. 4.8) have been disclosed in the Elan/Pharmacia patent literature (eg., **37–39**); from the stereochemistry shown, it suggests the secondary hydroxyl functionality could be *(S)*- or *(R)*- for acceptable BACE-1 activity [30]. A series of 1,2- and 1,3-diols (Fig. 4.9) are also described (e.g., **40–42**), albeit without reported activity [31]. And finally, the Elan/Pharmacia BACE team also published patent applications on numerous additional peptidomimetic scaffolds (Fig. 4.10) throughout the course of their collaboration, including, but not limited to: P_1-shifted

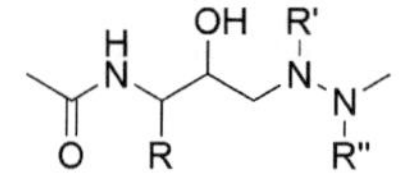

Aza-hydroxyethylamine

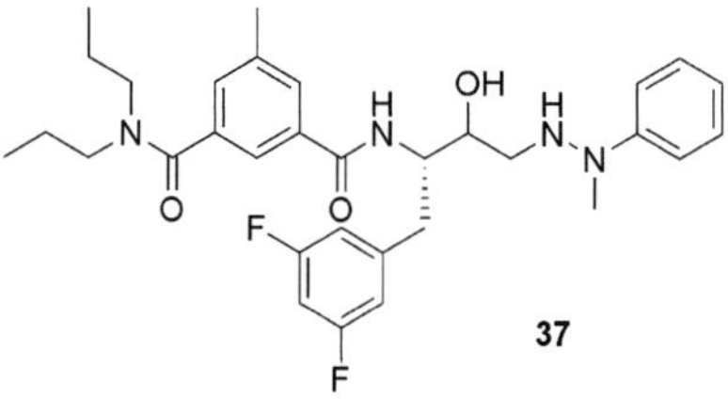

37

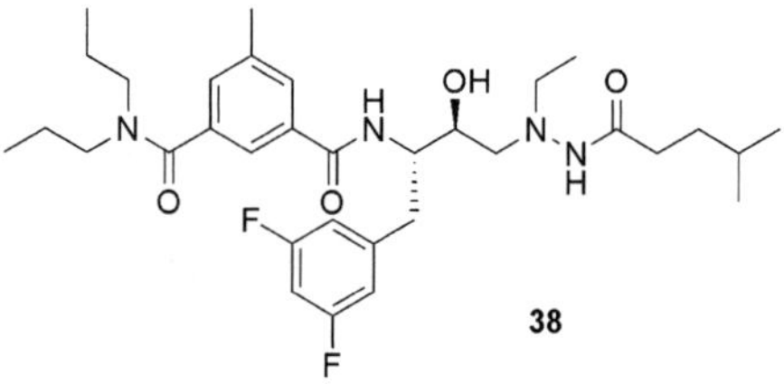

38

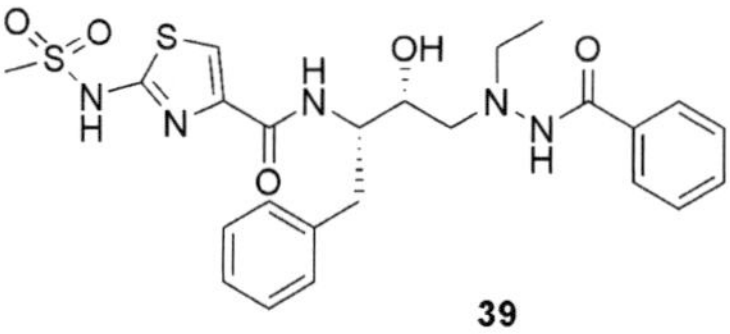

39

Figure 4.8 Elan/Pharmacia BACE inhibitors.

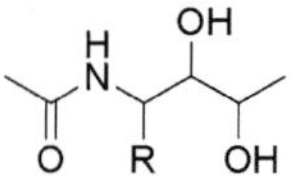

Diols

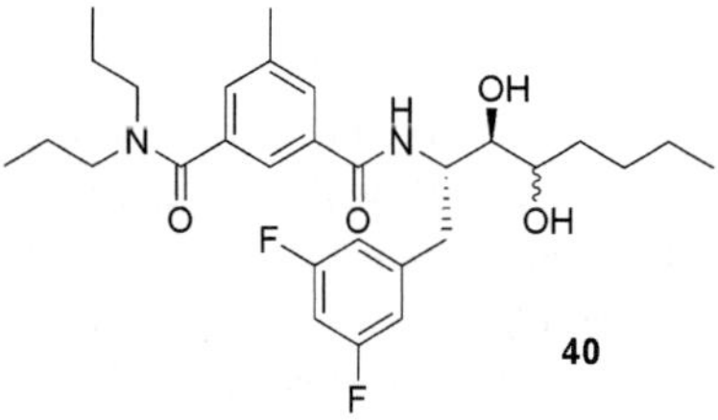

40

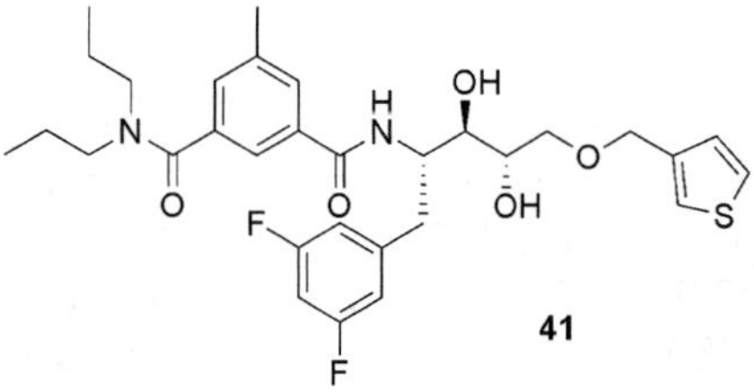

41

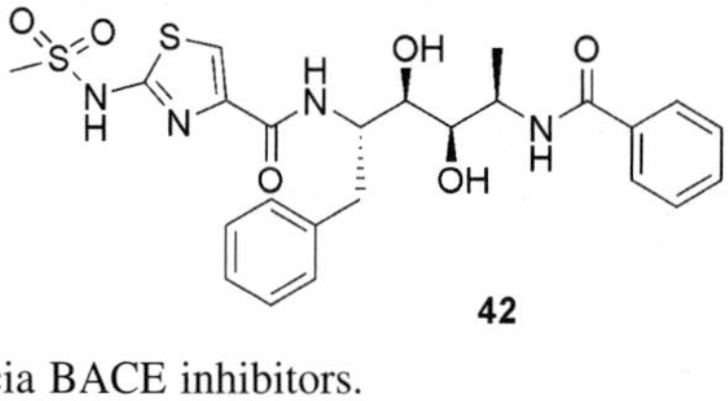

42

Figure 4.9 Elan/Pharmacia BACE inhibitors.

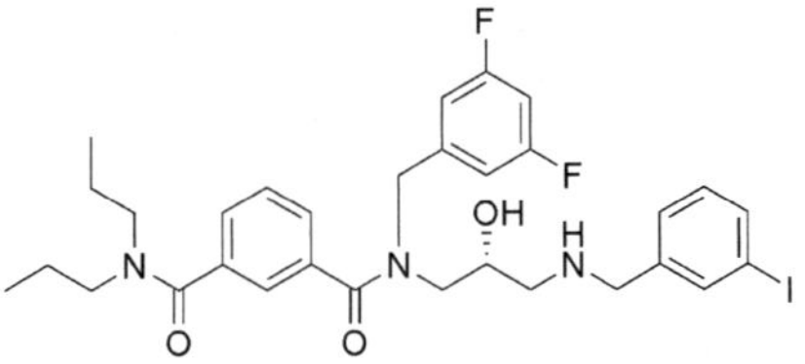

43, P1-shifted hydroxyethylamine

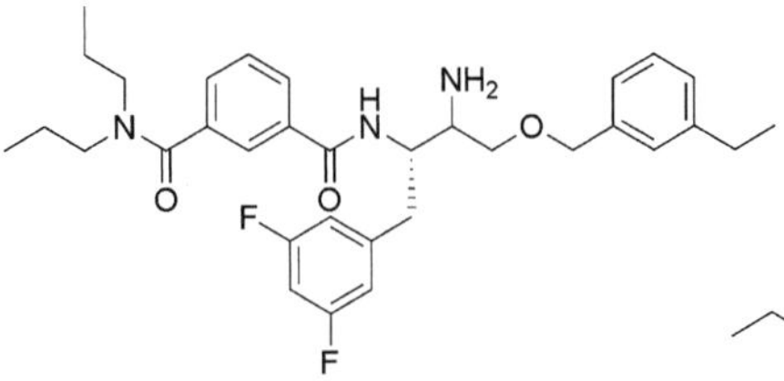

44, Aminomethyl ether

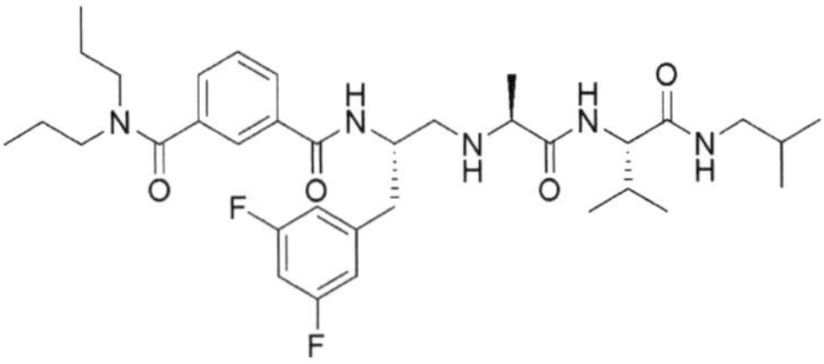

45, Reduced amide

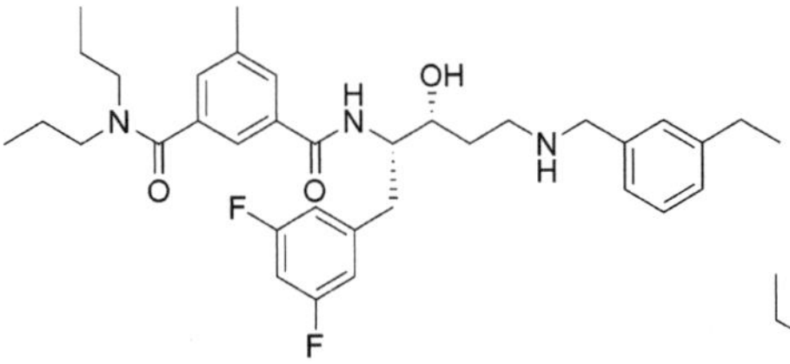

46, Hydroxypropylamine

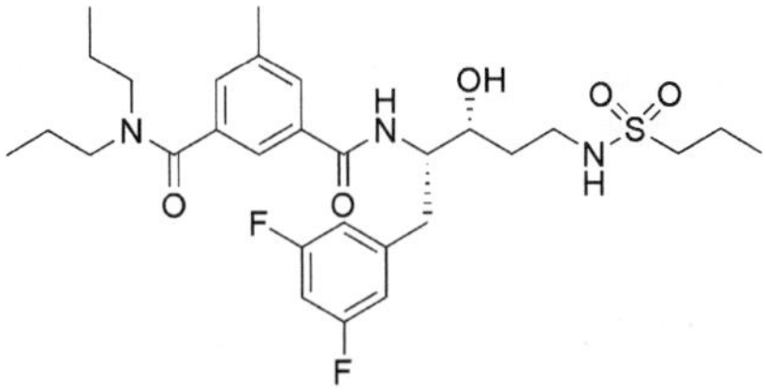

47, Hydroxypropyl sulfonamide

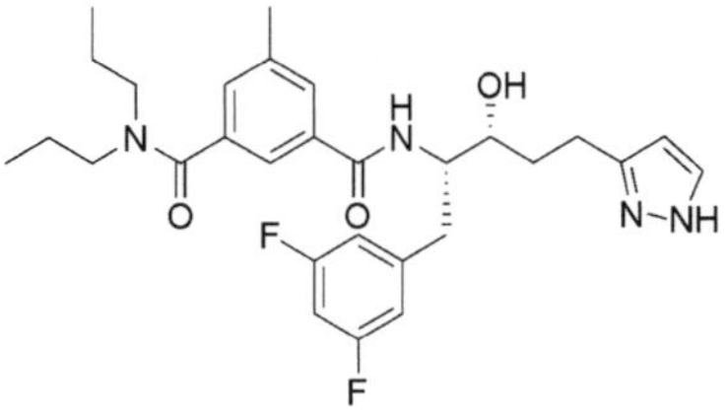

48, Hydroxypropyl heteroaryl

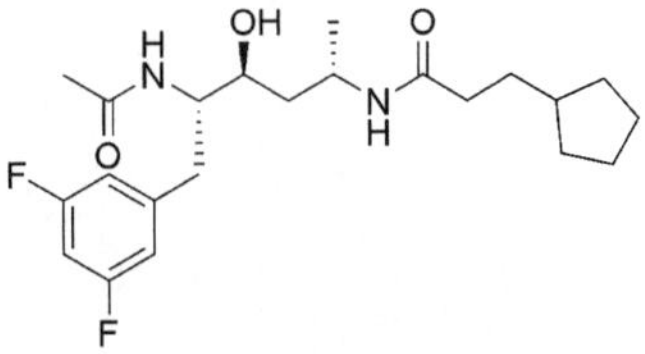

49, N-terminal truncated hydroxyethylene

Figure 4.10   Elan/Pharmacia BACE inhibitors.

HEAs (Fig. 4.10, **43**) [32], aminomethyl ethers (Fig. 4.10, **44**) [33], reduced amides (Fig. 4.10, **45**) [34], hydroxypropyl amines (Fig. 4.10, **46**) [35], hydroxypropyl sulfonamides (Fig. 4.10, **47**) [36], hydroxypropyl heteroaryl (Fig. 4.10, **48**) [37], and N-terminal truncated hydroxyethylene (Fig. 4.10, **49**) inhibitors [38]. Specific details of BACE-1 activity for these diverse scaffolds were not disclosed.

4.3 OKLAHOMA MEDICAL RESEARCH FOUNDATION (OMRF)/MULTIPLE COLLABORATORS

Tang and colleagues at the Oklahoma Medical Research Foundation (OMRF) – in an ongoing and highly productive collaboration with Ghosh and coworkers – reported on the design and synthesis of inhibitor **OM-99-2** (Fig. 4.11, **50**) [39]. An octapeptide with a BACE-1 IC_{50} = 2 nM, **OM-99-2** was based on the cleavage site of Swedish-mutant APP (EVNL/DAEF); **OM-99-2** incorporates the Leu-based hydroxyethylene (HE) peptide isostere and an Asp to Ala mutation at P_1'. Along with the milestone of publishing the first crystal structures of BACE-1 inhibitors bound to enzyme [40], combinatorial libraries and additional SAR were initiated to afford

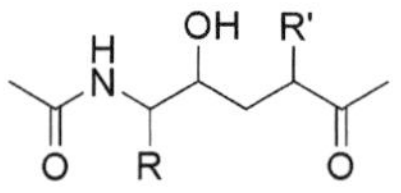

Hydroxyethylene

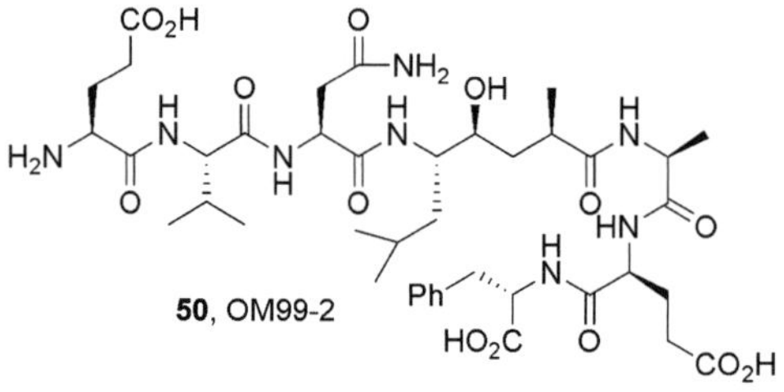

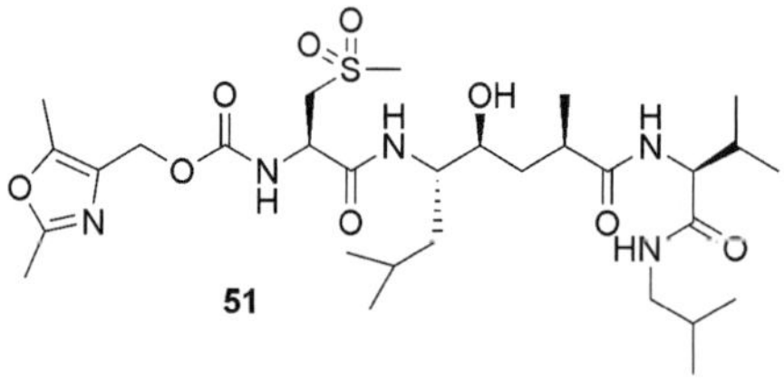

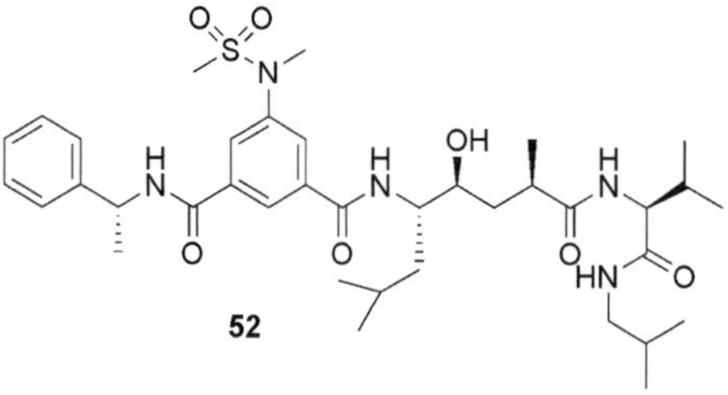

	BACE Ki	Cell IC_{50}
50, OM99-2	0.0016 µM	>10 µM
51	0.00012 µM	1.4 µM
52	0.0011 µM	0.039 µM

Figure 4.11   Oklahoma Medical Research Foundation/University of Oklahoma Health Science Center/University of Illinois at Chicago/Purdue University/Zapac Inc.

the N-terminal oxazole containing inhibitor **51** (Fig. 4.11) [41–43]. One realized advantage of truncating the peptidic character of **OM-99-2** was the demonstration of cellular activity for **51** (Fig. 4.11) ($IC_{50} = 1.4\,\mu M$). The cellular activity was further improved by 35-fold when P_1-P_3 was modified by incorporation of the previously demonstrated (*vide supra*) isophthalamide functionality to give **52** (Fig. 4.11) [44]. A significant evolution in the design of the Tang/Ghosh peptidomimetics came with replacement of the hydroxyethylene with HEA transition-state isostere. As was previously demonstrated in the Elan/Pharmacia HEAs, cellular potency was immediately improved; inhibitor **GRL-8234** (Fig. 4.12, **53**) was published on in 2008 with a BACE-1 $IC_{50} = 1.8\,nM$ and with a cellular $IC_{50} = 1.0\,nM$ [45]. Importantly, when **GRL-8234** was dosed by intraperitoneal administration (8 mg/kg) to Tg2576 mice, a 65% reduction of plasma Aβ40 production was observed 3h post dosing. As evidenced by recently published patent applications, Tang, Ghosh et al. continue

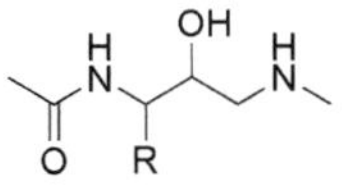

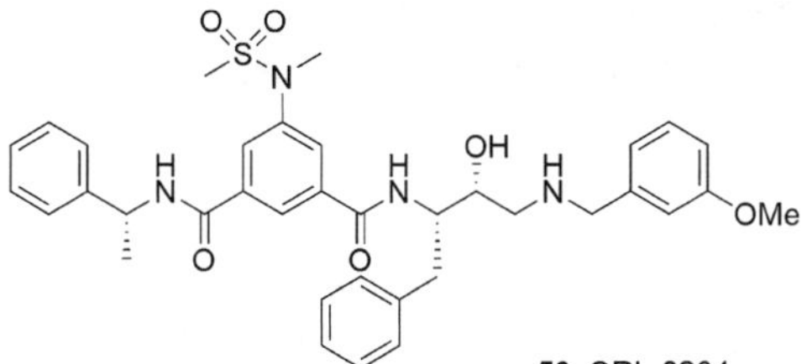

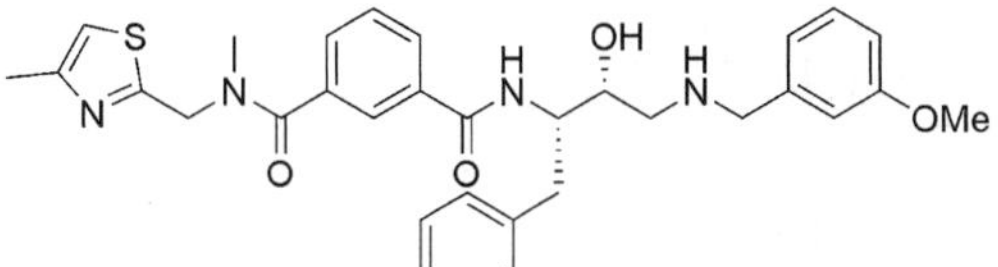

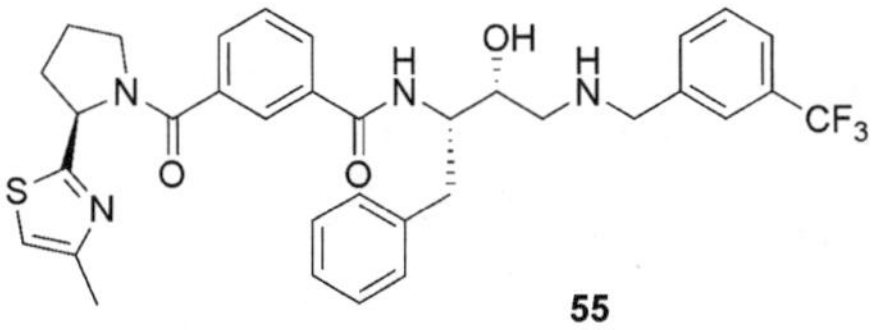

Figure 4.12 Oklahoma Medical Research Foundation/University of Oklahoma Health Science Center/University of Illinois at Chicago/Purdue University/Zapac, Inc.

to optimize HEA inhibitors (e.g., Fig. 4.12, **54,55**) [46]. Recently, the biotech company CoMentis has announced the entry of the first BACE-1 inhibitor **CTS-21166** (structure unpublished) into early human clinical trials for disease-modifying treatment for Alzheimer's disease [47]. CoMentis is codeveloping **CTS-21166** with Astellas Pharma. Pharmacodynamic proof of activity in humans (sustained, dose-dependent reductions in plasma $A\beta$ levels in both AUC reduction and peak reduction over 72 h) has been described upon IV dosing with excellent pharmacokinetic properties consistent with once a day dosing.

4.4   ELI LILLY

Eli Lilly and Company has published efforts toward the development of several TSI classes of BACE inhibitors, including statines, hydroxyethylenes, hydroxyethylene-containing macrocycles, and HEAs. In 2003, Hu et al. reported on a series of inhibitors designed based on the statine TSI [48]. Lilly researchers started from a heptapeptide scaffold and systematically removed amino acid residues to determine how large the scaffold needed to be to remain a potent BACE-1 inhibitor. These efforts ultimately resulted in a new scaffold with four peptide components. Further optimization of this scaffold was aided by computational docking studies and resin-bound peptide synthesis. Various P_3, P_2, and P_2' groups were explored resulting in potent BACE-1 inhibitors exemplified by **56** (Fig. 4.13), BACE $IC_{50} = 86$ nM). X-ray co-crystal structures for several related inhibitors were obtained and were to be used for subsequent structure-based improvement on molecules such as **56** (Fig. 4.13).

In 2003 and 2004 Lilly disclosed its efforts toward the design of BACE-1 inhibitors containing the HE TSI [49]. The stated goal of these studies was the generation of BACE-1 inhibitors that displayed better whole cell activity. The Lilly group hypothesized that improving the aqueous solubility of HE BACE-1 inhibitors

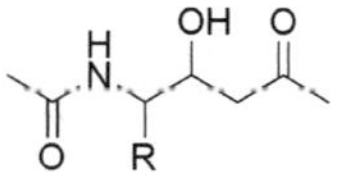

Statine

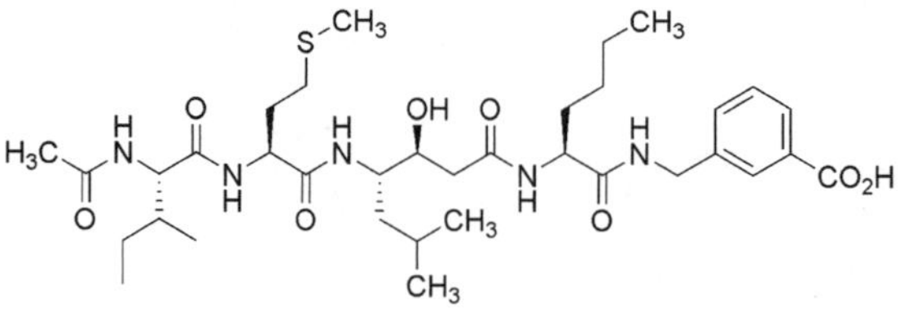

	BACE IC_{50}	Cell IC_{50}
	86 nM	NA

56

Figure 4.13   Eli Lilly & Company BACE inhibitors.

would result in improved cellular potency. Initial work was focused on modifications to the C-terminus of inhibitors such as **57** (Fig. 4.14). Ultimately, it was found that replacement of the C-terminal phenyl group with a pyridine moiety led to inhibitor **58** (Fig. 4.14), which displayed improved cellular potency. Subsequent inhibitors were then prepared based on **58** (Fig. 4.14), and this included a series of pentapeptides in which variations were made in the P$_2$ and P$_3$ groups. These efforts culminated in the discovery of inhibitor **59** (Fig. 4.14), in which the P$_2$-P$_3$ combination of Val-Met had been replaced with Ile-Ala. Inhibitor **59** displayed increased enzyme activity and an improved ratio of whole cell to enzyme activity (10-fold for **59** [Fig. 4.14] vs. 25-fold for **58** [Fig. 4.14]). Furthermore, structural analysis of a structurally related inhibitor indicated that the C-terminal pyridine moiety could be further modified without a detrimental impact on potency. Additional SAR on the N-terminal moiety of related molecules has also been disclosed [50].

More recently, Lilly has described efforts toward macrocyclic variants of HE TSI inhibitors of BACE-1 [51]. The goal was to further optimize a potent BACE-1 inhibitor **60** (Fig. 4.15) through intramolecular attachment of appropriate residues. Lilly scientists surmised that a macrocyclic variant of **60** (Fig. 4.15) would achieve increased potency through stabilization of the bound conformation, have improved absorption properties, and be more resistant to gastric degradation. Based on analysis of X-ray data, P$_1$-P$_3$ and P$_1$-N$_2$ were identified as suitable points for cyclization. A series of P$_1$-P$_3$ macrocycles displayed reduced BACE-1 enzyme inhibition. However, a P$_1$-N$_2$ macrocycle **61** (Fig. 4.15) containing a P$_3$-Ile group exhibited potency both enzymatic potency (65 nM) and whole cell activity (880 nM). BACE X-ray

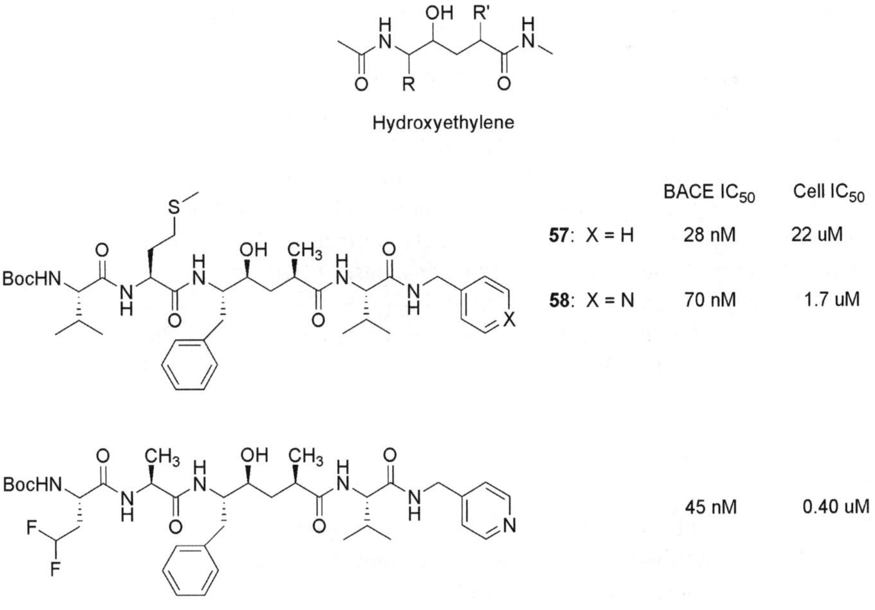

Figure 4.14 Eli Lilly & Company BACE inhibitors.

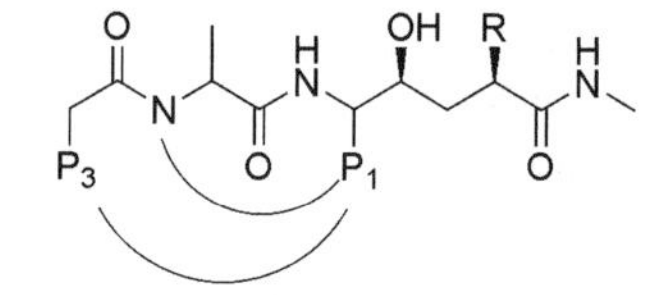

Hydroxyethylene
macrocycles

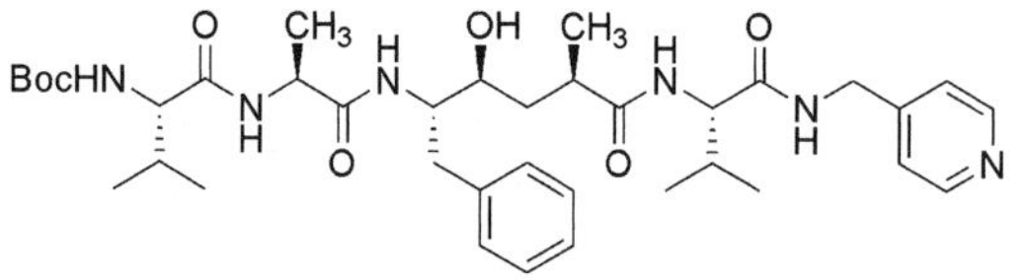

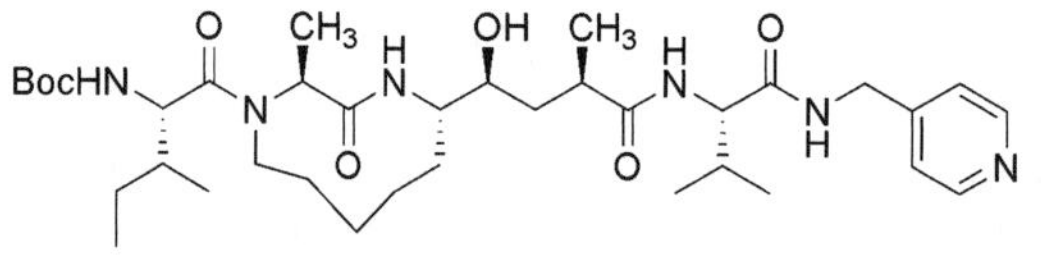

	BACE IC_{50}	Cell IC_{50}
60	0.082 μM	2.8 μM
61	0.065 μM	0.88 μM

Figure 4.15   Eli Lilly & Company BACE inhibitors.

co-crystallization of **61** (Fig. 4.15) indicated that the molecule bound with the main chain peptide groups adopting a very similar conformation to acyclic analogs, suggesting that the macrocycle present in **61** (Fig. 4.15) had helped to stabilize the bound conformation. Furthermore, the data suggest that the N_2-H in the monocyclic peptide may not be a required for potency.

Lilly has also published several HEA BACE inhibitors in the patent literature [52, 53]. These include pyrrolidine, piperidine, and morpholine derivatives (Fig. 4.16). Disclosed data for these compounds span a wide range of enzyme activity. For example, pyrrolidine **62** (Fig. 4.16) is a potent BACE-1 inhibitor and displays excellent cellular activity. Morpholine inhibitor **63** (Fig. 4.16) is also quite potent against BACE-1 and in cells. Encouragingly, **63** (Fig. 4.16) has also demonstrated *in vivo* efficacy. In the transgenic PDAPP mouse *in vivo* efficacy experiment, in which **63** (Fig. 4.16) was dosed subcutaneously at 100 mg/kg, 39%, 40%, and 25% reductions of Aβ levels were observed in plasma, cerebrospinal fluid (CSF), and cortex, respectively [1f, 53].

4.5   MERCK

Merck has also published extensively on the development of BACE-1 inhibitors. In 2004, Merck published efforts toward development of their own hydroxyethylene (HE) inhibitor that was selective for BACE-1 over other aspartyl proteases such as Cat-D and renin [54]. The initial SAR screening efforts focused on replacement of typical hydrophobic P_1' groups with polar groups. These efforts led to potent HE

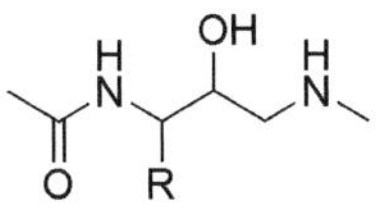

Hydroxyethylamine
(Piperidine and morpholine)

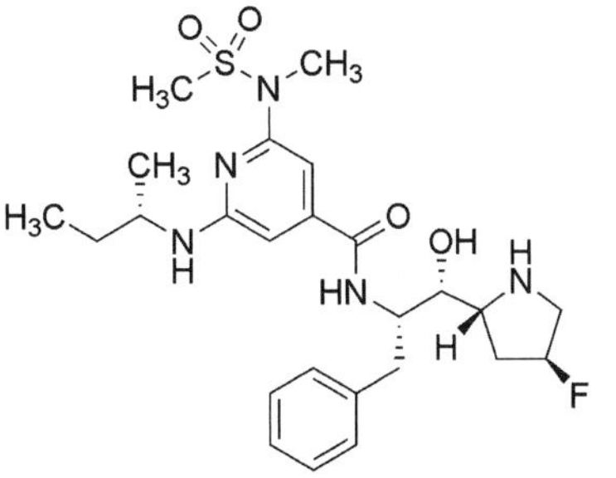

	BACE IC$_{50}$	Cell IC$_{50}$
62	4 nM	13 nM
63	78 nM	95 nM

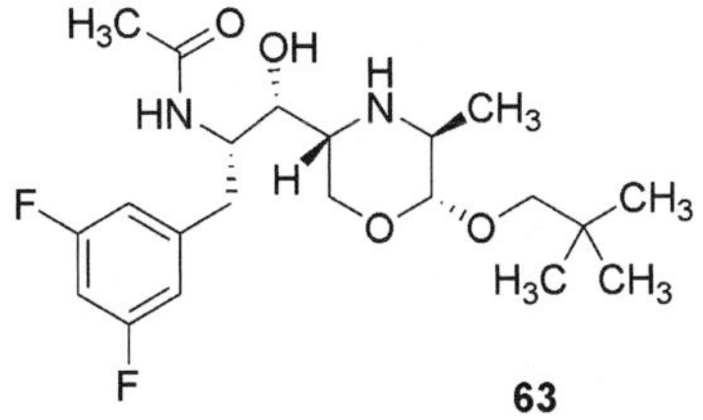

Figure 4.16   Eli Lilly & Company BACE inhibitors.

BACE inhibitor **64** (Fig. 4.17), which displayed 47-fold selectivity against Cat-D and 44-fold selectivity against renin. These structural modifications did not improve selectivity over BACE-2 and cellular activity was not reported.

Attempts across the pharmaceutical industry to identify BACE-1 inhibitors through conventional high throughput screening campaigns have met with significant challenge. In 2004, Merck published their results of an extensive screening effort toward BACE-1. Merck employed the Automated Ligand Identification System technology, developed by NeoGenesis, to screen a multimillion compound library against BACE-1 [55]. A single compound, **65** (Fig. 4.18), was identified from this screening effort. Follow-up studies supported active site inhibition as the mechanism of action for **65** (Fig. 4.18). SAR optimization of **65** (Fig. 4.18) then led to inhibitor **66** (Fig. 4.18). Interestingly, X-ray co-crystallization of **66** (Fig. 4.18) with a BACE-1 variant suggested that **66** (Fig. 4.18) does not directly interact with the two catalytic aspartic acid residues but rather binds to a water molecule situated between these aspartic acids. Inhibitor **66** (Fig. 4.18) also displays good selectivity against Cat-D and renin (>500 μM) as well as BACE-2 (137 μM) A similar trisubstituted aromatic core seems to be retained in many of the BACE-1 inhibitors subsequently reported by Merck and independently identified by others.

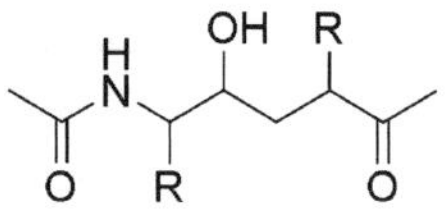

Hydroxyethylene

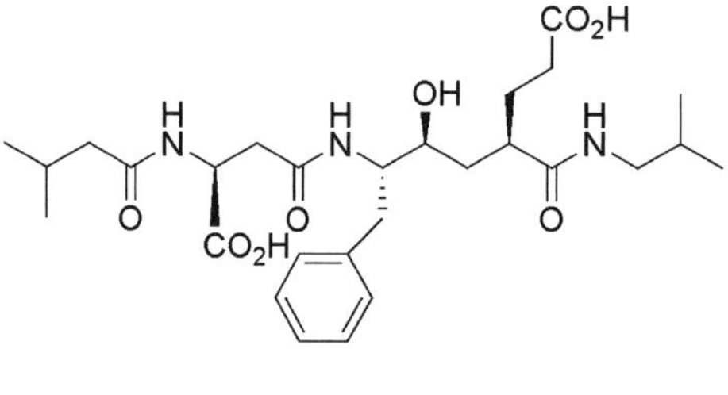

	BACE K_i	Cell IC_{50}
	1.7 μM	NA

64

Figure 4.17 Merck BACE inhibitors.

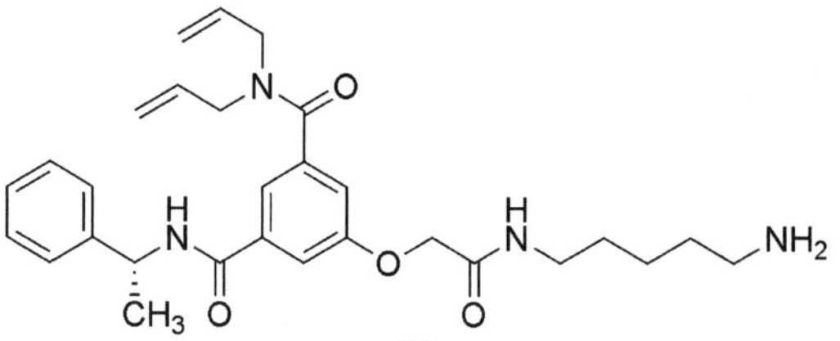

	BACE IC_{50}	Cell IC_{50}
65	25 μM	NA
66	1.4 μM	NA

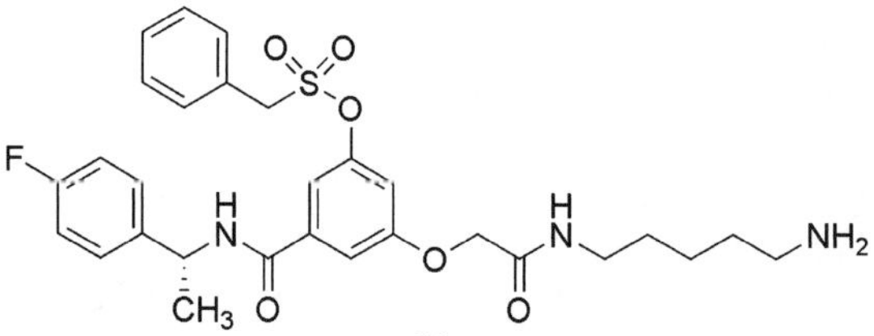

Figure 4.18 Merck BACE inhibitors.

Merck has reported on their development of HEA BACE-1 inhibitors [56]. These inhibitors were designed based on **65** (Fig. 4.18) and thus contained an N-terminal isophthalamide moiety. By incorporating the HEA TSI into this new inhibitor scaffold, Merck scientists hoped to improve the potency through direct interaction with the catalytic aspartic acids. This resulted in compound **67** (Fig. 4.19), which was considerably more potent both against the BACE-1 enzyme and

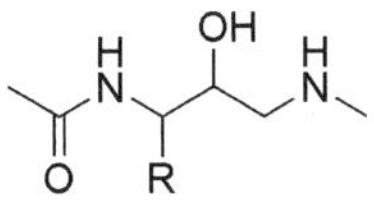

Hydroxyethylamine

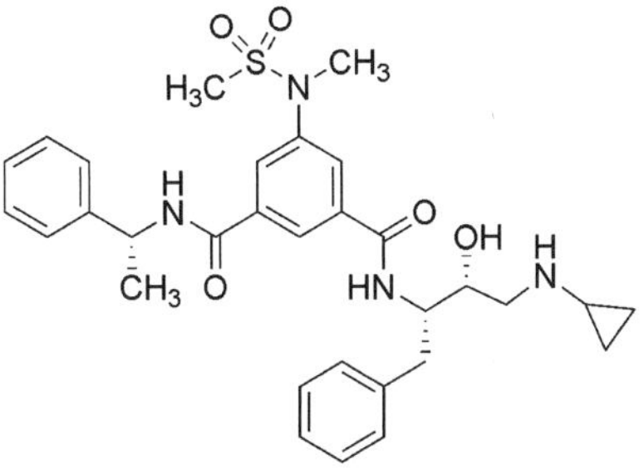

BACE IC_{50}	Cell IC_{50}
15 nM	29 nM

67

Figure 4.19   Merck BACE inhibitors.

in a cellular assay. Furthermore, this compound showed selectivity against renin (>50 μM), Cat-D (7.6 μM), and BACE-2 (230 nM). The authors attributed the selectivity to the P_1 sulfonamide groups.

Reduced amide inhibitors in combination with the structural motif (N-terminal isophthalamide) exemplified by screen hit **65** (Fig. 4.18) have been reported by Merck [57]. SAR focused on the P_1' and P_2' substituents, with the combination of $P_1' = $ Me and $P_2' = i$-Bu providing potent BACE-1 inhibitor **68** (Fig. 4.20). In addition to displaying both enzyme and cellular potency, **68** (Fig. 4.20) was selective against BACE-2 (5- to 10-fold) and renin (>20 μM). X-ray analysis of **68** bound to BACE-1 indicated that the reduced amide interacted with only one of the catalytic aspartic acid units (Asp228). Macrocyclic variants of these reduced amide BACE-1 inhibitors, such as **69** (Fig. 4.20), displayed both enzyme and functional activity against BACE-1 [58]. Furthermore, when transgenic APP-YAC mice were given an intravenous bolus of 100 mg/kg of **69** (Fig. 4.20), Aβ40 levels were reduced by 25% after 1 h.

Merck has also used a primary amine to bind to the catalytic aspartates in conjunction with either an isophthalimide core (in collaboration with Sunesis) or an isonicotinamide core [59]. Compound **70** (Fig. 4.21) emerged from these studies as a suitable candidate for *in vivo* study. Upon treatment of APP-YAC mice with **70** (intravenous bolus, 50 mg/kg) in a time-course study, statistically significant reduction of Aβ40 (34%) was observed out to 3 h. A dose response study with **70** (Fig. 4.21) (APP-YAC mice) was also performed, and 34% reduction of Aβ40 was observed after administration of an intravenous bolus of 50 mg/kg. Lower doses did not appear to produce statistically significant effects on Aβ40. While the authors

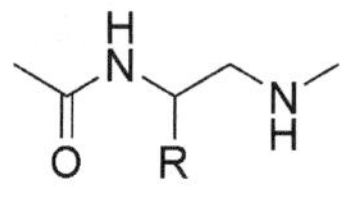

Reduced amide

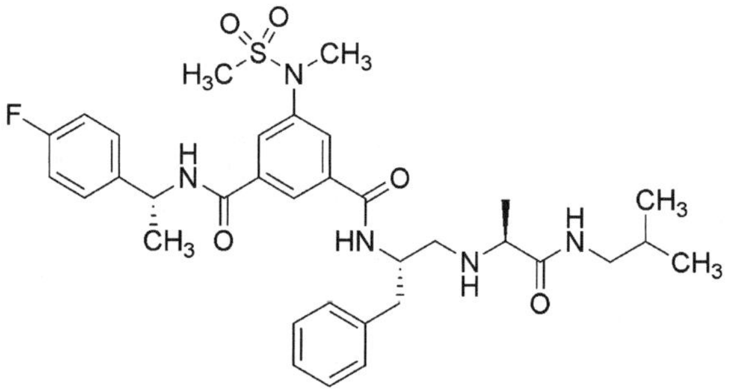

	BACE IC$_{50}$	Cell IC$_{50}$
68	8 nM	22 nM
69	4 nM	76 nM

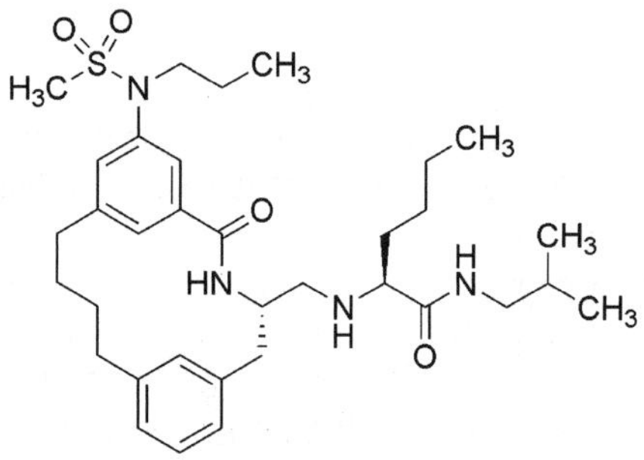

Figure 4.20   Merck BACE inhibitors.

were encouraged by the in vivo performance of **70** (Fig. 4.21), they also commented that **70** (Fig. 4.21) suffered from high clearance and volume of distribution in rat as well as poor bioavailability (%F = 13). An additional primary amine-based inhibitor (tertiary carbamine) containing the isonicotinamide core is inhibitor **71** (Fig. 4.21) [60]. Compound **71** (Fig. 4.21) is a potent inhibitor against isolated BACE enzyme and in a cellular environment. Furthermore, **71** (Fig. 4.21) is selective against Cat-D and renin (IC$_{50}$ > 100 μM). The authors also comment that **71** (Fig. 4.21) possesses excellent membrane permeability and does not suffer from p-glycoprotein (P-gp) transport. When APP-YAC mice were administered an intraperitoneal dose of 100 mg/kg of **71** (Fig. 4.21), brain Aβ40 was reduced by 26% at 2 h and 29% at 4 h. The pharmacodynamic effects of compound **71** (Fig. 4.21) were also investigated in Rhesus monkeys. The authors comment that **71** (Fig. 4.21) is both poorly bioavailable and highly metabolized in monkey. Consequently, monkeys were dosed with ritanovir 2 h prior to being dosed with **71** (Fig. 4.21). This protocol enabled sufficient

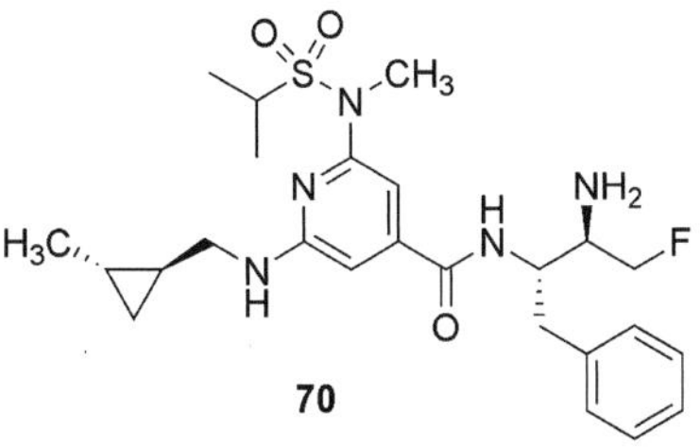

Figure 4.21 Merck BACE inhibitors.

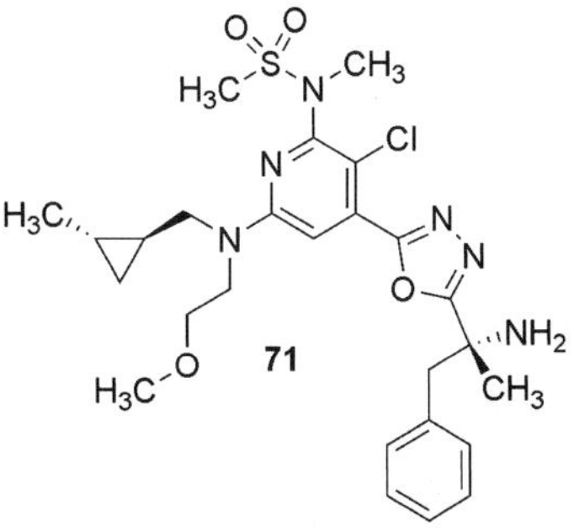

plasma exposure to be achieved. When monkeys were dosed orally with 15 mg/kg twice daily following the above protocol, an average plasma Aβ40 reduction of 61% was observed. Additionally, CSF Aβ40, Aβ42 and sAPPβ were reduced by 42%, 43%, and 41% respectively. The authors state that this is the first example of a BACE-1 inhibitor demonstrating significant reduction of both CSF and plasma Aβ levels in a nonhuman primate [60].

Merck has very recently disclosed several BACE-1 inhibitor classes that have emerged from their most recent high-throughput screening (HTS) efforts (Fig. 4.22). In 2008, Merck published that they identified a weak iminohydantoin BACE-1 inhibitor (Fig. 4.22, **72**; IC_{50} = 22 μM) from a high throughput screening at a compound test concentration of 100 μM [61]. Inhibitor **72** (Fig. 4.22) was optimized to inhibitor **73** (Fig. 4.22) resulting in a 200-fold improvement in BACE-1 activity. Unfortunately, **73** (Fig. 4.22) suffered from a 47-fold rightward shift in cellular activity and did not demonstrate statistically significant brain Aβ40 reductions in a transgenic mouse expressing hAPP. Efforts continue to improve upon the cellular activity, brain penetration, and in vivo performance of these HTS-derived BACE-1 inhibitors [62]. Most recently, Merck has also published on both small-molecule pyrimidines (Fig. 4.22, **74,75**) that appear to bind to BACE-1 without catalytic aspartate interaction [63] and on aminothiazoles (Fig. 4.22, **76,77**) and aminoinda-zoles (Fig. 4.22, **78**) that display a pH dependent effect on binding affinity [64]. For example, aminothiazole **76** (Fig. 4.22) was derived from high throughput screening at BACE enzyme assay at pH 4.5 and then optimized to aminoindazole **78** (Fig. 4.22) with a BACE-1 IC_{50} = 0.47 μM at pH 6.5. Gratifyingly, **78** (Fig. 4.22) also

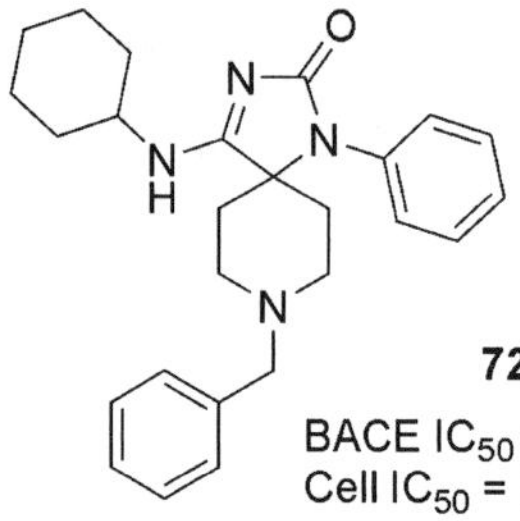

72
BACE IC_{50} = 22 μM
Cell IC_{50} = Inactive

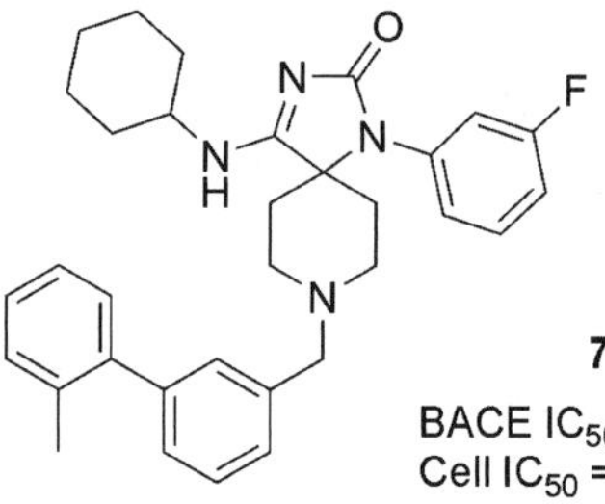

73
BACE IC_{50} = 0.11 μM
Cell IC_{50} = 5.2 μM

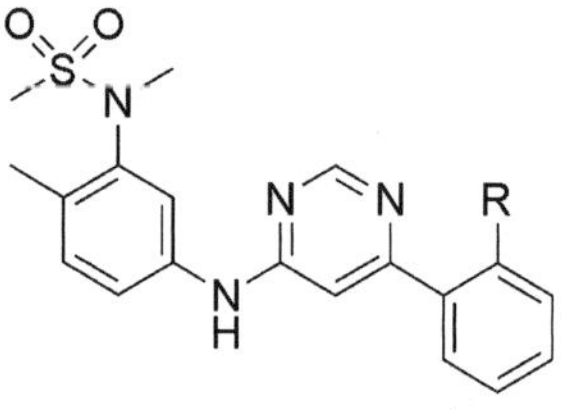

R = NMe$_2$, **74**, BACE IC_{50} = 317 μM
R = H, **75**, BACE IC_{50} = 25 μM

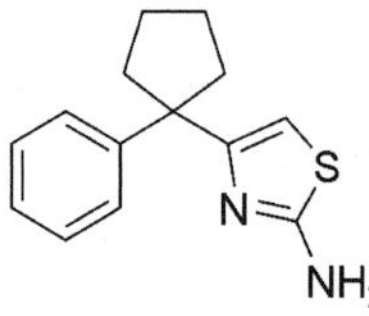

76, BACE IC_{50} = 217 μM   **77**, BACE IC_{50} = 32 μM   **78**, BACE IC_{50} = 0.47 μM
Cell IC_{50} = 1.8 μM

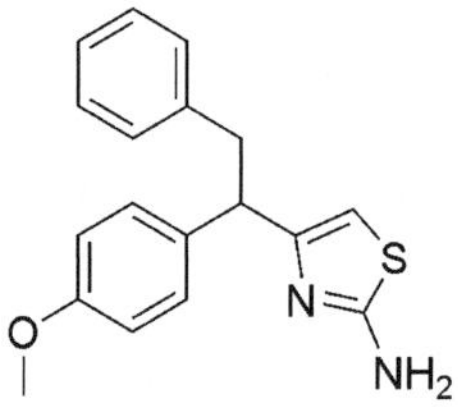

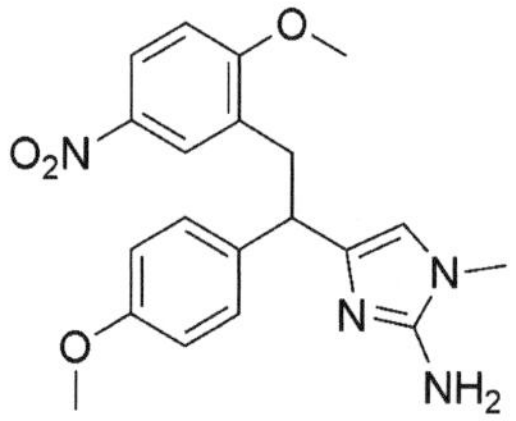

Figure 4.22   Merck HTS-based BACE inhibitors.

exhibited a cellular IC_{50} = 1.8 μM. *In vivo* efficacy was not disclosed for inhibitors **74–78** (Fig. 4.22).

4.6   GLAXOSMITHKLINE

GlaxoSmithKline began work toward developing a BACE-1 inhibitor by first explor-ing the hydroxyethylene series (Fig. 4.23, **79,80**) [65]; due to the same druggability challenges faced by their predecessors, they too switched to the HEA TSI. In 2008, GSK published their findings in a series of papers describing their own "1st-gener-ation" HEA inhibitors. Beginning with a P$_1'$-P$_2'$ C-terminal amide HEA inhibitor (Fig.

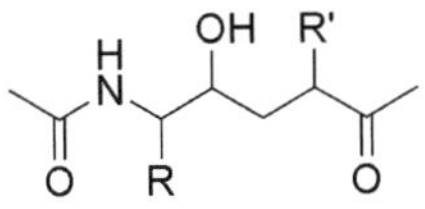

Hydroxyethylene

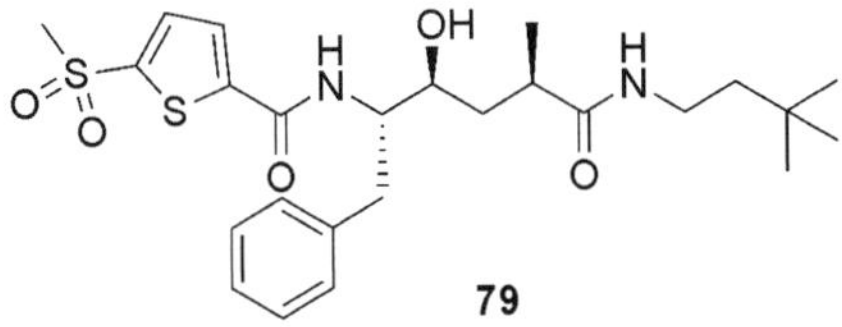

	BACE IC_{50}	Cell IC_{50}
79	180 nM	Not reported
80	1-200 nM	Not reported

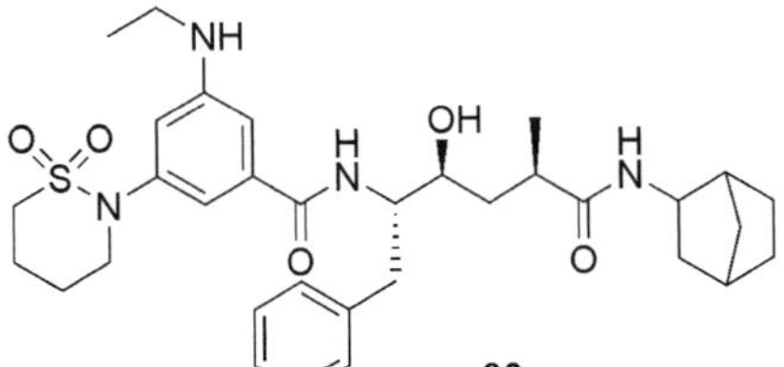

Figure 4.23 Glaxo-Smith Kline BACE inhibitors.

4.24, **81**) [66], GSK first elected to replace the amide through SAR as it was felt this strategy offered the higher probability to improve cell/enzyme ratios and improve oral bioavailability and brain penetration. Unfortunately, this SAR of 150 newly synthesized compounds afforded only four with acceptable in vitro activity (BACE-1 IC_{50}'s < 200 nM) [67] and best among the four was the previously known [9] P_2' occupying *meta*-substituted (in this case, CF_3) benzyl (Fig. 4.24, **82**). From this point, GSK's 1st-generation HEA SAR investigation turned to the non-prime side where it proved possible to replace the lactam with other H-bond acceptors (HBA), for example, a sultam group [68]. One such fluoro-substituted sultam derivative (Fig. 4.24, **83**, **GSK188909**) was found to be a nanomolar inhibitor in cells with a sufficient pharmacokinetic profile to demonstrate an *in vivo* pharmacodynamic effect. Oral administration (250 mg/kg twice daily for 5 days) of **GSK188909** to TASTPM mice reduced brain Aβ40 (18%) and Aβ42 (23%) [69]. Not surprisingly, greater pharmacodynamic effects were seen upon coadministration with a P-gp inhibitor. Further optimization by GSK researchers led to their "2nd-generation" HEA inhibitors incorporating a tricyclic non-prime side with a benzyl (Fig. 4.24, **84**) or a truncated cyclopropyl (Fig. 4.24, **85**) prime-side [70]; a full account of these findings have not yet been reported. The patent literature also describes GSKs work toward HEA [71] and related ketone-based [72] inhibitors of BACE-1.

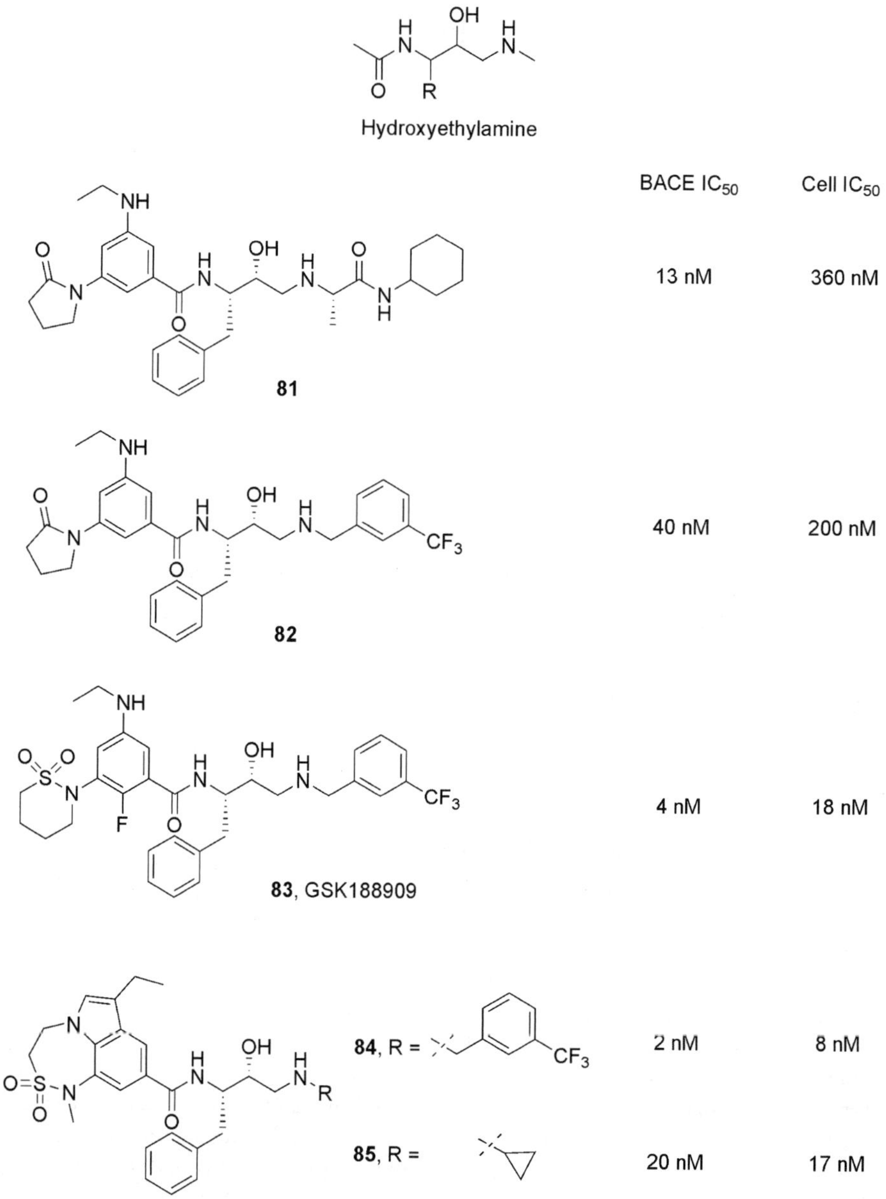

Hydroxyethylamine

	BACE IC$_{50}$	Cell IC$_{50}$

81 — 13 nM — 360 nM

82 — 40 nM — 200 nM

83, GSK188909 — 4 nM — 18 nM

84, R = [m-CF$_3$-benzyl] — 2 nM — 8 nM

85, R = [cyclopropylmethyl] — 20 nM — 17 nM

Figure 4.24   Glaxo-Smith Kline BACE inhibitors.

4.7   SCHERING PLOUGH

Schering Plough Corporation has now published their efforts to develop HEA BACE-1 inhibitors. In 2008, Schering published back-to-back reports on the development of conformationally constrained pyrrolidine and piperidine BACE-1 inhibi-

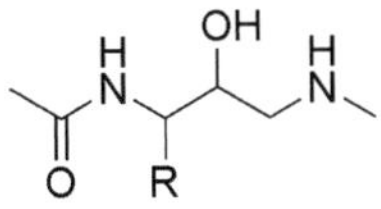

Hydroxyethylamine

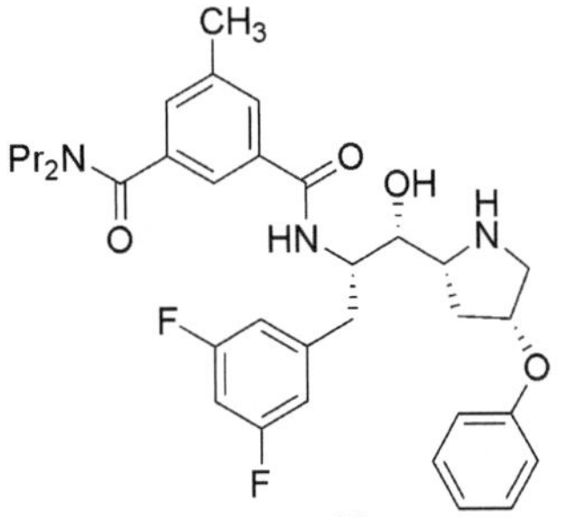

	BACE IC$_{50}$	Cell IC$_{50}$
86	3 nM	165 nM
87	0.7 nM (K$_i$)	21 nM

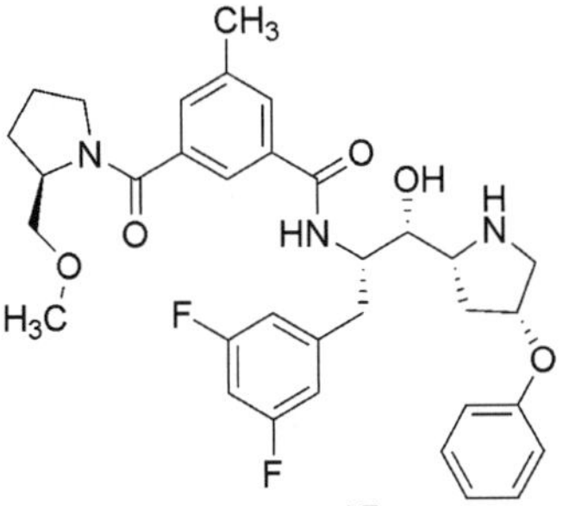

Figure 4.25 Schering Plough BACE inhibitors.

tors. The first paper described optimization of pyrrolidine and piperidine substituents intended to bind in the S$_2'$ pocket, which led to compounds such as **86** (Fig. 4.25), in which the phenoxy substituent occupied the S$_2'$ pocket as indicated by X-ray co-crystallization [73]. While **86** (Fig. 4.25) displayed potency both against the BACE-1 enzyme and in a cellular environment, it also possessed potent activity against Cat-D (291 nM) and Cat-E (24 nM). In a subsequent article, Schering described their efforts to optimize both the activity and pharmacokinetic profile of the pyrrolidine HEA BACE-1 inhibitors, which resulted in the discovery of inhibitor **87** (Fig. 4.25) [74]. In addition to being a potent BACE-1 inhibitor, **87** (Fig. 4.25) demonstrated improved selectivity against Cat-D (2.5 μM), Cat-E (170 nM), and renin (500 nM). Furthermore, the authors were encouraged that **87** (Fig. 4.25) did not inhibit CYP2D6, 3A4, and 2C9 up to 30 μM and demonstrated only 12% inhibition in a rubidium-efflux hERG assay at 5 μg/mL. When transgenic CRND8 mice were dosed orally with **87** (Fig. 4.25) at 10, 30, and 100 mg/kg, plasma Aβ40 levels were dose-dependently reduced by 4%, 25%, and 70%, respectively. Subcutaneous dosing at 10, 30, and 100 mg/kg resulted in greater levels of Aβ40 reduction (58%, 77%, and 88%, respectively). However, the authors state that no effect on cortical Aβ40 levels were observed in spite of the fact that **87** (Fig. 4.25) achieved brain exposure in excess of 50-fold the cellular IC_{50}. The authors note that compound **87** (Fig. 4.25) had a high efflux ratio in the Caco-2 P-gp assay.

Schering Plough has also reported on a series of piperizinone and imidazolidinone HEA inhibitors [75]. Using X-ray crystallography, the authors designed compounds containing a carbonyl group on the prime side-binding group to hydrogen bond with Thr72 and improve potency. These efforts led to piperazinone **88** (Fig. 4.26) and imidazolidinone **89** (Fig. 4.26), both of which were potent inhibitors of the BACE enzyme. However, both compounds were less potent in the BACE cellular assay. The authors reported on a variety of structural changes that could be made to improve cellular potency. Both **88** and **89** (Fig. 4.26) were tested in CRND8 mice (subcutaneous, 100 mg/kg) and showed modest reduction of Aβ40. However, the authors note that neither compound had an affect on brain Aβ40 levels owing

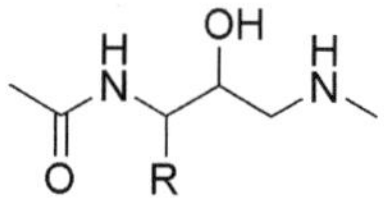

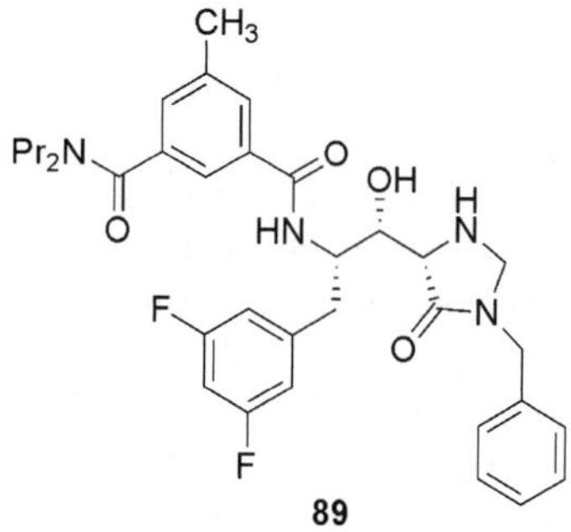

Hydroxyethylamine

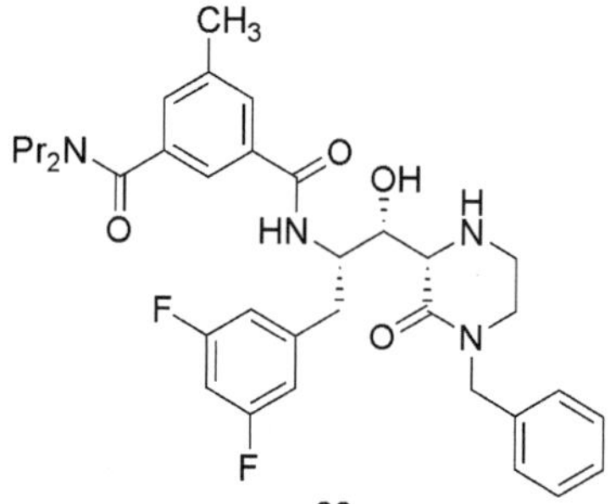

Figure 4.26   Schering Plough BACE inhibitors.

to low brain penetration. Also, both **88** and **89** (Fig. 4.26) showed only 1–15-fold selectivity against Cat-D, Cat-E, and pepsin. Schering has also disclosed macrocyclic variants of piperazinone inhibitors [76].

4.8 BRISTOL-MYERS SQUIBB

Bristol-Myers Squibb (BMS) has reported extensive studies on various TSIs as BACE inhibitors. Many of these disclosures have been via patent. For example, in 2004 BMS claimed a series of gamma-lactam HEA BACE inhibitors [77]. Several compounds were specified, with **90** (Fig. 4.27) serving as a representative example.

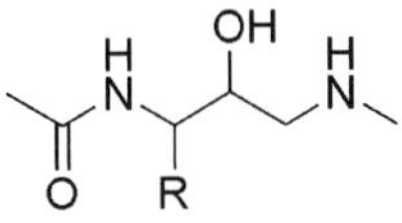

Hydroxyethylamine

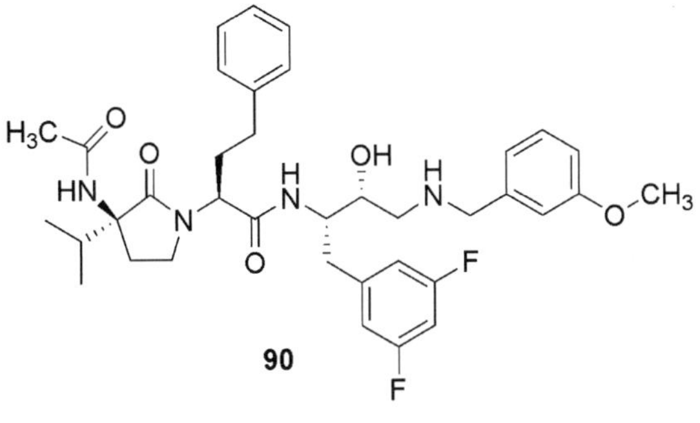

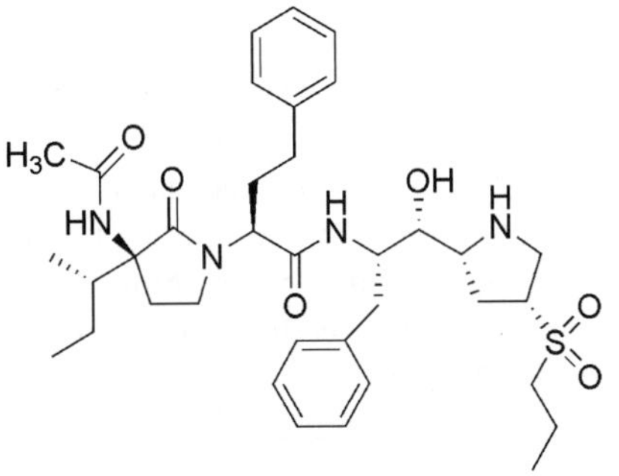

	BACE IC$_{50}$	Cell IC$_{50}$
90	<100 nM	NA
91	3.3 nM	5 nM

Figure 4.27   Bristol-Myer Squibb BACE inhibitors.

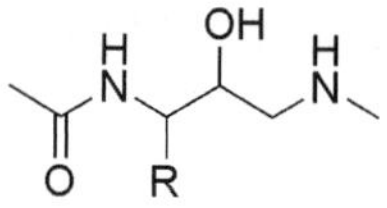

Hydroxyethylamine

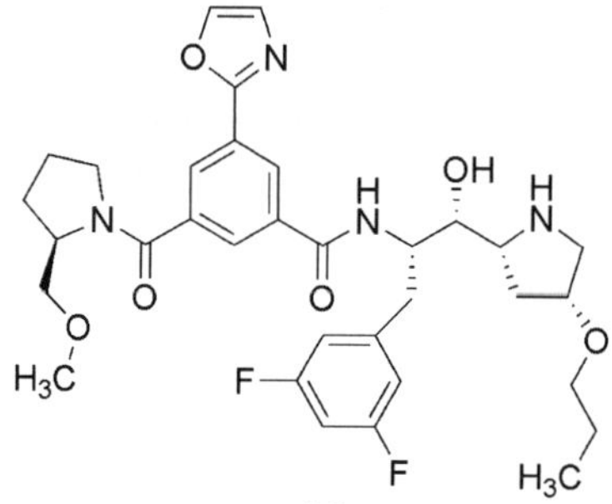

	BACE IC$_{50}$	Cell IC$_{50}$

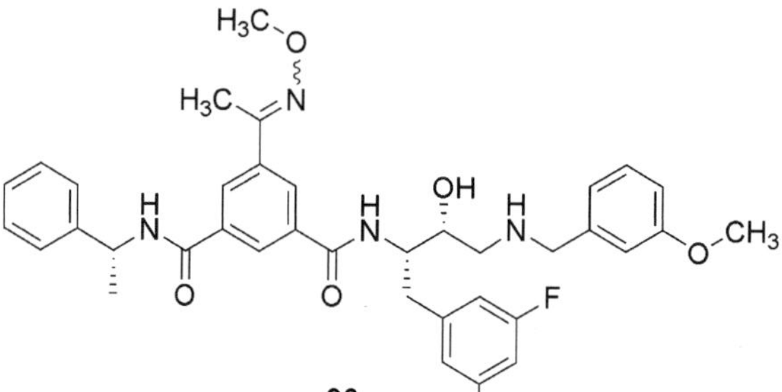

<100 nM   NA

92

32 nM   82 nM

93

Figure 4.28   Bristol-Myer Squibb BACE inhibitors.

Only BACE-1 enzyme inhibition data was reported for these compounds. Pyrrolidines such as **91** (Fig. 4.27) [78] and **92** (Fig. 4.28) [79] have also been reported. Compound **91** (Fig. 4.27) was potent both against the BACE-1 enzyme and in a cellular assay. Furthermore, **91** (Fig. 4.27) caused dose-dependent reduction of plasma Aβ40 in both wild-type and P-gp knockout mice as well as dose-dependent reduction of brain Aβ40 in P-gp knockout mice. However, **91** (Fig. 4.27) failed to reduce brain Aβ40 in wild-type mice. Compound **91** (Fig. 4.27) showed low selectivity against other aspartyl proteases (IC$_{50}$ = 130 nM for Cat-D, 29 nM for Cat-E, and 140 nM for pepsin). BMS has published additional studies on isophthalimides without conformational constraint imposed by the pyrrolidine ring system [80]. Compounds such as **93** (Fig. 4.28) are active both against the BACE-1 enzyme and in cells, while other compounds show varying intrinsic and cellular activity. The authors comment

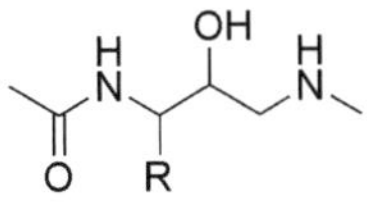

Hydroxyethylamine
macrocycle

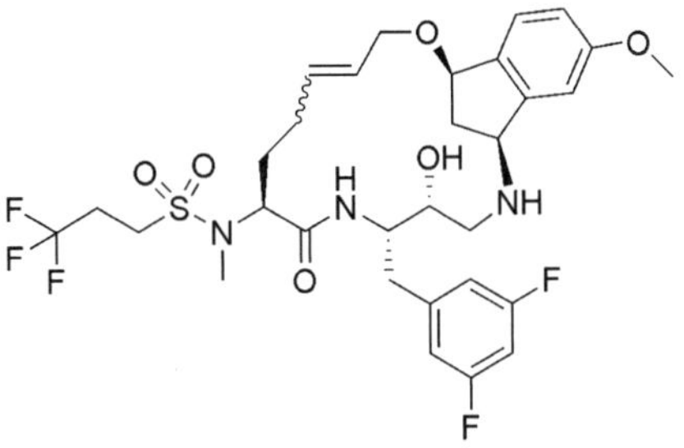

	BACE IC$_{50}$	Cell IC$_{50}$
	4.9 nM	NA

94

Figure 4.29   Bristol-Myer Squibb BACE inhibitors.

that additional studies are ongoing to address the P-gp and pharmacokinetic liabilities of these molecules. BMS has also disclosed macrocyclic HEA BACE inhibitors such as **94** (Fig. 4.29) [78]. Compound **94** (Fig. 4.29) was a potent BACE-1 inhibitor and displayed dose-dependent reduction of plasma Aβ40 in wild-type mice and brain Aβ40 in P-gp knockout mice. However, similarly to compound **91** (Fig. 4.27), macrocycle **94** (Fig. 4.29) failed to reduce brain Aβ40 in wild-type mice.

4.9   NOVARTIS

Novartis has also made contributions to the field of BACE-1 inhibitor design. Hydroxyethylene transition state mimetics were first explored to afford pyrrolidine spirocycles (Fig. 4.30, **95**) [81], macrocycles (Fig. 4.30, **96**) [82, 83], and non-prime side tricyclic hetereocycles (not shown) [84]. Modest enzyme activity and poor cellular activity was addressed by the common switch from the hydroxyethylene to HEA TSI to provide two macrocycles (Fig. 4.31, **97**, **NB-544** and Fig. 4.31, **98**, **NB-533**) with published in vivo efficacy data [85]. Specifically, **NB-544** was tested in APP51/16 transgenic mice expressing wild-type hAPP under a brain promoter [86]; upon intravenous administration (2 × 30 μmol/kg, ~15 mg/kg) a modest but statistically significant reduction (20%) of Aβ42 in forebrain extracts was demonstrated. Testing of **NB-533** in APP51/16 mice upon oral administration (1 × 100 μmol/kg or 2 × 100 μmol/kg) did not produce a statistically significant Aβ reduction in brain extracts, despite a slightly lower P-gp efflux liability for **NB-533** compared with **NB-544** (BA/AB = 9.4 and 15, respectively). Novartis also continues to explore a wide diversity within the HEA framework, including examples of additional

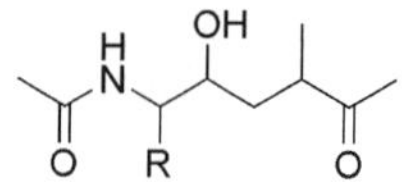

Hydroxyethylene

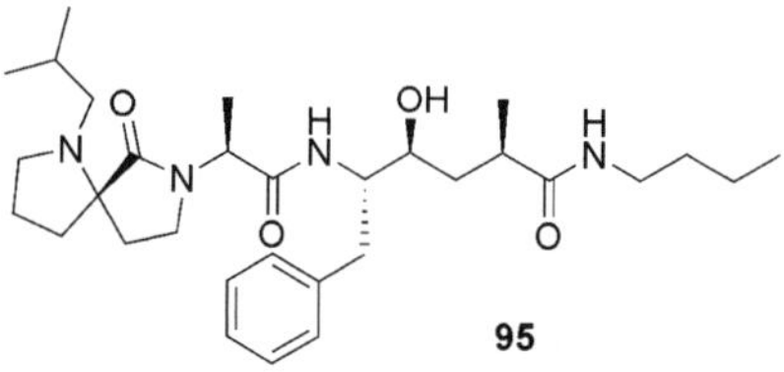

	BACE IC$_{50}$	Cell IC$_{50}$
95	<20 μM	Not reported
96	0.15 μM	8.7 μM

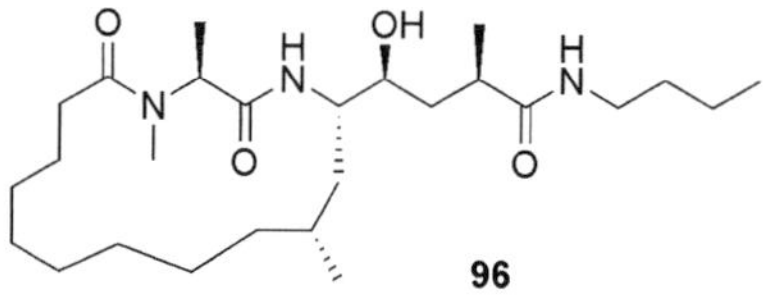

Figure 4.30   Novartis BACE inhibitors.

macrocycles (Fig. 4.31, **99**) [87], cyclohexyl carboxamides (Fig. 4.31, **100**) [88], N-terminal truncated P$_1$-P$_3$ (Fig. 4.31, **101**) [89], and the very unique HEA contained in the backbone of an amino-benzyl substituted cyclic sulfone (Fig. 4.31, **102**) [90].

4.10   AMGEN

Focused on HEAs exclusively, Amgen has recently forged ahead with their own BACE-1 inhititor project. Combining unique and diverse prime and non-prime-side SAR, Amgen has disclosed examples of substituted prime-side chromane-containing inhibitors (Fig. 4.32, **103–107**) including pyridyl substituted benzamides (**103**) [91], pyridones (**104**) [92], acetamides (**105**) [93] and (**106**) [94], and oxiranes (**107**) [95] on the non-prime side. While these previously published examples report general IC$_{50}$ < 5 μM activity in both BACE FRET and cell assay systems, a very recent report of HEA inhibitors with non-prime side pyrimidinyl and [1,2,4]-triazolo[4,3-a]pyrazinyl functionality describes activity down to IC$_{50}$ < 0.10 μM [96].

4.10.1   Kyoto Pharmaceutical University/University of Tokyo

Researchers at the Kyoto Pharmaceutical University, in collaboration with the University of Tokyo, have previously and recently continued to publish on their work to develop BACE-1 inhibitors containing the hydroxymethylcarbonyl (HMC)

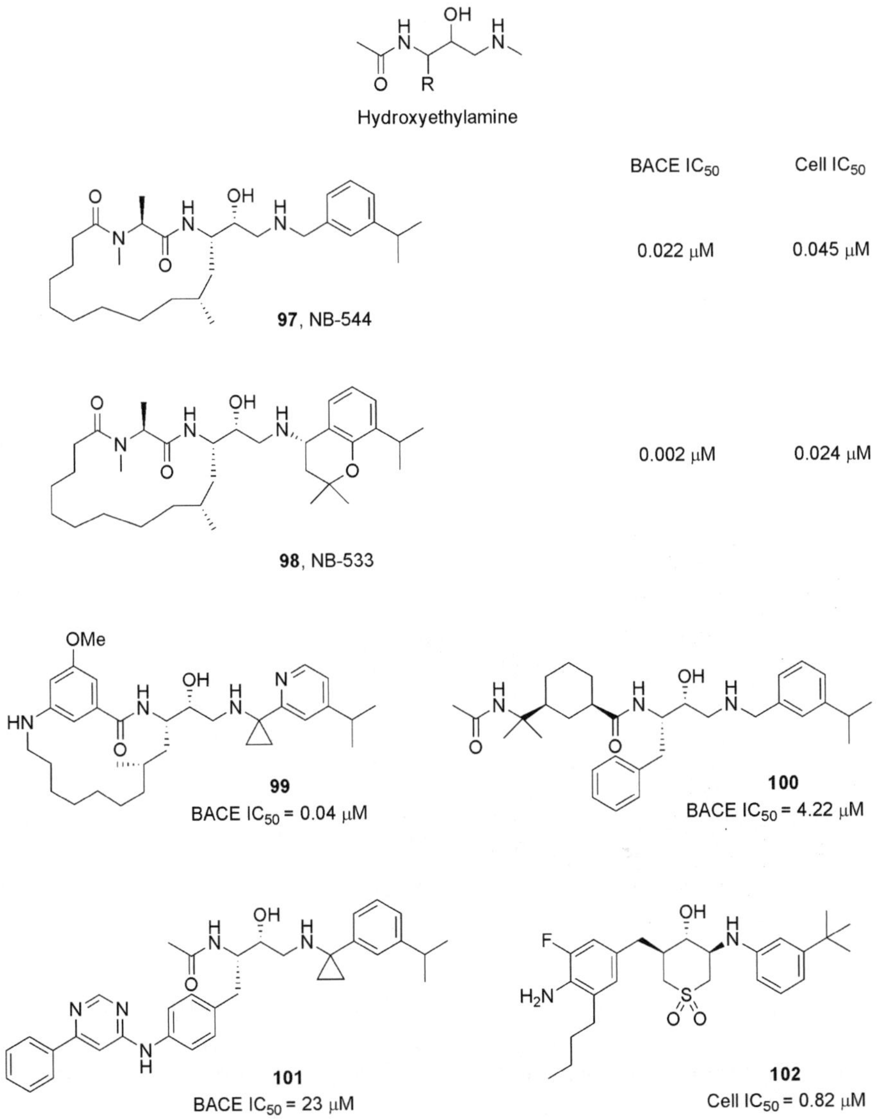

Hydroxyethylamine

	BACE IC$_{50}$	Cell IC$_{50}$

97, NB-544 — 0.022 μM — 0.045 μM

98, NB-533 — 0.002 μM — 0.024 μM

99
BACE IC$_{50}$ = 0.04 μM

100
BACE IC$_{50}$ = 4.22 μM

101
BACE IC$_{50}$ = 23 μM

102
Cell IC$_{50}$ = 0.82 μM

Figure 4.31   Novartis BACE inhibitors.

isostere as a substrate transition-state mimic (Fig. 4.33) [97]. As a prototypical example, **KMI-429** (Fig. 4.33, **108**) has also reportedly shown significant reduction of Aβ production in vivo by direct administration into the hippocampus of APP transgenic and wild-type mice [98]. Most recently, this work has resulted in the optimization of the P$_1'$ functionality with nonacidic moieties (Fig. 4.33, **109**, **KMI-758**) [99], and continued focus on the P$_2$ pyridine scaffold (Fig. 4.33, **110**, **KMI-1283**) to optimize interactions with S$_2$ and S$_3$ of BACE-1 [100].

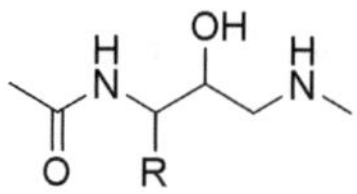

Hydroxyethylamine

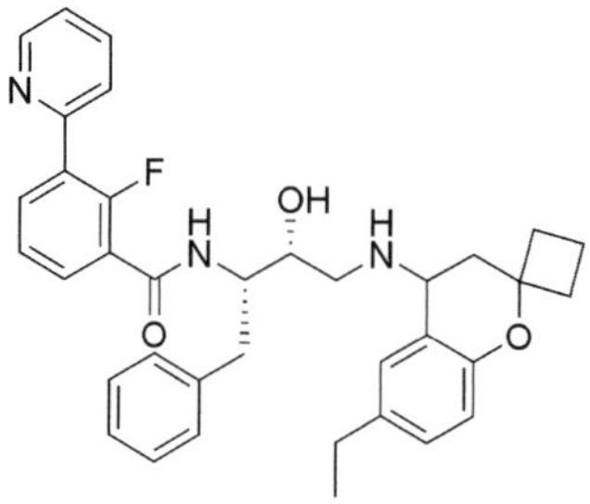

103 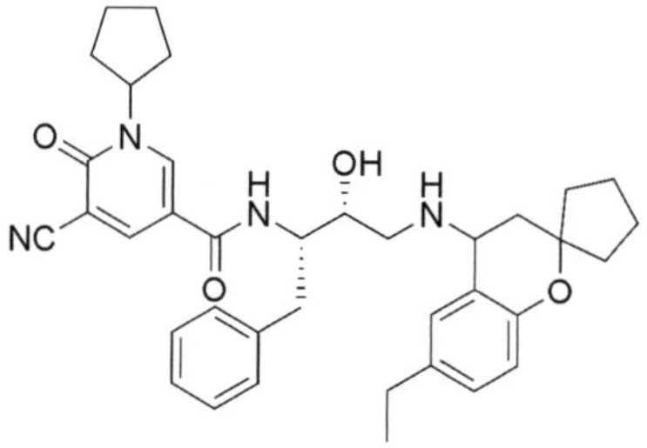   104

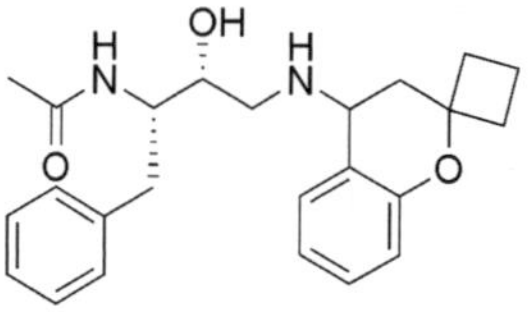

105 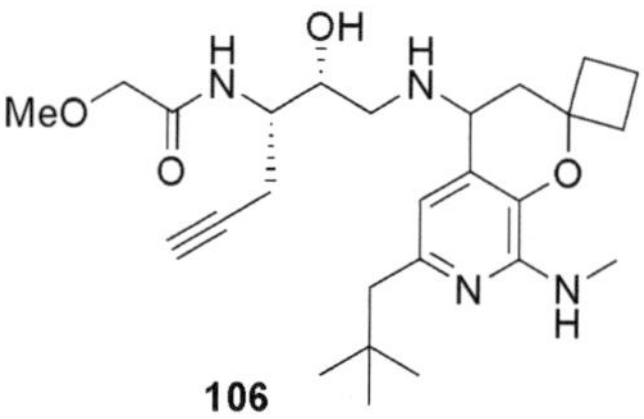   106

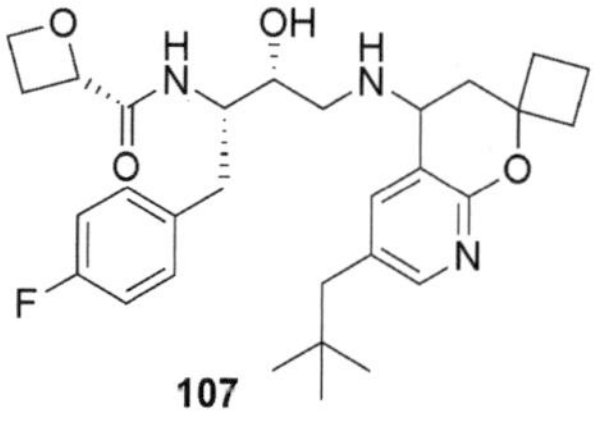

107

Figure 4.32   Amgen BACE inhibitors.

4.11   WYETH

Another noteworthy exception to the limited success of identifying BACE-1 inhibitors from HTS is from researchers at Wyeth who did identify N-[2-(2,5-diphenyl-pyrrol-1-yl)-acetyl]guanidine (Fig. 4.34, **111, WY-25105**) as an inhibitor of BACE-1 [101]. Using a fluorescence resonance energy (FRET) assay, **WY-25105** displayed a BACE-1 $IC_{50} = 3.7\,\mu M$ and inhibited Aβ formation in a cellular assay with an $IC_{50} = 8.9\,\mu M$. Dose-dependent reduction in βCTF and Aβ levels in a radiolabeled immunoprecipitation cellular assay confirmed BACE-1 mediated inhibition (no effect on α-sAPP). Initial SAR efforts to fill the lipophilic S_1 pocket led to modest

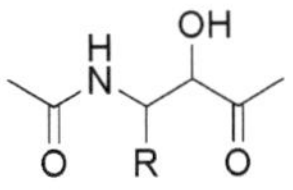

Norstatine (hydroxymethylcarbonyl)

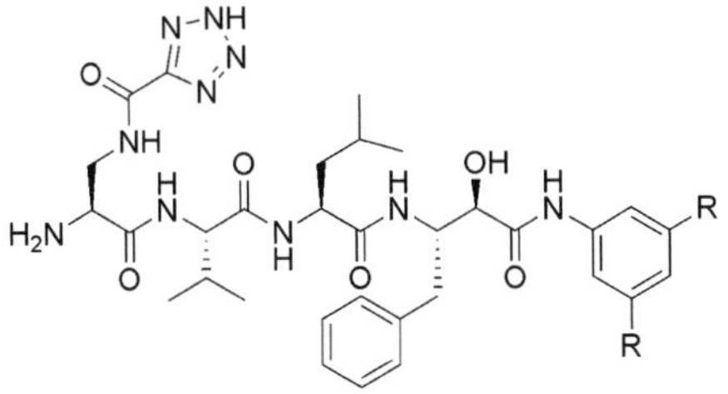

108 (KMI-429), R = CO$_2$H, BACE IC$_{50}$ = 3.9 nM

109 (KMI-758), R = Cl, BACE IC$_{50}$ = 14.0 nM

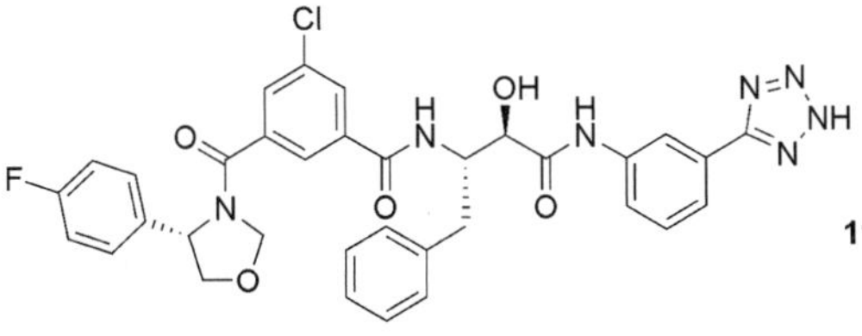

110 (KMI-1283), BACE IC$_{50}$ = 13.0 nM

Figure 4.33   Kyoto Pharmaceutical University/University of Tokyo BACE inhibitors.

improvements in BACE-1 activity (Fig. 4.34, **112**, IC$_{50}$ = 1.3 µM). Further optimiza-tion incorporated guanidine nitrogen substituents terminating in polar functionalities to access the S$_1'$ pocket with concomitant decrease in size (phenyl to propyl) of the P$_1$ substitution [102]. Acylguanidine **113** (Fig. 4.34) was identified to have a BACE IC$_{50}$ = 0.12 µM and a cellular IC$_{50}$ = 1.2 µM. Wyeth has also reported on the substitu-tion with a thiophene ring for the key pyrrole nucleus (Fig. 4.34, **114**). Further reports from Wyeth are anticipated describing the optimization of these inhibitors [103] and related masked amino-pyrimidines [104].

Also originating from HTS at Wyeth was **WY-24454** (Fig. 4.35, **115**) with a BACE FRET IC$_{50}$ = 38 µM. Removal of the solvent-exposed tetrahydropyri-midine ring gave 2-amino-3,5-dihydro-4H-imidazol-4-one (Fig. 4.35, **116**) having a 10-fold improvement in activity (IC$_{50}$ = 3.6 µM) [105]. Later developments included optimizing to a 2-fluoro-3-pyridyl group to occupy the S$_3$ pocket which was then conserved in an exploration of the P$_1'$ where it was found that a wide diversity of substitution at P$_2'$ was tolerated. For example, suitable P$_2'$ substitution included keto-piperidines (**117**) [106], pyrroles (**118**) [107], pyrazoles (not shown) [108], thiophenes (not shown) [109], piperidines (not shown) [110], and pyridines (**119**) [111]. In the aminohydantoin series, Wyeth has shown that a single enantiomer (e.g., *(S)*-**119**) is preferred. It has also been shown that the two phenyl rings may be tethered via an ethylene bridge with retention of BACE enzyme activity [112].

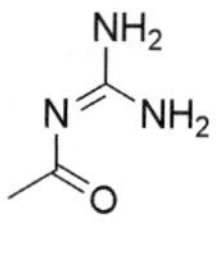

Acylguanidine

	BACE IC$_{50}$	Cell IC$_{50}$
111, **WY-25105**	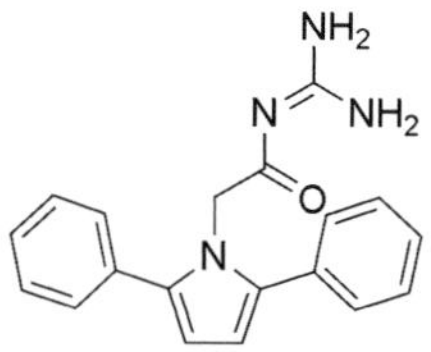 3.7 μM	8.9 μM
112	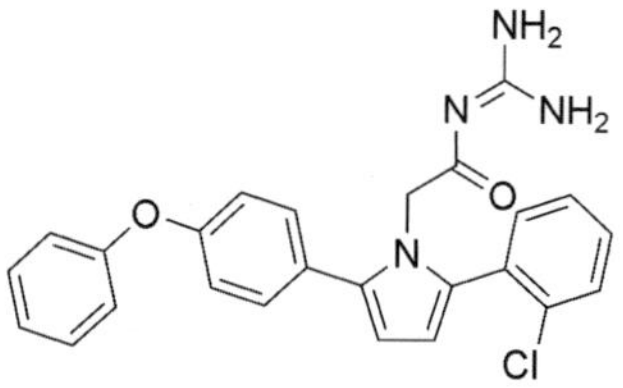 1.3 μM	13 μM
113	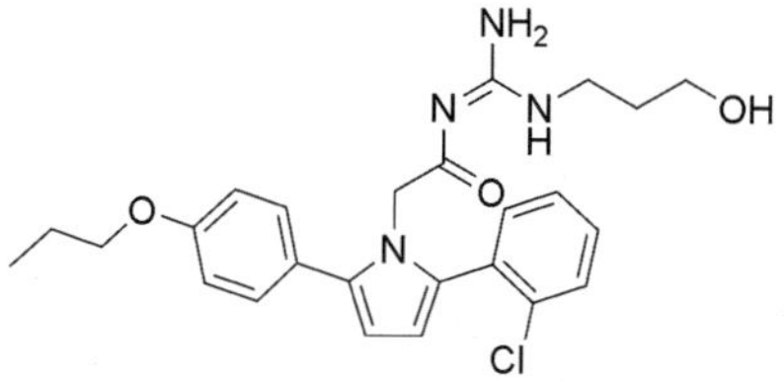 0.12 μM	1.2 μM
114	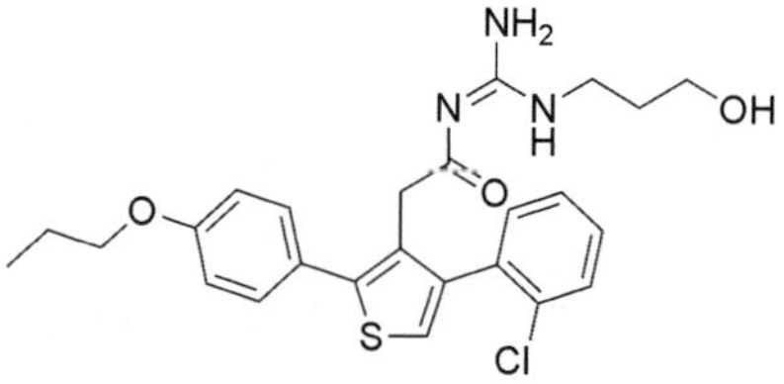 0.15 μM	2.2 μM

Figure 4.34 Wyeth HTS-based BACE inhibitors.

Highlighting the progress of the Wyeth aminohydantoin SAR was the disclosure of potent inhibitor **WY-258131**, *(R)*-**120** (Fig. 4.35) [105b]. **WY-258131** demonstrates good enzyme and cell activity (BACE IC$_{50}$ = 10 nM, cellular ED$_{50}$ = 20 nM) with both a BACE-2/BACE-1 and Cat-D/BACE-1 ratio equal to 82. In Tg2576 mice, **WY-258131** dose dependently decreased Aβ40 in plasma with 10 and 30 mg/kg showing significant decreases upon oral administration (BID, 7 days). Brain Aβ40 and Aβ42 were also dose dependently decreased upon oral administration (BID, 14

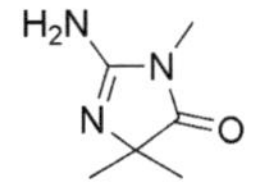

Aminohydantoins

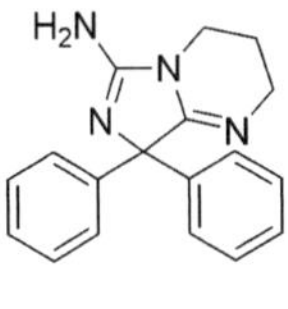

115, WY-24454
BACE IC$_{50}$ = 38 μM

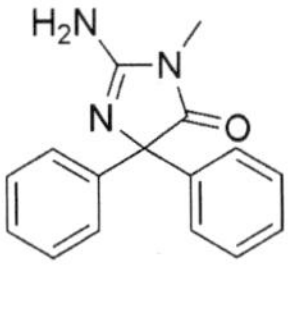

116
BACE IC$_{50}$ = 3.6 μM

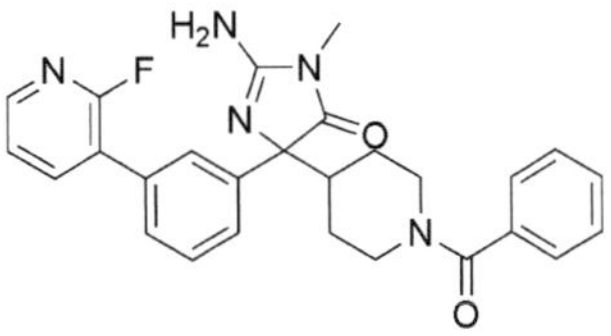

117
BACE IC$_{50}$ = 0.48 μM

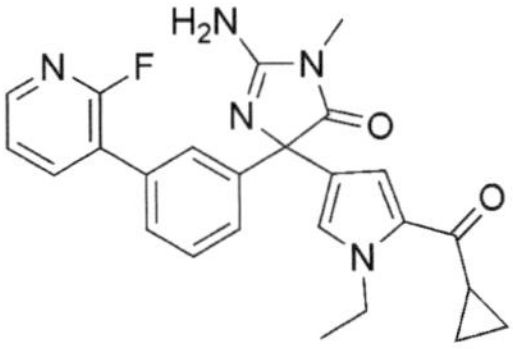

118
BACE IC$_{50}$ = 0.019 μM

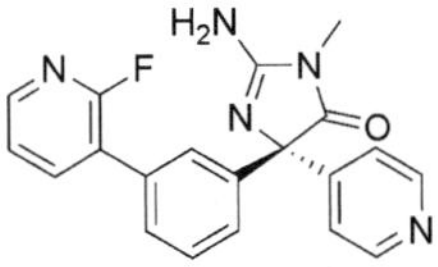

(R,S)-119
BACE IC$_{50}$ = 0.03 μM
(S)-119
BACE IC$_{50}$ = 0.007 μM

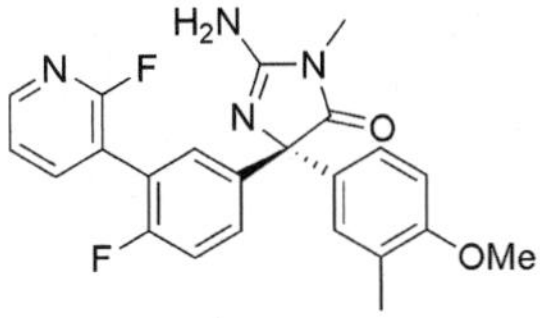

(R,S)-120
BACE IC$_{50}$ = 0.040 μM
ELISA ED$_{50}$ = 0.060 μM
(R)-120, WY-258131
BACE IC$_{50}$ = 0.010 μM
ELISA ED$_{50}$ = 0.020 μM

Figure 4.35   Wyeth HTS-based BACE inhibitors.

days) in Tg2576 mice (3, 10 mg/kg), however a plateauing of effect was seen at the highest dose (30 mg/kg), and the maximal decrease was approximately 30%. Finally, **WY-258131** was shown to produce a significant and dose dependent increase in contextual memory (reversal of cognitive deficits) in the transgenic animals and the inhibitor did not have a significant effect on wild-type performance. Wyeth has published several patent applications covering their progress in the aminohydantoin SAR [113], and also covering indolylalkylpyrimin-2-amines as BACE-1 inhibitors [114].

4.12   FINAL REMARKS

The substantial resources and effort that have been applied to development of peptide, peptidomimetic, and HTS-derived BACE-1 inhibitors have resulted in significant advances to aspartyl protease design over the past several years. The field has progressed from initial substrate mimics to a variety of smaller and truncated (C- or N-terminus) peptidomimetics that have demonstrated *in vivo* efficacy in multiple preclinical species. CoMentis has even advanced a BACE inhibitor into clinical trials with positive reports of pharmacodynamic effect. But, challenges still remain for these efforts to deliver a first-in-class, best-in-class BACE-1 inhibitor for disease modification of Alzheimer's disease. These challenges still include cell permeability, blood–brain barrier penetration, oral bioavailability, and sustained duration of action. Between 2004 up to the present (~5.5 years), more than 550 BACE-1 patent citations appear in SciFinder, indicative of the extraordinary effort being applied to overcome these challenges. In the coming years, it will be interesting to see how researchers in the field of BACE-1 inhibitor design will attempt to address these challenges with unique and creative strategies.

REFERENCES

1. (a) Silvestri, R. 2009. Boom in the development of non-peptidic β-secretase (BACE1) inhibitors for the treatment of Alzheimer's disease. *Med Res Rev* **29**:295–338; (b) Stachel, S.J. 2009. Progress toward the development of a viable BACE-1 inhibitor. *Drug Dev Res* **70**:101–110; (c) Tomita, T. 2009. Secretase inhibitors and modulators for Alzheimer's disease treatment. *Expert Rev Neurother* **9**:661–679; (d) Ghosh, A.K., Kumaragurubaran, N., Hong, L., Koelsh, G., and Tang, J. 2008. Memapsin 2 (beta-secretase) inhibitors: drug development. *Curr Azlheimer Res* **5**:121–131; (e) Ghosh, A.K., Gemma, S., and Tang, J. 2008. β-Secretase as a therapeutic target for Alzheimer's disease. *Neurotherapeutics* **5**:399–408; (f) Durham, T.B. and Shepherd, T.A. 2006. Progress toward the discovery and development of efficacious BACE inhibitors. *Curr Opin Drug Discov Devel* **9**:776–791; (g) John, V. 2006. Human β-secretase (BACE) and BACE inihibitors: progress report. *Curr Top Med Chem* **6**:569–578; (h) Ziora, Z., Kimura, T., and Kiso, Y. 2006. Small-sized BACE1 inhibitors. *Drugs of the Future* **31**:53–63; (i) John. V., Beck, J.P., Bienkowski, M.J., Sinha, S., and Heinrikson, R.L. 2003. Human β-secretase (BACE) and BACE inhibitors. *J Med Chem* **46**: 4625–4630.
2. Tung, J.S., Davis, D.L., Anderson, J.P., Walker, D.E., Mamo, S., Jewett, N., Hom, R.K., Sinha, S., Thorsett, E.D., and John, V. 2002. Design of substrate-based inhibitors of human β-secretase. *J Med Chem* **45**:259–262.
3. Hom, R.K., Fang, L.Y., Mamo, S., Tung, J.S., Guinn, A.C., Walker, D.E., Davis, D.L., Gailunas, A.F., Thorsett, E.D., Sinha, S., Knopps, J.E., Jewett, N.E., Anderson, J.P., and John, V. 2003. Design and synthesis of statine-based cell-permeable peptidomimetic inhibitors of human β-secretase. *J Med Chem* **46**:1799–1802.
4. (a) John, V., Tung, J., Fang, L., and Mamo, S.S. 2000. Preparation of statine-derived tetrapeptides as inhibitors of β-secretase. PCT Int Appl WO2000077030; (b) Schostarez, H.J. and Chrusciel, R.A. 2003. Preparation of statine derivatives for the treatment of Alzheimer's disease. PCT Int Appl WO2003006021.
5. Kaldor, S.W., Dressman, B.A., Hammond, M., Appelt, K., Burgess, J.A., Lubbehusen, P.P., Muesing, M.A., Hatch, S., Wiskerchen, M.A., and Baxter, A.J. 1995. Isophthalic acid derivatives: amino acid surrogates for the inhibition of HIV-1 protease. *Bioorg Med Chem Lett* **5**:721–726.
6. Hom, R.K., Gailunas, A.F., Mamo, S., Fang, L.Y., Tung, J.S., Walker, D.E., Davis, D., Thorsett, E.D., Jewett, N.E., and John, V. 1995. Design and synthesis of hydroxyethylene-based peptidomimetic inhibitors of human β-secretase. *J Med Chem* **47**:158–164.

7. (a) Gailunas, A., Tucker, J.A., and John, V. 2003. Preparation of phenethylamines for the treatment of Alzheimer's disease. PCT Int Appl WO2003027068; (b) John, V., Hom, R., and Tucker, J. 2003. Preparation of β-hydroxyamine derivatives for the treatment of Alzheimer's disease. PCT Int Appl WO2003002122; (c) Maillard, M. and Tucker, J.A. 2002. Substituted aminoalcohols useful in treatment of Alzheimer's disease. PCT Int Appl WO2002100820; (d) Hom, R., Mamo, S., Tung, J., Gailunas, A., John, V., and Fang, L. 2001. Preparation of hydroxyethylenes with peptide subunits for pharmaceutical use in the treatment of Alzheimer's disease. PCT Int Appl WO2001070672.

8. (a) Beck, J.P., Gailunas, A., Hom, R., Jagodzinska, B., John, V., and Maillaird, M. 2002. Preparation of disubstituted amines for treating Alzheimer's disease. PCT Int Appl WO2002002520; (b) Maillaird, M., Hom, R., Gailunas, A., Jagodzinska, B., Fang, L.Y., John, V., Freskos, J.N., Pulley, S.R., Beck, J.P., and Tenbrink, R.E. 2002. Preparation of substituted amines to treat Alzheimer's disease. PCT Int Appl WO2002002512; (c) Fang, L.Y., Hom, R., John, V., and Maillaird, M. 2002. Preparation of substituted amines for treating Alzheimer's disease. PCT Int Appl WO2002002505.

9. Maillard, M.C., Hom, R.K., Benson, T.E., Moon, J.B., Shumeye, M., Bienkowski, M., Tomasselli, A.G., Woods, D.D., Prince, D.B., Paddock, D.J., Emmons, T.L., Tucker, J.A., Dappen, M.S., Brogley, L., Thorsett, E.D., Jewett, N., Sinha, S., and John, V. 2007. Design, synthesis, and crystal structure of hydroxyethyl secondary amine-based peptidomimetic inhibitors of human β-secretase. *J Med Chem* **50**:776–781.

10. Kortum, S.W., Benson, T.E., Bienkowski, M.J., Emmons, T.L., Prince, D.B., Paddock, D.J., Tomasselli, A.G., Moon, J.B., LaBorde, A., and Tenbrink, R.E. 2007. Potent and selective isophthalamide S2 hydroxyethylamine inhibitors of BACE1. *Bioorg Med Chem Lett* **17**:3378–3383.

11. Chirapu, S.R., Pachaiyappan, B., Nural, H.F., Cheng, X., Yuan, H., Lankin, D.C., Abdul-Hay, S.O., Thatcher, G.R.J., Shen, Y., Kozikowski, A.P., and Petukhov, P.A. 2009. Molecular modeling, synthesis, and activity studies of novel biaryl and fused-ring BACE1 inhibitors. *Bioorg Med Chem Lett* **19**:264–274.

12. Freskos, J.N., Fobian, Y.M., Benson, T.E., Bienkowski, M.J., Brown, D.L., Emmons, T.L., Heintz, R., LaBorde, A., McDonald, J.J., Mischke, B.V., Molyneaux, J.M., Moon, J.B., Mullins, P.B., Prince, D.B., Pakkock, D.J., Tomasselli, A.G., and Winterrowd, G. 2007. Design of potent inhibitors of human β-secretase. Part 1. *Bioorg Med Chem Lett* **17**:73–77.

13. Freskos, J.N., Fobian, Y.M., Benson, T.E., Moon, J.B., Bienkowski, M.J., Brown, D.L., Emmons, T.L., Heintz, R., LaBorde, A., McDonald, J.J., Mischke, B.V., Molyneaux, J.M., Mullins, P.B., Prince, D.B., Paddock, D.J., Tomasselli, A.G., and Winterrowd, G. 2007. Design of potent inhibitors of human β-secretase. Part 2. *Bioorg Med Chem Lett* **17**:78–81.

14. Freskos, J., Aquino, J., Brown, D.L., Fang, L., Fobian, Y.M., Gailunas, A., Guinn, A., Varghese, J., Romero, A.G., Tucker, J., Tung, J., and Walker, D. Preparation of peptide-related hydroxyalkylamines for pharmaceutical use in the treatment of Alzheimer's disease. 2002. PCT Int Appl WO2002098849.

15. (a) Pulley, S.R., Beck, J.P., and Tenbrink, R.E. 2002. Macrocycles useful in the treatment of Alzheimer's disease. PCT Int Appl WO2002100856; (b) Pulley, S.R., Beck, J.P., Tenbrink, R.E., and Jacobs, J.S. 2002. Preparation of macrocycles useful in the treatment of Alzheimer's disease. PCT Int Appl WO2002100399.

16. Varghese, J., Jagodzinska, B., Maillard, M., Beck, J.P., Tenbrink, R.E., and Getman, D. 2003. Preparation of substituted amines prodrugs useful in treating Alzheimer's disease. PCT Int Appl WO2003072535.

17. Fobian, Y.M., Freskos, J.N., and Jagodzinska, B.A. 2004. Preparation of 1,3-diamino-2-hydroxypropane derivatives as beta-secretase enzyme inhibitors. PCT Int Appl WO2004022523.

18. Hurley, T.R., Colson, C.E., Hicks, G., and Ryan, M.J. 1993. Orally active water-soluble N, O-acyl transfer products of a β, γ-bishydroxyl amide containing renin inhibitor. *J Med Chem* **36**:1496–1498.

19. Hamada, Y., Ohtake, J., Sohma, Y., Kimura, T., Hayashi, Y., and Kiso, Y. 2002. New water-soluble prodrugs of HIV protease inhibitors based on O → N intramolecular acyl migration. *Bioorg Med Chem Lett* **10**:4155–4167.

20. John, V., Maillard, M., Jagodzinska, B., Beck, J.P., Gailunas, A., Fang, L., Sealy, J., Tenbrink, R., Freskos, J., Mickelson, J., Samala, L., and Hom, R. 2003. Preparation of N,N'-substituted-1,3-diamino-2-hydroxypropanes for treating Alzheimer's disease. PCT Int Appl WO2003040096.

21. Gailunas, A., Hom, R., John, V., Maillard, M., Chrusciel, R.A., Fisher, J., Jacobs, J., Freskos, J.N., Brown, D.L., and Fobian, Y.M. 2003. Preparation of N-(3-amino-2-hydroxy-propyl) substituted alkanamides as inhibitors of the beta secretase enzyme for treating Alzheimer's disease. PCT Int Appl WO2003006423.

22. Pully, S.R. and Tucker, J.A. 2004. Preparation of peptide-related substituted ureas and carbamates for the treatment of Alzheimer's disease. PCT Int Appl WO2004050609.

23. Maillard, M.C., Baldwin, E.T., Beck, J.P., Hughes, R., John, V., Pulley, S.R., and Tenbrink, R. 2004. Preparation of ring-containing N-acetyl 2-hydroxy-1,3-diaminoalkanes as β-secretase inhibitors for treating Alzheimer's disease and other diseases characterized by deposition of Aβ-peptide. PCT Int Appl WO2004024081.

24. (a) Bembenek, S.D., Tounge, B.A., and Reynolds, C.H. 2009. Ligand efficiency and fragment-based drug discovery. *Drug Discov Today* **14**:278–283; (b) Reynolds, C.H., Tounge, B.A., and Bembenek, S.D. 2008. Ligand binding efficiency: trends, physical basis and implications. *J Med Chem* **51**:2432–2438.

25. (a) John, V., Hom, R., Sealy, J., Tucker, J. 2006. Methods of treatment of amyloidosis using bi-aryl aspartyl protease inhibitors. US Pat Appl Publ US2006014737; (b) John, V., Maillard, M., Fang, L., Tucker, J., Brogley, L., Aquino, J., Bowers, S., Probst, G., and Tung, J. 2005. Preparation of bicyclic compounds as aspartyl protease and β-secretase inhibitors for treating conditions associated with amyloidosis such as Alzheimer's disease. PCT Int Appl WO2005087714; (c) John, V., Hom, R., Sealy, J., Aquino, J., Probst, G., Tung, J., and Fang, L. 2005. Preparation of N-(3-amino-2-hydroxypropyl)acetamides as aspartyl protease and beta secretase inhibitors for treating conditions associated with amyloidosis such as Alzheimer's disease. PCT Int Appl WO2005070407.

26. (a) Neitz, R.J., Tisdale, E., Jagodzinska, B., Truong, A., and Tung, J.S. 2007. Preparation of cyclopropyl fluorophenyl aminohydroxybutylamides as aspartyl protease inhibitors for treatment of amyloidosis. PCT Int Appl WO2007047305; (b) Hom, R., Toth, G., Probst, G., Bowers, S., Truong, A., and Tung, J.S. 2007. Preparation of aryl cyclopropyl (heterocyclyl) aminohydroxybutylamides as aspartyl protease inhibitors for treatment of amyloidosis. PCT Int Appl WO2007047306; (c) Hom, R., Fang, L., and John, V. 2006. Preparation of ethanol cyclic amine selective β-secretase inhibitors for treatment of amyloidosis. PCT Int Appl WO2006026533; (d) Hom, R., Fang, L., and John, V. 2006. Methods of treatment of amyloidosis using substituted ethanolcyclicamine aspartyl protease inhibitors. PCT Int Appl WO2006026532; (e) Sealy, J., Hom, R., John, V., Probst, G., and Tung, J.S. 2006. Preparation of oxime-containing N-(3-amino-1-arylmethyl-2-hydroxypropyl) carboxamide and related selective β-secretase inhibitors for treating amyloidosis. PCT Int Appl WO2006010094; (f) John, V., Maillard, M., Jagodzinska, B., Aquino, J., Probst, G., and Tung, J.S. 2006. Preparation of oxime, hydrazone and other derivative substituted hydroxyethylamine selective β-secretase inhibitors for treating amyloidosis. PCT Int Appl WO2006010095; (g) Hom, R., Tucker J., John V., and Shah N. 2005. Preparation of 2-amino-and 2-thio-substituted 1,3-diaminopropanes as β-secretase inhibitors for treating Alzheimer's disease and other diseases characterized by deposition of Aβ-peptide. PCT Int Appl WO2005095326; (h) John, V., Maillard, M., Tucker, J., Aquino, J., Jagodzinska, B., Brogley, L., Tung, J., Bowers, S., Dressen, D., Probst, G., and Shah, N. 2005. Preparation of hydroxyethylamines as aspartyl protease inhibitors for treatment of amyloidosis. PCT Int Appl WO2005087751.

27. Tenbrink, R., Maillard, M., and Warpehoski, M. 2003. Preparation of substituted hydroxyethylamines as β-secretase inhibitors. PCT Int Appl WO2003050073.

28. (a) Aquino, J.R., John, V., Tucker, J.A., Hom, R., Pulley, S., and Tenbrink, R. 2004. Preparation of phenacyl-substituted 2-hydroxy-3-diaminoalkanes as inhibitors of β-secretase. PCT Int Appl WO2004094413; (b) Aquino, J., John, V., Tucker, J.A., Hom, R., Pulley, S., Tenbrink, R. 2004. Preparation of 2-hydroxy-3-aminoalkylbenzamides as β-secretase inhibitors for the treatment of Alzheimer's disease. PCT Int Appl WO2004094384.

29. John, V., Maillard, M., Tucker, J., Aquino, J., Hom, R., Tung, J., Dressen, D., Shah, N., and Neitz, R.J. 2005. Preparation of substituted urea and carbamate, phenacyl-2-hydroxy-3-

diaminoalkane, and benzamide-2-hydroxy-3-diaminoalkane aspartyl protease and β-secretase inhibitors for treating conditions associated with amyloidosis such as Alzheimer's disease. PCT Int Appl WO2005087215.

30. (a) Schostarez, H.J. and Chrusciel, R.A. 2002. Preparation of peptide-related hydrazine derivatives for treating Alzheimer's disease. PCT Int Appl WO2002100410; (b) Schostarez, H.J., Chrusciel, R.A., and Centko, R.S. 2002. Acylaminopropylhydrazines as β-secretase inhibitors. PCT Int Appl WO2002094768; (c) Fang, L.Y. and John, V. 2002. Compounds to treat Alzheimer's disease. PCT Int Appl WO2002002506.

31. (a) Romero, A.G., Schostarez, H.J., and Roels, C.M. 2003. Preparation of amine 1,2- and 1,3-diol aldols and their use for treatment of Alzheimer's disease. PCT Int Appl WO2003043975; (b) Schostarez, H.J. and Hanson, G.J. 2003. Aminodiols useful in the treatment of Alzheimer's disease and similar diseases. PCT Int Appl WO2003043618; (c) Schostarez, H.J. and Chrusciel, R.A. 2003. Preparation of amine diols as β-secretase inhibitors for the treatment of Alzheimer's disease. PCT Int Appl WO2003006453; (d) Schostarez, H.J. and Chrusciel, R.A. 2003. Preparation of diamine diols as β-secretase inhibitors for the treatment of Alzheimer's disease. PCT Int Appl WO2003006013; (e) Schostarez, H.J. and Chrusciel, R.A. 2002. Preparation of aminediols as β-secretase inhibitors for the treatment of Alzheimer's and other diseases characterized by deposition of Aβ peptide. PCT Int Appl WO2002100818.

32. Hom, R. and Varghese, J. 2004. Preparation of hydroxyaminopropylbenzamides for the treatment of Alzheimer's disease. PCT Int Appl WO2004029019.

33. Beck, J.P., Drowns, M., and Warpehoski, M.A. 2004. Preparation of ring-containing aminoether carboxamides as β-secretase inhibitors for treating Alzheimer's disease and other diseases characterized by deposition of Aβ-peptide. PCT Int Appl WO2004024675.

34. Jagodzinska, B. and Warpehoski, M.A. 2003. Preparation of substituted amino carboxamides for the treatment of Alzheimer's disease. PCT Int Appl WO2003057721.

35. Fisher, J.F., Jacobs, J.S., and Scherer, B.A. 2003. Preparation of arylhydroxypropylamines used for treatment of Alzheimer's disease and to reduce amyloid beta peptide formation. PCT Int Appl WO2003029169.

36. Tucker, J.A., Sherer, B.A., Xu, Y.Z., Brogley, L., Pulley, S.R., Jacobs, J.S., Beck, J.P., and John, V. 2004. Preparation of hydroxypropyl benzamides as β-secretase inhibitors for the treatment of Alzheimer's disease. US Pat Appl Publ US2004039034.

37. Gailunas, A., Tucker, J.A., and John, V. 2003. Preparation of phenethylamines for the treatment of Alzheimer's disease. PCT Int Appl WO2003027068.

38. Tucker, J.A. 2005. Preparation of hydroxypropyl amide peptide analogs for the treatment of Alzheimer's disease. PCT Int Appl WO2005042472.

39. (a) Ghosh, A.K., Shin, D., Downs, D., Koelsch, G., Lin, X., Ermolieff, J., and Tang, J. 2000. Design of potent inhibitors for human brain memapsin 2 (β-secretase). *J Am Chem Soc* **122**:3522–3523; (b) Tang, J.J.N., Hong, L., and Ghosh, A.K. 2001. Inhibitors of memapsin 2 and use thereof. PCT Int Appl WO2001000665.

40. (a) Hong, L., Koelsch, G., Lin, X., Wu, S., Terzyan, S., Ghosh, A.K., Zhang, X.C., and Tang, J. 2000. Structure of the protease domain of memapsin 2 (β-secretase) complexed with inhibitor. *Science* **290**:150–153; (b) Tang, J.J.N., Lin, X., and Koelsch, G. 2001. Catalytically active recombinant memapsin 2, 3D crystal structure-based inhibitor design, synthesis, and screening, for Alzheimer's disease treatment. PCT Int Appl WO2001000663; (c) Hong, L., Turner, R.T. III, Koelsch, G., Shin, D., Ghosh, A.K., and Tang, J. 2002. Crystal structure of memapsin 2 (β-secretase) in complex with an inhibitor OM00-3. *Biochemistry* **41**:10963–10967; (d) Hong, L. and Tang, J. 2004. Flap position of free memapsin 2 (β-secretase), a model for flap opening in aspartic protease catalysis. *Biochemistry* **43**:4689–4695.

41. Ghosh, A.K., Kumaragurubaran, N., Hong, L., Lei, H., Hussain, K.A., Liu, C.-F., Devasamudram, T., Weerasena, V., Turner, R., Koelsch, G., Bilcer, G., and Tang, J. 2006. Design, synthesis and X-ray structure of protein-ligand complexes: important insight into selectivity of memapsin 2 (β-secretase) inhibitors. *J Am Chem Soc* **128**:5310–5311.

42. (a) Ghosh, A., Lei, H., Devasamudram, T., Lui, C., Tang, J., and Bilcer, G. 2006. Preparation of pseudopeptides which inhibit β-secretase activity. PCT Int Appl WO2006034296; (b) Ghosh, A., Lei, H., Devasamudram, T., Liu, C., Tang, J., and Bilcer, G. 2006. Preparation of pseudopeptides

which inhibit β-secretase activity. PCT Int Appl WO2006034277; (c) Ghosh, A.K., Tang, J., Bilcer, G., Chang, W., Hong, L., Koelsch, G.E., Loy, J.A., Turner, R.T., and Devasumadram, T. 2004. Compounds which inhibit beta-secretase activity and methods of use thereof. U.S. Pat Appl Publ US2004121947; (d) Ghosh, A.K., Tang, J., Bilcer, G., Chang, W., Hong, L., Koelsch, G., Loy, J., and Turner, R.T. III. 2003. Design of β-secretase inhibitors for treatment of Alzheimer's disease based on crystal structures of β-secretase and side chain interactions in inhibitor complexes. PCT Int Appl WO2003039454; (e) Tang, J., Koelsch, G., and Ghosh, A.K. 2002. Inhibitors of memapsin 2 and their use in Alzheimer's disease treatment. PCT Int Appl WO2002053594; (f) Ghosh, A.K., Devasamudram, T., Hong, L., DeZutter, C., Xu, X., Weerasena, V., Koelsch, G., Bilcer, G., and Tang, J. 2005. *J Bioorg Med Chem Lett* **15**:15–20.

43. (a) Turner, R.T. III, Koelsch, G., Hong, L., Castenheira, P., Ghosh, A., and Tang, J. 2001. Subsite specificity of memapsin 2 (β-secretase): implications for inhibitor design. [Erratum for **40**(34): 10001–10006]. *Biochemistry* **40**:12230; (b) Turner, R.T. III, Koelsch, G., Hong, L., Castenheira, P., Ghosh, A., and Tang, J. 2001. Subsite specificity of memapsin 2 (β-secretase): implications for inhibitor design. *Biochemistry* **40**:10001–10006; (c) Ghosh, A.K., Bilcer, G., Harwood, C., Kawahama, R., Shin, D., Hussain, K.A., Hong, L., Loy, J.A., Nguyen, C., Koelsch, G., Ermolieff, J., and Tang, J. 2001. Structure-based design: potent inhibitors of human brain memapsin 2 (β-secretase). *J Med Chem* **44**:2865–2868.

44. Ghosh, A.K., Kumarahurubaran, N., Hong, L., Kulkarni, S.S., Xu, X., Chang, W., Weerasena, V., Turner, R., Koelsch, G., Bilcer, G., and Tang, J. 2007. Design, synthesis, and X-ray structure of potent memapsin 2 (β-secretase) inhibitors with isophthalamide derivatives as the PP-ligands. *J Med Chem* **50**:2399–2407.

45. Ghosh, A.K., Kumaragurubaran, N., Hong, L., Kulkarni, S., Xu, X:, Miller, H.B., Reddy, D.S., Weerasena, V., Turner, R., Chang, W., Koelsch, G., and Tang, J. 2008. Potent memapsin 2 (β-secretase) inhibitors: design, synthesis, protein-ligand X-ray structure, and in vivo evaluation. *Bioorg Med Chem Lett* **18**:1031–1036.

46. (a) Ghosh, A.K., Liu, C., Devasamudram, T., Lei, H., Swanson, L.M., Ankala, S.V., Lilly, J.C., and Bilcer, G.M. 2009. Preparation of (3-hydroxy-4-amino-butan-2-yl)-3-[2-(thiazol-2-yl)pyrro-lidine-1-carbonyl]benzamide derivatives and related compounds as selective beta-secretase inhibitors. PCT Int Appl WO2009042694; (b) Ghosh, A.K., Liu, C., Devasamudram, T., Lei, H., Swanson, L.M., Ankala, V.S., Lilly, J.C., and Bilcer, G.M. 2009. Isophthalamide compounds which inhibit beta-secretase activity and their preparation, pharmaceutical compositions and use in the treatment of Alzheimer's disease. PCT Int Appl WO2009015369; (c) Ghosh, A.K., Kumaragurubaran, N., Liu, C., Devasamudram, T., Lei, H., Swanson, L., Ankala, S., Tang, J., and Bilcer, G. 2006. Preparation of benzene-1,3-dicarboxamides which inhibit β-secretase activity. PCT Int Appl WO2006110668.

47. See www.comentis.com.

48. Hu, J., Cwi, C.L., Smiley, D.L., Timm, D., Erickson, J.A., McGee, J.E., Yang, H.-C., Mendel, D., May, P.C., Shapiro, M., and McCarthy, J.R. 2003. Design and synthesis of statine-containing BACE inhibitors. *Bioorg Med Chem Lett* **13**:4335–4339.

49. Lamar, J., Hu, J., Bueno, A.B., Yang, H.-C., Guo, D., Copp, J.D., McGee, J., Gitter, B., Timm, D., May, P., McCarthy, J., and Chen, S.-H. 2004. Phe*-ala-based pentapeptide mimetics are BACE inhibitors: P2 and P3 SAR. *Bioorg Med Chem Lett* **14**:239–243.

50. Chen, S.–H., Lamar, J., Guo, D., Kohn, T., Yang, H.–C., McGee, J., Timm, D., Erickson, J., Yip, Y., May, P., and McCarthy, J. 2004. P3 cap modified Phe*-ala series BACE inhibitors. *Bioorg Med Chem Lett* **14**:245–250.

51. Rojo, I., Martin, J.A., Broughton, H., Timm, D., Erickson, J., Yang, H.-C., and McCarthy, J.R. 2006. Macrocyclic peptidomimetic inhibitors of β-secretase (BACE): first X-ray structure of a macrocyclic peptidomimetic-BACE complex. *Bioorg Med Chem Lett* **16**:191–195.

52. Dally, R.D., Shepherd, T.A., Bender, D.M., and Rojo Garcia, M.I. 2005. BACE inhibitors. PCT Int Appl WO2005108358.

53. Durham, T.B., Hahn, P.J., Kohn, T.J., McCarthy, J.R., Broughton, H.B., Dally, R.D., Gonzalez-Garcia, M.R., Henry, K.J. Jr., Shepherd, T.A., Erickson, J.A., and Bueno-Melendo, A.B. 2006. BACE inhibitors. PCT Int Appl WO2006034093.

54. Brady, S.F., Singh, S., Crouthamel, M.-C., Holloway, M.K., Coburn, C.A., Garsky, V.M., Bogusky, M., Pennington, M.W., Vacca, J.P., Hazuda, D., and Lai, M.-T. 2004. Rational design and synthesis of selective BACE-1 inhibitors. *Bioorg Med Chem Lett* **14**:601–604.

55. Coburn, C.A., Stachel, S.J., Li, Y.-M., Rush, D.M., Steele, T.G., Chen-Dodson, E., Holloway, M.K., Xu, M., Huang, Q., Lai, M.-T., DiMuzio, J., Crouthamel, M.-C., Shi, X.-P., Sardana, V., Chen, Z., Munshi, S., Kuo, L., Makara, G.M., Annis, D.A., Tadikonda, P.K., Nash, H.M., Vacca, J.P., and Wang, T. 2004. Identification of a small molecule nonpeptide active site β-secretase inhibitor that displays a nontraditional binding mode for aspartyl proteases. *J Med Chem* **47**:6117–6119.

56. Stachel, S.J., Coburn, C.A., Steele, T.G., Jones, K.G., Loutzenhiser, E.F., Gregro, A.R., Rajapakse, H.A., Lai, M.-T., Crouthamel, M.-C., Xu, M., Tugusheva, K., Lineberger, J.E., Pietrak, B.L., Espeseth, A.S., Shi, X.-P., Chen-Dodson, E., Holloway, M.K., Munshi, S., Simon, A.J., Kuo, L., and Vacca, J.P. 2004. Structure-based design of potent and selective cell-permeable inhibitors of human β-secretase (BACE-1). *J Med Chem* **47**:6447–6450.

57. Coburn, C.A., Stachel, S.J., Jones, K.G., Steele, T.G., Rush, D.M., DiMuzio, J., Pietrak, B.L., Lai, M.-T., Huang, Q., Lineberger, J., Jin, L., Munshi, S., Holloway, M.K., Espeseth, A., Simon, A., Hazuda, D., Graham, S.L., and Vacca, J.P. 2006. BACE-1 inhibition by a series of ψ[CH$_2$NH] reduced amide isosteres. *Bioorg Med Chem Lett* **16**:3635–3638.

58. Stachel, S.J., Coburn, C.A., Sankaranarayanan, S., Price, E.A., Pietrak, B.L., Huang, Q., Lineberger, J., Espeseth, A., Jin, L., Ellis, J., Holloway, M.K., Munshi, S., Allison, T., Hazuda, D., Simon, A.J., Graham, S.L., and Vacca, J.P. 2006. Macrocyclic inhibitors of β-secretase: functional activity in an animal model. *J Med Chem* **49**:6147–6150.

59. (a) Yang, W., Lu, W., Lu, Y., Zhong, M., Sun, J., Thomas, A., Wilkinson, J.M., Fucini, R.V., Lam, M., Randal, M., Shi, X.-P., Jacobs, J.W., McDowell, R.S., Gordon, E.M., and Ballinger, M.D. 2006. Aminoethylenes: a tetrahedral intermediate isostere yielding potent inhibitors of the aspartyl protease BACE-1. *J Med Chem* **49**:839–842. (b) Stanton, M.G., Stauffer, S.R., Gregro, A.R., Steinbeiser, M., Nantermet, P., Sankaranarayanan, S., Price, E.P., Wu, G., Crouthamel, M.-C., Ellis, J., Lai, M.-T., Espeseth, A.S., Shi, X.-P., Jin, L., Colussi, D., Pietrak, B., Huang, Q., Xu, M., Simon, A.J., Graham, S.L., Vacca, J.P., and Selnick, H. 2007. Discovery of isonicotinamide derived β-secretase inhibitors: in vivo reduction of β-amyloid. *J Med Chem* **50**:3431–3433.

60. (a) Nantermet, P.G., Rajapakse, H.A., Stanton, M.G., Stauffer, S.R., Barrow, J.C., Gregro, A.R., Moore, K.P., Steinbeiser, M.A., Swestock, J., Selnick, H.G., Graham, S.L., McGaughey, G.B., Colussi, D., Lai, M.-T., Sankaranarayanan, S., Simon, A.J., Munshi, S., Cook, J.J., Holahan, M.A., Michener, M.S., and Vacca, J.P. 2009. Evolution of tertiary carbinamine BACE-1 inhibitors: Ab reduction in Rhesus CSF upon oral dosing. *ChemMedChem* **4**:37–40. (b) Sankaranarayanan, S., Holahan, M.A., Colussi, D., Crouthamel, M.-C., Devanarayan, V., Ellis, J., Espeseth, A., Gates, A.T., Gram, S.L., Gregro, A.R., Hazuda, D., Hochman, J.H., Holloway, K., Jin, L., Kahana, J., Lai, M.-T., Lineberger, J., McGaughey, G., Moore, K.P., Nantermet, P., Pietrak, B., Price, E.A., Rajapakse, H., Stauffer, S., Steinbeiser, M.A., Seabrook, G., Selnick, H.G., Shi, X.-P., Stanton, M.G., Swestock, J., Tugusheve, K., Tyler, K.X., Vacca, J.P., Wong, J., Wu, G., Xu, M., Cook, J.J., and Simon, A.J. 2009. First demonstration of cerebrospinal fluid and plasma Aβ lowering with oral administration of a β-site amyloid precursor protein-cleaving enzyme 1 inhibitor in nonhuman primates. *J Pharm Exper Ther* **328**:131–140.

61. Barrow, J.C., Stauffer, S.R., Rittle, K.E., Ngo, P.L., Yang, Z.Q., Selnick, H.G., Graham, S.L., Munshi, S., McGaughey, G.B., Holloway, M.K., Simon, A.J., Price, E.A., Sankaranarayanan, S., Colussi, D., Tugusheva, K., Lai, M.-T., Espeseth, A.S., Xu, M., Huang, Q., Wolfe, A., Pietrack, B., Zuck, P., Levorse, D.A., Hazuda, D., and Vacca, J.P. 2008. Discovery and X-ray crystallographic analysis of a spiropiperidine iminohydantoin inhibitor of β-secretase. *J Med Chem* **51**:6259–6262.

62. (a) Stauffer, S.R. and Graham, S.L. 2008. Bicyclic spiropiperidine β-secretase inhibitors for the treatment of Alzheimer's disease. PCT Int Appl WO2008085509; (b) Stauffer, S.R., Hills, I.D., and Nomland, A. 2008. Spiropiperidine β-secretase inhibitors for the treatment of Alzheimer's disease. PCT Int Appl WO2008054698; (c) Nantermet, P.G., Holloway, M.K., Moore, K.P., and Stauffer, S.R. 2008. Preparation of macrocyclic spiropiperidine as β-secretase inhibitors. PCT Int Appl

WO2008045250; (d) Egbertson, M.S., Stauffer, S.R., Coburn, C.A., Barrow, J.C., Yang, W., Lu, W., Fahr, B., Neilson, L.A., and Wai, J.M. 2008. Preparation of aryldiazaspiro [4.5]decanone derivatives for use as anti-Alzheimer's agents. PCT Int Appl WO2008030412.

63. Steele, T.G., Hills, I.D., Nomland, A.A., de León, P., Allison, T., McGaughey, G., Colussi, D., Tugusheva, K., Haugabook, S.J., Espeseth, A.S., Zuck, P., Graham, S.L., and Stachel, S.J. 2009. *Bioorg Chem Med Lett* **19**:17–20.

64. Stachel, S.J., Coburn, C.A., Rush, D., Jones, K.L.G., Zhu, H., Rajapakse, H., Graham, S.L., Simon, A., Holloway, M.K., Allison, T.J., Munshi, S.K., Espeseth, A.S., Zuck, P., Colussi, D., Wolfe, A., Pietrak, B.L., Lai, M.-T., and Vacca, J.P. 2009. *Bioorg Med Chem Lett* **19**:2977–2980.

65. (a) Demont, E.H. Redshaw, S., and Walter, D.S. 2004. Preparation of 3-(1,1-dioxotetrahydro-1,2-thiazin-2-yl) or 3-(1,1-dioxo-isothiazolidin-2-yl) substituted benzamide compounds for treatment of Alzheimer's disease. PCT Int Appl WO2004111022; (b) Faller, A., MacPherson, D.T., Milner, P.H., Stanway, S.J., and Trouw, S.S. 2003. Preparation of benzamide derivatives as inhibitors of Asp-2. PCT Int Appl WO2003045913; (c) Faller, A., Milner, P.H., and Ward, J.G. 2003. N-carbamoylalkylcarboxamides and -sulfonamides with Asp-2 inhibitory activity. PCT Int Appl WO2003045903.

66. Clarke, B., Demont, E., Dingwall, C., Dunsdon, R., Faller, A., Hawkins, J., Hussain, I., MacPherson, D., Maile, G., Matico, R., Milner, P., Mosley, J., Naylor, A., O'Brien, A., Redshaw, S., Riddell, D., Rowland, P., Soleil, V., Smith, K.J., Stanway, S., Stemp, G., Sweitzer, S., Theobald, P., Vesey, D., Walter, D.S., Ward, J., and Wayne, G. 2008. *Bioorg Med Chem Lett* **18**:1011–1016.

67. Clarke, B., Demont, E., Dingwall, C., Dunsdon, R., Faller, A., Hawkins, J., Hussain, I., MacPherson, D., Maile, G., Matico, R., Milner, P., Mosley, J., Naylor, A., O'Brien, A., Redshaw, S., Riddell, D., Rowland, P., Soleil, V., Smith, K.J., Stanway, S., Stemp, G., Sweitzer, S., Theobald, P., Vesey, D., Walter, D.S., Ward, J., and Wayne, G. 2008. *Bioorg Med Chem Lett* **18**:1017–1021.

68. Beswick, P., Charrier, N., Clarke, B., Demont, E., Dingwall, C., Dunsdon, R., Faller, A., Gleave, R., Hawkins, J., Hussain, I., Johnson, C.N., MacPherson, D., Maile, G., Matico, R., Milner, P., Mosley, J., Naylor, A., O'Brien, A., Redshaw, S., Riddell, D., Rowland, P., Skidmore, J., Soleil, V., Smith, K.J., Stanway, S., Stemp, G., Stuart, A., Sweitzer, S., Theobald, P., Vesey, D., Walter, D.S., Ward, J., and Wayne, G. 2008. *Bioorg Med Chem Lett* **18**:1022–1026.

69. Hussain, I., Hawkins, J., Harrison, D., Hille, C., Wayne, G., Cutler, L., Buck, T., Walter, D., Demont, E., Howes, C., Naylor, A., Jeffrey, P., Gonzalez, M.I., Dingwall, C., Michel, A., Redshaw, S., and Davis, J.B. 2007. *J Neurochem* **100**:802–809.

70. Charrier, N., Clarke, B., Cutler, L., Demont, E., Dingwall, C., Dunsdon, R., East, P., Hawkins, J., Howes, C., Hussain, I., Jeffrey, P., Maile, G., Matico, R., Mosley, J., Naylor, A., O'Brien, A., Redshaw, S., Rowland, P., Soleil, V., Smith, K.J., Sweitzer, S., Theobald, P., Vesey, D., Walter, D.S., and Wayne, G. 2008. *J Med Chem* **51**:3313–3317.

71. (a) Demont, E.H., Redshaw, S., and Walter, D.S. 2006. Novel hydroxyethylamine and ketone compounds having Asp2 inhibitory activity. PCT Int Appl WO2006103088; (b) Demont, E.H., Redshaw, S., and Walter, D.S. 2006. Preparation of substituted hydroxyethylamine compounds for treating Alzheimer's disease. PCT Int Appl WO2006040151; (c) Demont, E.H., Redshaw, S., and Walter, D.S. 2005. Preparation of N,N'-substituted-1,3-diamino-2-oxopropane derivatives as Asp2 inhibitors for use against diseases characterized by elevated β-amyloid levels or β-amyloid deposits, particularly Alzheimer's disease. PCT Int Appl WO2005113525; (d) Redshaw, S., Demont, E.H., and Walter, D.S. 2005. Preparation of tricyclic indole hydroxyethylamine derivatives and their use in the treatment of Alzheimer's disease. PCT Int Appl WO2005058915; (e) Demont, E.H., Redshaw, S., and Walter, D.S. 2004. Preparation of hydroxydiaminopropyl tricyclic indolecarboxamides for treatment of β-amyloid related disease. PCT Int Appl WO2004094430; (f) Demont, E.H., Redshaw, S., and Walter, D.S. 2004. Preparation of hydroxyethylamine derivatives for the treatment of Alzheimer's disease. PCT Int Appl WO2004080376; (g) Demont, E.H., Faller, A., MacPherson, D.T., Milner, P.H., Naylor, A., Redshaw, S., Stanway, S.J., Vesey, D.R., and Walter, D.S. 2004. Preparation of hydroxyethylamine derivatives for the treatment of Alzheimer's disease. PCT Int Appl WO2004050619.

72. (a) Demont, E.H., Redshaw, S., and Walter, D.S. 2006. Tricyclic indole derivatives for use in the treatment of Alzheimer's disease. PCT Int Appl WO2006040148; (b) Demont, E.H., Redshaw, S.,

and Walter, D.S. 2006. Heterocyclic ketone compounds for treating Alzheimer's disease. PCT Int Appl WO2006040149.

73. Iserloh, U., Wu, Y., Cumming, J.N., Pan, J., Wang, L.Y., Stamford, A.W., Kennedy, M.E., Kuvelkar, R., Chen, X., Parker, E.M., Strickland, C., and Voigt, J. 2008. Potent pyrrolidine- and piperidine-based BACE-1 inhibitors. *Bioorg Med Chem Lett* **18**:414–417.

74. Iserloh, U., Pan, J., Stamford, A.W., Kennedy, M.E., Zhang, Q., Zhang, L., Parker, E.M., McHugh, N.A., Favreau, L., Strickland, C., and Voigt, J. 2008. Discovery of an orally efficacious 4-phenoxy-pyrrolidine-based BACE-1 inhibitor. *Bioorg Med Chem Lett* **18**:418–422.

75. Cumming, J.N., Le, T.X., Babu, S., Carroll, C., Chen, X., Favreau, L., Gaspari, P., Guo, T., Hobbs, D.W., Huang, Y., Iserloh, U., Kennedy, M.E., Kuvelkar, R., Li, G., Lowrie, J., McHugh, N.A., Ozgur, L., Pan, J., Parker, E.M., Saionz, K., Stamford, A.W., Strickland, C., Tadesse, D., Voigt, J., Wang, L., Wu, Y., Zhang, L., and Zhang, Q. 2008. Rational design of novel, potent piperazinone and imidazolidinone BACE1 inhibitors. *Bioorg Med Chem Lett* **18**:3236–3241.

76. Stamford, A.W., Huang, Y., Li, G., Strickland, C.O., and Voigt, J.H. 2006. Preparation of macrocyclic β-secretase inhibitors. PCT Int Appl WO2006014944.

77. Decicco, C.P., Tebben, A.J., Thompson, L.A., and Combs, A.P. 2004. Preparation of novel α-amino-γ-lactams as β-secretase inhibitors. PCT Int Appl WO2004013098.

78. Meredith, J.E. Jr., Thompson, L.A., Toyn, J.H., Marcin, L., Barten, D.M., Marcinkeviciene, J., Kopcho, L., Kim, Y., Lin, A., Guss, V., Burton, C., Iben, L., Polson, C., Cantone, J., Ford, M., Drexler, D., Fiedler, T., Lentz, K.A., Grace, J.E. Jr., Kolb, J., Corsa, J., Pierdomenico, M., Jones, K., Olson, R.E., Macor, J.E., and Albright, C.F. 2008. P-glycoprotein efflux and other factors limit brain amyloid β reduction by β-site amyloid precursor protein-cleaving enzyme 1 inhibitors in mice. *J Pharm Exper Ther* **326**:502–512.

79. Thompson, L.A., Boy, K.M., Shi, J., and Macor, J.E. 2006. Preparation of isophthalates as β-secretase inhibitors. PCT Int Appl WO2006099352.

80. Wu, Y.J., Zhang, Y., Good, A.C., Burton, C.R., Toyn, J.H., Albright, C.F., Macor, J.E., and Thompson, L.A. 2009. Synthesis and SAR of hydroxyethylamine based phenylcarboxyamides as inhibitors of BACE. *Bioorg Med Chem Lett* **19**:2654–2660.

81. Auberson, Y., Glatthar, R., Salter, R., Simic, O., and Tintelnot-Blomley, M. 2005. Preparation of substituted spirocyclic lactams as inhibitors of proteinase BACE1. PCT Int Appl WO2005035535.

82. (a) Machauer, R., Veenstra, S., Rondeau, J.-M., Tintelnot-Blomley, M., Betschart, C., Paganetti, P., and Neumann, U. 2009. Structure-based design and synthesis of macrocyclic peptidomimetic β-secretase (BACE-1) inhibitors. [Erratum for **19**:1361–1365] *Bioorg Med Chem Lett* **19**:2366; (b) Machauer, R., Veenstra, S., Rondeau, J.-M., Tintelnot-Blomley, M., Betschart, C., Paganetti, P., and Neumann, U. 2009. Structure-based design and synthesis of macrocyclic peptidomimetic β-secretase (BACE-1) inhibitors. *Bioorg Med Chem Lett* **19**:1361–1365.

83. Betschart, C. and Tintelnot-Blomley, M. 2005. Macrocyclic compounds having aspartic protease inhibiting activity and pharmaceutical uses thereof. PCT Int Appl WO2005003106.

84. Auberson, Y., Betschart, C., Flohr, S., Glatthar, R., Simic, O., Tintelnot-Blomley, M., Troxler, T.J., Vangrevelinghe, E., and Veenstra, S.J. 2005. A preparation of dibenz[b,f]oxepincarboxamide derivatives, useful for the treatment of neurological and vascular disorders related to β-amyloid generation and aggregation. PCT Int Appl WO2005014517.

85. Machauer, R., Laumen, K., Veenstra, S., Rondeau, J.-M., Tintelnot-Blomley, M., Betschart, C., Jaton, A.-L., Desrayaud, S., Staufenbiel, M., Rabe, S., Paganetti, P., and Neumann, U. 2009. Macrocyclic peptidomimetic β-secretase (BACE-1) inhibitors with activity in vivo. *Bioorg Med Chem Lett* **19**:1366–1370.

86. Abramowski, D., Wiederhold, K.-H., Furrer, U., Jaton, A.-L., Neuenschwander, A., Runser, M.J., Danner, S., Reichwald, J., Ammaturo, D., Staab, D., Stoeckli, M., Rueeger, H., Neumann, U., and Staufenbiel, M.D. 2008. Dynamics of Aβ turnover and deposition in different β-amyloid precursor protein transgenic mouse models following γ-secretase inhibition. *J Pharmacol Exp Ther* **327**:411–424.

87. (a) Laumen, K., Machauer, R., Tintelnot-Blomley, M., and Veenstra, S.J. 2008. Preparation of macrocyclic compounds useful as BACE inhibitors. PCT Int Appl WO2008009750; (b) Machauer, R. 2008. Preparation of macrocyclic compounds useful as BACE inhibitors. PCT Int Appl WO2008009734; (c) Betschart, C., Koller, M., Laumen, K., Lerchner, A., Machauer, R., McCarthy,

C., Tintelnot-Blomley, M., and Veenstra, S.J. 2007. Preparation of macrocyclic lactam compounds useful as β-site APP-cleaving enzyme (BACE) inhibitors. PCT Int Appl WO2007077004; (d) Betschart, C., Lerchner, A., Machauer, R., Rueeger, H., Tintelnot-Blomley, M., and Veenstra, S.J. 2006. Preparation of macrocyclic lactones for treatment of β-amyloid related disease. PCT Int Appl WO2006074950; (e) Lerchner, A., Machauer, R., Simic, O., and Tintelnot-Blomley, M. 2006. Preparation of macrocyclic compounds as BACE inhibitors for treating vascular and neurological disorders related to β-amyloid generation. PCT Int Appl WO2006074940; (f) Auberson, Y., Betschart, C., Glatthar, R., Laumen, K., Machauer, R., Tintelnot-Blomley, M., Troxler, T.J., and Veenstra, S.J. 2005. Preparation of macrocyclic lactams for treatment of neurological or vascular disorders related to β-amyloid generation and/or aggregation. PCT Int Appl WO2005049585.

88. Hanessian, S., Maji, D.K., Shao, Z., Subramaniyan, G., Tintelnot-Blomley, M., Yang, G., and Yun, H. 2009. Preparation of substituted cyclohexanecarboxamides useful as β-site APP-cleaving enzyme (BASE) inhibitors. PCT Int Appl WO2009013293.

89. Frederiksen, M., Lueoend, R.M., McCarthy, C., Moebitz, H., Rondeau, J.-M., Roy, B.L., and Rueeger, H. 2008. Preparation of 2-hydroxy-1,3-diaminopropane derivatives for the treatment of neurological or vascular disorders. PCT Int Appl WO2008062044.

90. (a) Briard, E., Lueoend, R.M., Machauer, R., Moebitz, H., Rogel, O., Rondeau, J.-M., Rueeger, H., Tintelnot-Blomley, M., and Veenstra, S.J. 2009. Preparation of aminobenzyl substituted cyclic sulfones as BACE inhibitors. PCT Int Appl WO2009024615; (b) Rueeger, H., Mccarthy, C., Moebitz, H., Rondeau, J.-M., and Tintelnot-Blomley, M. 2007. Preparation of cyclic sulfones useful as β-secretase (bace) inhibitors. PCT Int. Appl WO2007093621.

91. Xue, Q., Albrecht, B.K., Andersen, D.L., Bartberger, M., Brown, J., Brown, R., Chaffee, S.C., Cheng, Y., Croghan, M., Graceffa, R., Harried, S., Hitchcock, S., Hungate, R., Judd, T., Kaller, M., Kreiman, C., La, D., Lopez, P., Masse, C.E., Monenschein, H., Nguyen, T., Nixey, T., Patel, V.F., Pennington, L., Weiss, M., Yang, B., and Zhong, W. 2007. Preparation of 2-hydroxy-1,3-diamino-alkanes including spiro substituted chroman derivatives as β-secretase modulators and their use for treatment Alzheimer' disease and related condition. PCT Int Appl WO2007061930.

92. Albrecht, B.K., Andersen, D.L., Bartberger, M., Brown, J., Brown, R., Chaffee, S.C., Cheng, Y., Croghan, M., Graceffa, R., Harried, S., Hitchcock, S., Hungate, R., Judd, T., Kaller, M., Kreiman, C., La, D., Lopez, P., Masse, C.E., Monenschein, H., Nguyen, T., Nixey, T., Patel, V.F., Pennington, L., Weiss, M., Xue, Q., Yang, B., and Zhong, W. 2007. Preparation of 2-hydroxy-1,3-diaminoalkanes including spiro substituted chroman derivatives as β-secretase modulators and their use for treatment Alzheimer's disease and related condition. PCT Int Appl WO2007062007.

93. Zhong, W., Hitchcock, S., Albrecht, B.K., Bartberger, M., Brown, J., Brown, R., Chaffee, S.C., Cheng, Y., Croghan, M., Graceffa, R., Harried, S., Hickman, D., Horne, D., Hungate, R., Judd, T., Kaller, M., Kreiman, C., La, D., Lopez, P., Masse, C.E., Monenschein, H., Nguyen, T., Nixey, T., Patel, V.F., Pennington, L., Weiss, M., Xue, Q., and Yang, B. 2007. Preparation of 2-hydroxy-1,3-diaminoalkanes including spiro substituted chroman derivatives as β-secretase modulators and their use for treatment Alzheimer's disease and related condition. PCT Int Appl WO2007061670.

94. Zhong, W., Hitchcock, S., Patel, V.F., Croghan, M., Dineen, T., Horne, D., Kaller, M., Kreiman, C., Lopez, P., Monenschein, H., Nguyen, T., Pennington, L., Xue, Q., and Yang, B. 2008. Substituted hydroxyethyl amine compounds as beta-secretase modulators and their preparation and use in the treatment of Alzheimer's disease and related conditions. PCT Int Appl WO2008147544.

95. Zhong, W., Hitchcock, S., Patel, V.F., Croghan, M., Dineen, T., Harried, S., Horne, D., Judd, T., Kaller, M., Kreiman, C., Lopez, P., Monenschein, H., Nguyen, T., Weiss, M., Xue, Q., and Yang, B. 2008. Substituted hydroxyethyl amine compounds as beta-secretase modulators and their preparation and use in the treatment of Alzheimer's disease and related conditions. PCT Int Appl WO2008147547.

96. Graceffa, R., Kaller, M., La, D., Lopez, P., Patel, V.F., and Zhong, W. 2009. Substituted hydroxyethyl amine compounds as beta-secretase modulators and methods of use. PCT Int Appl WO2009064418.

97. Hamada, Y., Igawa, N., Ikari, H., Ziora, Z., Nguyen, J.-T., Yamani, A., Hidaka, K., Kimura, T., Saito, K., Hayashi, Y., Ebina, M., Ishiura, S., and Kiso, Y. 2006. *Bioorg Med Chem Lett* **16**:4354–4359; and references therein.

98. Asai, M., Hattori, C., Iwata, N., Saido, T.C., Sasagawa, N., Szabó, B., Hashimoto, Y., Maruyama, K., Tanuma, S., Kiso, Y., and Ishiura, S. 2006. *J Neurochem* **96**:533–540.

99. Hamada, Y., Abdel-Rahman, H., Yamani, A., Nguyen, J.-N., Stochaj, M., Hidaka, K., Kimura, T., Hayashi, Y., Saito, K., Ishiura, S., and Kiso, Y. 2008. *Bioorg Med Chem Lett* **18**:1649–1653.

100. Hamada, Y., Ohta, H., Miyamoto, N., Sarma, D., Hamada, T., Nakanishi, T., Yamasaki, M., Yamani, A., Ishiura, S., and Kiso, Y. 2009. *Bioorg Med Chem Lett* **19**:2435–2439.

101. Cole, D.C., Manas, E.S., Stock, J.R., Condon, J.S., Jennings, L.D., Aulabaugh, A., Chopra, R., Cowling, R., Ellingboe, J.W., Fan, K.Y., Harrison, B.L., Hu, Y., Jacobsen, S., Jin, G., Lin, L., Lovering, F.E., Malamas, M.S., Stahl, M.L., Strand, J., Sukhdeo, M.N., Svenson, K., Turner, M.J., Wagner, E., Wu, J., Zhou, P., and Bard, J. 2006. Acylguanidines as small molecule β-secretase inhibitors. *J Med Chem* **49**:6158–6161.

102. (a) Jennings, L.D., Cole, D.C., Stock, J.R., Sukhdeo, M.N., Ellingboe, J.W., Cowling, R., Jin, G., Manas, E.S., Fan, K.Y., Malamas, M.S., Harrison, B.L., Jacobsen, S., Chopra, R., Lohse, P.A., Moore, W.J., O'Donnell, M.-M., Hu, Y., Robichaud, A.J., Turner, M.J., Wagner, E., and Bard, J. 2008. Acylguanidine inhibitors of β-secretase: optimization of the pyrrole ring substituents extending into the S′₁ substrate binding pocket. *Bioorg Med Chem Lett* **18**:767–771; (b) Cole, D.C., Stock, J.R., Chopra, R., Cowling, R., Ellingboe, J.W., Fan, K.Y., Harrison, B.L., Hu, Y., Jacobsen, S., Jennings, L.D., Jin, G., Lohse, P.A., Malamas, M.S., Manas, E.S., Moore, W.J., O'Donnell, M.-M., Olland, A.M., Robichaud, A.J., Svenson, K., Wu, J., Wagner, E., and Bard, J. 2008. Acylguanidine inhibitors of β-secretase: optimization of the pyrrole ring substituents extending into the S₁ and S₃ substrate binding pockets. *Bioorg Med Chem Lett* **18**:1063–1066.

103. Fobare, W.F., Solvibile, W.R., Robichaud, A.J., Malamas, M.S., Manas, E., Turner, J., Hu, Y., Wagner, E., Chopra, R., Cowling, R., Jin, G., and Bard, J. 2008. Thiophene substituted acylguanidines as BACE1 inhibitors. *Bioorg Med Chem Lett* **17**;5353–5356.

104. Malamas, M.S., Fobare, W.F., Solvibile, W.R., Lovering, F.E., Condon, J.S., and Robichaud, A.J. 2006. Amino-pyridines as inhibitors of β-secretase and their preparation, and pharmaceutical compositions. US Pat Appl Publ US2006173049.

105. (a) Nowak, P., Aulabaugh, A., Chen, J., Cole, D.C., Chopra, R., Cowling, R., Dar, M., Ellingboe, J.W., Fan, K.Y., Hu, B., Jacobsen, S., Jani, M., Jin, G., Lo, M.-C., Malamas, M.S., Manas, E.S., Narasimhan, R., Robichaud, A., Sabus, C., Stock, J.R., Tischler, M., Turner, J., Wagner, E., Zhou, P., and Bard, J. 2007. Hit-to-lead optimization of aminohydantoins as β-secretase inhibitors. 233rd ACS National Meeting, Chicago, IL, United States, March 25–29, MEDI-307; (b) Malamas, M.S., Erdei, J., Gunawan, I., Pawel, N., Chlenov, M., Robichaud, A.J., Turner, J., Hu, Y., Wagner, E., Aschmies, S., Comery, T., Di, L., Fan, K., Chopra, R., Oganesian, A., Huselton, C., and Bard, J. 2007. Aminohydantoins as highly potent, selective and orally active BACE1 inhibitors. 233rd ACS National Meeting, Chicago, IL, March 25–29, MEDI-234.

106. Yan, Y., Zhou, P., Malamas, M., Aschmies, S., Bard, J., Comery, T., Hu, Y., Oganesian, A., Turner, J., Wagner, E., Reinhart, P., and Robichaud, A. 2008. Syntheses and biological properties of carbocyclic substituted aminohydantoin derivatives. 235th ACS National Meeting, New Orleans, LA, April 6–10, MEDI-258.

107. (a) Zhou, P., Yan, Y., Fobare, W.F., Malamas, M., Solvibile, W.R., Chopra, R., Fan, K.Y., Hu, Y., Turner, J., Wagner, E., Magolda, R.L., Abougharbia, M.A., Reinhart, P., Pangalos, M., Bard, J., and Robichaud, A. 2008. Substituted-pyrrole 2-amino-3,5-dihyro-4H-imidazol-4-ones as highly potent BACE1 inhibitors: optimization of the S3 pocket. 235th ACS National Meeting, New Orleans, LA, April 6–10, MEDI-259; (b) Solvibile, W.R., Fobare, W.F., Abou-Gharbia, M., Andrae, P.M., Aschmies, S., Chopra, R., Fan, K.Y., Hu, Y., Magolda, R.L., Pangalos, M., Quagliato, D.A., Turner, J., Wagner, E., Yan, Y., Zhou, P., Bard, J., Malamas, M., and Robichaud, A. 2008. 2-Substituted-pyrrole 2-amino-3,5-dihydro-4H-imidazol-4-ones: highly potent, and selective BACE1 inhibitors. 235th ACS National Meeting, New Orleans, LA, April 6–10, MEDI-256; (c) Erdei, J., Gunawan, I., Quagliato, D.A., Yan, Y., Fobare, W.F., Solvibile, W.R., Fan, K., Robichaud, A., Turner, J., Wagner, E., Hu, Y., Aschmies, S., Chopra, R., Bard, J., and Malamas, M. 2008. N-Alkyl substituted-pyrrole 2-amino-3,5-dihydro-4H-imidazol-4-ones as potent, and selective BACE1 inhibitors. 235th ACS National Meeting, New Orleans, LA, April 6–10, MEDI-255; (d) Fobare, W.F., Malamas, M., Robichaud, A., Solvibile, W.R., Zhou, P., Quagliato, D.A., Erdei, J., Gunawan, I., Yan, Y., Andrae, P.M., Turner, J., Wagner, E., Hu, Y., Fan, K.Y., Aschmies, S.,

Chopra, R., and Bard, J. 2008. Substituted-pyrrole 2-amino-3,5-dihydro-4H-imidazol-4-ones as highly potent and selective BACE1 inhibitors. 235th ACS National Meeting, New Orleans, LA, April 6–10, MEDI-182.

108. Yan, Y., Zhou, P., Malamas, M.S., Li, Y., Aschmies, S., Bard, J., Bernotas, R.C., Chopra, R., Comery, T., Fan, K.Y., Hu, Y., Oganesian, A., Turner, J., Wagner, E., Wang, Z., Reinhart, P., and Robichaud, A.J. 2007. Piperidinyl-2-aminohydantoin derivatives for the inhibition of beta-secretase. 233rd ACS National Meeting, Chicago, IL, March 25–29, MEDI-309.

109. Malamas, M.S., Erdei, J., Gunawan, I., Barnes, K., Johnson, M., Robichaud, A., Turner, J., Hui, Y., Hu, Y., Chopra, R., Fan, K., and Bard, J. 2008. Thienyl aminohydantoins as potent BACE1 inhibitors. 236th ACS National Meeting, Philadelphia, PA, August 17–21, MEDI-297.

110. Yan, Y., Zhou, P., Malamas, M.S., Li, Y., Aschmies, S., Bard, J., Bernotas, R.C., Chopra, R., Comery, T., Fan, K.Y., Hu, Y., Oganesian, A., Turner, J., Wagner, E., Wang, Z., Reinhart, P., and Robichaud, A.J. 2007. Piperidinyl-2-aminohydantoin derivatives for the inhibition of beta-secretase. 233rd ACS National Meeting, Chicago, IL, March 25–29, MEDI-309.

111. (a) Zhou, P., Bard, J., Chopra, R., Fan, K.Y., Hu, Y., Li, Y., Magolda, R.L., Malamas, M.S., Pangalos, M., Reinhart, P., Turner, J., Wang, Z., and Robichaud, A.J. 2007. Pyridinylaminohydantoins as small molecule BACE1 inhibitors: Exploration of the S3 pocket. 234th ACS National Meeting, Boston, MA, August 19–23, MEDI-294; (b) Malamas, M.S., Barnes, K., Hui, Y., Zhou, P., Robichaud, A.J., Bard, J., Turner, J., Hu, Y., Fan, K.Y., Chopra, R., and Johnson, M. 2007. Substituted-pyridine 2-amino-3,5-dihydro-4H-imidazol-4-ones as highly potent, and selective BACE1 inhibitors. 234th ACS National Meeting, Boston, MA, August 19–23, MEDI-236; (c) Malamas, M.S., Barnes, K., Hui, Y., Zhou, P., Robichaud, A.J., Bard, J., Turner, J., Hu, Y., Fan, K.Y., Chopra, R., and Johnson, M. 2007. Substituted-pyridine 2-amino-3,5-dihydro-4H-imidazol-4-ones as highly potent, and selective BACE1 inhibitors. 234th ACS National Meeting, Boston, MA, August 19–23, MEDI-236.

112. Quagliato, D.A., Andrae, P., Chlenov, M., Fan, K., Li, D., Robichaud, A., Turner, J., Wagner, E., Bard, J., and Malamas, M. 2008. Rigid analogs of 4,4-diaryl-iminohydantoins as potent inhibitors of beta-secretase. 235th ACS National Meeting, New Orleans, LA, April 6–10, MEDI-257.

113. (a) Malamas, M.S., Robichaud, A.J., Porte, A.M., Morris, K.M., Solvibile, W.R., and Kim, J.-L. 2008. Preparation of amino-5-[4-(difluoromethoxy)phenyl]-5-phenylimidazolone derivatives as inhibitors of β-secretase. PCT Int Appl WO2008118379; (b) Malamas, M.S., Robichaud, A.J., Porte, A.M., Solvibile, W.R., Morris, K.M., Antane, S.A., Kim, J.-L., and Mcdevitt, R.E. 2008. Amino-5-[substituted-4-(difluoromethoxy)phenyl]-5- phenylimidazolone compounds as β-secretase inhibitors and their preparation, and use in the treatment of β-amyloid deposits and neurofibrillary tangles. PCT Int Appl WO2008115552; (c) Malamas, M.S., Barnes, K.D., and Johnson, M.R. 2008. Imidazole amines as inhibitors of beta-secretase and their preparation, pharmaceutical compositions and use in the treatment of diseases associated with elevated β-amyloid deposits and β-amyloid levels. PCT Int Appl WO2008022024; (d) Malamas, M.S., Erdei, J.J., Fobare, W.F., Quagliato, D.A., Antane, S.A., and Robichaud, A.J. 2007. Preparation of imidazolone derivatives as inhibitors of β-secretase. US Pat Appl Publ. US2007072925; (e) Malamas, M.S., Gunawan, I.S., Erdei, J.J., Nowak, P.W., Stock, J.R., and Yan, Y. 2007. Cycloalkyl amino-hydantoin compounds and use thereof for β-secretase modulation and treatment of diseases with β-amyloid deposits and neurofibrillary tangles. US Pat Appl Publ. US2007027199; (f) Malamas, M.S., Zhou, P., Fobare, W.F., Solvibile, W.R., Gunawan, I.S., Erdei, J.J., Yan, Y., Andrae, P.M., and Quagliato, D.A. 2007. Preparation of amino-5-(5-membered)hetero-arylimidazolone compounds as β-secretase modulators for treating diseases involving β-amyloid deposits and neurofibrillary tangles. US Pat Appl Publ. US2007004786; (g) Zhou, P., Malamas, M.S., Li, Y., Robichaud, A.J., and Quagliato, D.A. 2007. Preparation of aminoheteroarylimidazolone compounds for use as β-secretase modulators to treat β-amyloid and neurofibrillary tangle associated diseases. US Pat Appl Publ. US2007004730; (h) Malamas, M.S., Erdei, J.J., Gunawan, I.S., Nowak, P., and Harrison, B.L. 2006. Preparation of 8,8-diphenyl-2,3,4,8-tetrahydroimidazo[1,5-a]pyrimidin-6-amines as β-secretase inhibitors for the treatment of Alzheimer's disease and related disorders. PCT Int Appl WO2006076284; (i) Malamas, M.S., Erdei, J.J., Gunawan, I.S., Barnes, K.D., Johnson, M.R., and Hui, Y. 2005. Preparation of diphenylimidazopyrimidine and -imidazole amines as selective inhibitors of β-secretase for use against Alzheimer's disease and other disorders. US Pat Appl Publ. US2005282826; (j) Malamas,

M.S., Erdei, J.J., Gunawan, I.S., Zhou, P., Yan, Y., and Quagliato, D.A. 2005. Preparation of amino-5,5-diphenylimidazolone derivatives for inhibition of beta-secretase and treatment of β-amyloid-related diseases. US Pat Appl Publ. US2005282825.

114. Yan, Y., Zhou, P., Fan, Y., Robichaud, A.J., and Malamas, M.S. 2008. Preparation of indolylalkyl pyridin-2-amines for the inhibition of β-secretase. PCT Int Appl WO2008036196.

CHAPTER 5

FRAGMENT-BASED APPROACHES FOR IDENTIFICATION OF BACE INHIBITORS

Andreas Kuglstatter[1] and Michael Hennig[2]

[1]Roche Palo Alto LLC, Palo Alto, CA and [2]F. Hoffmann-La Roche Ltd., Basel, Switzerland

5.1 INTRODUCTION

Fragment screening methods have been developed to complement established technologies for the generation of information to inspire medicinal chemistry efforts for a particular target [1–4]. In contrast to screening methods of random compound libraries like high-throughput screening (HTS), fragment screening uses a compound library that contains substances which are selected to follow three basic rules – a molecular weight of less than about 300 Da, no more than three hydrogen bonding donors or acceptors, and clogP less than three [4]. Additional properties like no more than three rotatable bonds and a polar surface of less than 60 Å^2 may be added. The small size of the fragments leads to a great diversity of potential binding modes to the target of pharmacological interest. Consequently, compared to HTS, a much smaller number of compounds is required to explore the chemical space of a binding site. This limits the screening effort to hundreds or a few thousand compounds. The advantage of fragments for the start of optimization toward a drug molecule is their favorable physicochemical properties and low chemical complexity. Also, the ligand efficiency (LE) as defined by binding energy per non-hydrogen atom [5, 6] is typically higher for fragments than for HTS hits. The disadvantage is the psychological and technological hurdle to work with ligand affinities in the micromolar (μM) to millimolar (mM) range. The advances in biophysical methods like surface plasmon resonance (SPR), nuclear magnetic resonance (NMR) spectroscopy, X-ray crystallography, and others have diminished the technological challenge regarding screening for low affinity ligand binding. A key element of all fragment-screening efforts is the visualization of the ligand to protein interaction by X-ray crystallography as

---

this information enables a directed medicinal chemistry effort to gain binding affinity while keeping the favorable physicochemical properties.

Exploration of fragments for drug discovery has been applied to many drug targets across the pharmaceutical industry. There appears to be a tendency to apply fragment screening methods to drug targets of low anticipated druggability or in discovery projects that suffer of limited chemical space. Along this line, the lack of good leads for the discovery of potent yet drug-like lead molecules favored application of fragment screening for β-site APP cleaving enzyme (BACE), and reports from at least three companies have been published.

5.2   BIOPHYSICAL METHODS APPLIED TO BACE FRAGMENT SCREENS

Besides the availability of a fragment library and screening technologies, purified protein of quality and quantity suitable for biophysical methods is a prerequisite for a successful fragment screen. Two main routes for protein production have been published for human BACE: (1) expression of the ectodomain in inclusion bodies of *Escherichia coli* with subsequent refolding [7] and (2) expression of the ectodomain or full length sequence in mammalian expression systems like human embryonic kidney (HEK)-293 [8] or insect cells [9]. Comparison of the published fragment screening procedures shows a remarkable diversity (Table 5.1). Roche used surface plasmon resonance (Biacore) for primary screening of 300 fragments, hit confirmation, and affinity measurement. Subsequently, X-ray structure determination facilitated exploration of the discovered tyramine by structure-guided chemistry [10]. Astex screened a library of 347 compounds complemented by 65 substances derived from virtual screening by soaking of BACE crystals with cocktails of six compounds. In a second step, the identified hits were characterized by IC50 measurements in two distinct biochemical assays to reduce false positive readout due to autofluorescence of compounds [11, 12]. AstraZeneca applied 1D NMR to evaluate competitive binding of 2000 compounds against the peptide **OM99-2** [7] (Fig. 5.1) which binds to the BACE active site (Fig. 5.2). After hit confirmation by SPR, crystals of the aspartic acid protease endothiapepsin were soaked with fragments. This surrogate X-ray system was used to avoid great discrepancies in the experimental conditions in screening and crystallography, especially with regard to the pH values of the buffer that could lead to differences in the protonation state, with implications for the binding properties as well as solubility of the molecules [13,14].

Beside the great differences in the methods used for BACE fragment screening and follow-up activities, all approaches delivered new hits that were characterized with binding affinity or enzyme inhibition data, and the binding mode of a few fragments could be visualized by X-ray crystallography. It is interesting to note that the number of BACE X-ray structures with compounds identified in hit expansion efforts was much higher than the number of crystal structures with compounds identified in the primary fragment screens. This demonstrates both the feasibility and the high value of hit expansion in a fragment-to-lead workflow. The high uncer-

TABLE 5.1 Overview of Conditions Applied to Fragment Screening of BACE

Company	Roche [10]	Astex [11, 12]	AstraZeneca [13, 14]
Protein for screening (expression host)	BACE-1, full-length protein (SF9)	BACE-1, residues 14–453 (*E. coli*)	BACE-1, residues 1–400 (HEK-293)
Primary screening method and buffer	Surface plasmon resonance (Biacore) 50 mM acetate pH 4.6, 150 mM NaCl, 3 mM EDTA, 4% DMSO	X-ray crystallography	1D-NMR, 50 mM acetate pH 4.6, 1.2–1.8% DMSO
No. of compounds screened	300	347 & 65 (virtual screening library)	2000
Secondary screening method	Surface plasmon resonance (Biacore)	Biochemical assay (FRET)	Surface plasmon resonance (Biacore) & NMR
X-ray crystallography system (soaking conditions)	BACE-1 ectodomain, K246A mutant (100 mM acetate pH 4.5, 2.5 M formate, 10% DMSO), P6122, a = b = 103 Å; c = 169 Å	BACE-1, residues 14–453 (citrate pH 6.6, 220 mM ammonium iodide, 33% PEG 5000 MME) P6122, a = b = 103 Å; c = 169 Å	Endothiapepsin, 100 mM acetate pH 4.6, 27.5% PEG 4000, 200 mM NH₄Ac, 15% glycerol, P21, a = 45.5 Å; b = 73.6 Å; c = 53.4 Å, β = 110.3°
No. of reported X-ray structures			
Initial fragment screen	1	2	0
Fragment hit expansion	2	8	1
Compound class with further chemistry exploration	Tyramines	Aminoquinolines	Isocytosines

tainty of computational methods to predict fragment binding modes in combination with the high experimental error of affinity data at the low affinity range typical for fragments usually results in weak structure–activity relationship. This emphasizes the importance of structural information, which provides guidance on exit vectors for the exploration of neighboring binding sites. In all three examples where crystal structures of BACE-fragment complexes were determined, medicinal chemists successfully established a more detailed structure–activity relationship and achieved increased activity for the inhibition of BACE.

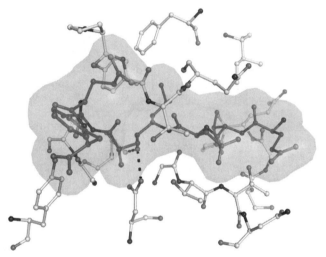

OM99-2

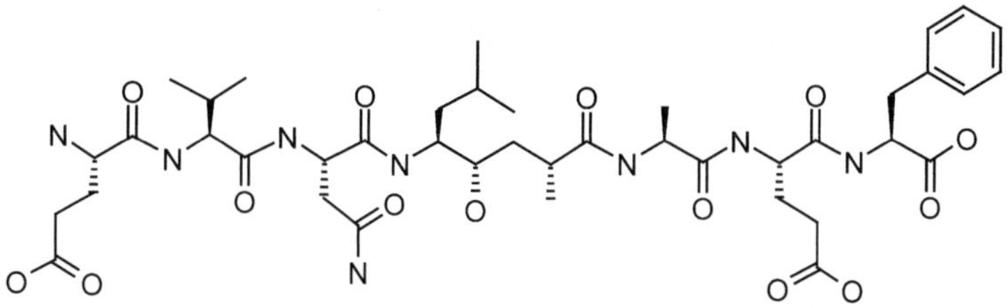

KD = 0.04 µM, LE = 0.16

Figure 5.1   Structure formula of the peptidic inhibitor **OM99-2**.

Figure 5.2   X-ray crystal structure of BACE protease domain in complex with **OM99-2** (PDB accession number 1FKN). **OM99-2** and its molecular surface are indicated in green. BACE flap residues are drawn in yellow, all other residues in the proximity of the ligand are drawn in grey. (See color insert.)

5.3   BACE INHIBITORS IDENTIFIED BY FRAGMENT SCREENING

In this paragraph, we summarize the optimization efforts for different series of BACE inhibitors that have been discovered based on fragment screening approaches. First, the discovery of inhibitor series that resulted from computational fragment screens is outlined. Then, inhibitor series based on experimental screens and backed by X-ray crystal structures are discussed. The order in which compounds are presented in this Chapter has been chosen to provide clarity of the structure–activity relationship and does therefore not necessarily reflect the order in which the compounds were synthesized according to the original publications.

1

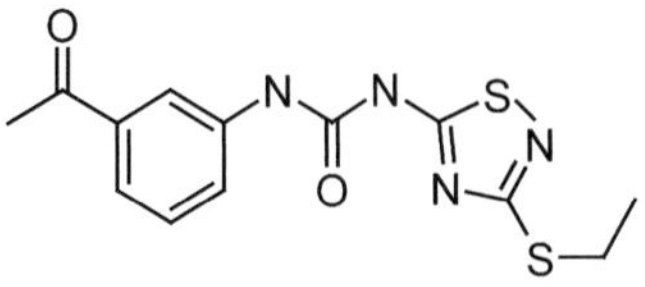

IC50 > 25 µM, LE < 0.3

2

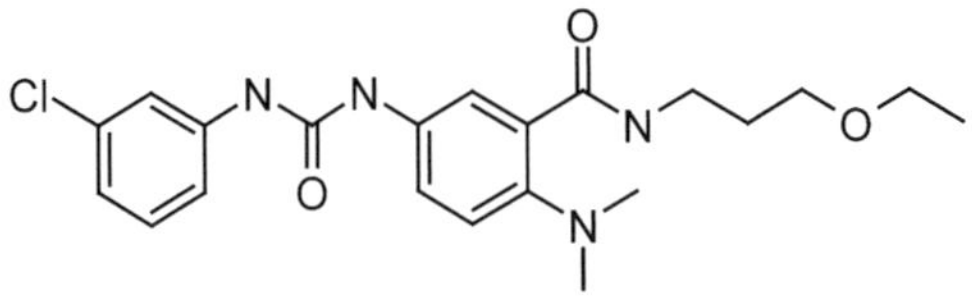

IC50 = 97 µM, LE = 0.19

3

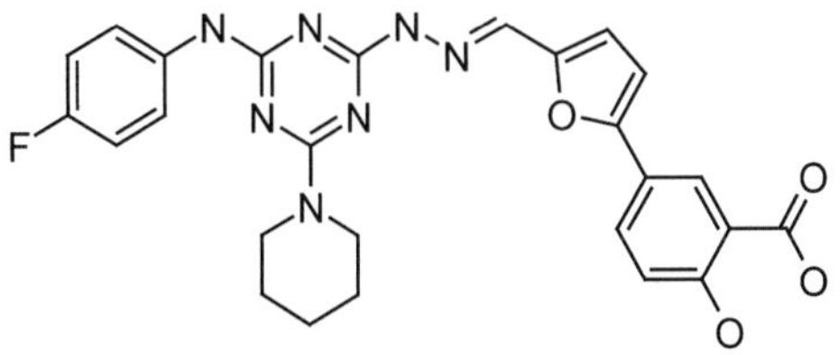

IC50 = 28 µM, LE = 1.6

Figure 5.3   Fragment-based BACE inhibitors reported by the Caflisch group.

5.3.1   Phenylureas

Phenylurea derivatives like compounds **1** and **2** (Fig. 5.3) were identified as BACE inhibitors by *in-silico* high-throughput docking of generic and focused fragment libraries into the BACE active site followed by continuum electrostatic calculations [15]. Even though the BACE enzyme IC50 of compound **1** in a fluorescence resonance energy transfer (FRET) assay was >25 µM, it showed an EC50 of 2.6 ± 0.9 µM in a cell-based assay measuring Aβ peptide secretion. Compound **2** inhibits BACE activity in the enzyme assay with IC50 = 97 ± 21 µM and in the cellular assay with IC50 = 2.6 ± 1.1 µM [15].

Two alternative binding modes to BACE were suggested for the phenylurea derivative **1** based on minimization in a flexible binding site [15]. In the first binding mode, both urea NH groups form hydrogen bonds to the side chain of the catalytic residue Asp32 (Fig. 5.4a). The compound **1** phenyl ring is occupying the S1 pocket and its 3-acetyl substituent is reaching into the adjacent S3 pocket. In this binding mode, the thiadiazole ring of compound **1** serves as a linker to position the 3-ethylsulfanyl moiety in the S2′ pocket of the BACE active site. In the alternative binding mode, both urea NH groups of compound **1** are in hydrogen bonding distance to the side chain of Asp228, the second catalytic residue (Fig. 5.4b). The entire ligand is

(a)   (b)

(c)

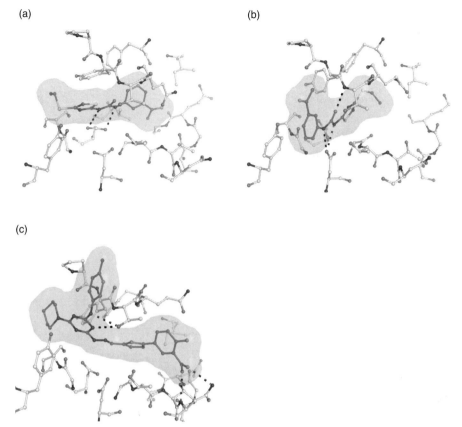

Figure 5.4   Binding modes of compounds **1** and **3** as derived by molecular docking. Two preferred docking modes have been reported for compound **1** (a, b) and one for compound **2** (c). (See color insert.)

flipped end-to-end compared with the first binding mode so that the phenyl ring is placed in the BACE S1′ pocket and the 3-acetyl substituent is pointing toward the solvent exposed S3′ area. The thiadiazole moiety is occupying the S1 pocket and its 3-ethyl-sulfanyl substituent is partially filling the S3 pocket.

Given the low molecular weight of the phenylureas **1** (322 Da) and **2** (419 Da), these compounds could serve as starting point for the discovery of novel therapeutically active BACE inhibitors. An X-ray crystal structure of BACE complexed with a phenylurea derivative would likely accelerate this process.

5.3.2   (1,3,5-Triazin-2-yl)Hydrazones

A series of (1,3,5-triazin-2-yl)hydrazone BACE inhibitors was discovered by docking over 300,000 small molecules in the 200–700 Da molecular weight rage into the BACE active site followed by ligand conformational searches and binding energy evaluation [16]. One representative, compound **3** (Fig. 5.3), inhibits the BACE enzyme with IC50 = 28 ± 4. Its cellular potency, EC50 = 17 ± 2 μM, was determined in an Aβ secretion assay.

The predicted binding mode of compound **3** [16] is shown in Fig. 5.4c. The (1,3,5-triazin-2-yl) hydrazone and furan moieties of the ligand are overlaying with the central part of the peptidic backbone of **OM-99** (Fig. 5.2). The hydrazone NH group is within about 4.5 Å and 5.0 Å of carboxy oxygen atoms of the catalytic residues Asp228 and Asp32, respectively. It has been suggested that the ligand hydrazone NH is forming water-mediated hydrogen bonds with both protein side chains [16]. The ligand 2-hydroxy-benzoic acid, piperidine, and 4-fluoro-phenyl moieties are occupying the BACE S2, S2′, and S3′ pockets, respectively.

The molecular weight of the (1,3,5-triazin-2-yl)hydrazones identified in this study is in the 460–650 range and therefore on the high end of what is generally considered fragment-like. Perhaps replacing the central hydrazonomethyl moiety with a group that interacts more closely with the catalytic Asp side chains will result in BACE inhibitors with higher ligand efficiency.

5.3.3   From Aminoquinolines to Aminopyridines

High-throughput X-ray crystallography was used to screen a library of 347 fragments for binding to the BACE protease domain [12]. The identified hits, aminoquinolines **4** and **5** (Fig. 5.5), are of very low molecular weight (144 Da) and therefore represented ideal starting points for further optimization irrespective of their low reported potency (IC50 ≈ 2 mM) as determined in FRET assay. The fragment screening hits **4** and **5** bind to the catalytic center of BACE essentially in the same way [12]. The amino group is located between and forming hydrogen bonds to the two carboxy side chains of the catalytic residues Asp32 and Asp228 (Fig. 5.6a,b). The pyridine ring is most likely protonated, which allows it to form another hydrogen bond to the Asp32 side chain. The fused benzyl ring of **4** is pointing toward the S3 pocket, while the fused benzyl ring of **5** is stacking edge-to-face with the aromatic side chain of the flap residue Tyr71.

The 6-substituted 2-aminopyridines **6** (Fig. 5.5) was designed based on the fragment screening hits **4** and **5** with the goal to gain additional binding energy in the lipophilic S1 pocket [11]. While this modification alone was not sufficient to increase BACE inhibition potency (IC50 > 2 mM), it allowed the structure-based design of compound **7** which inhibits BACE with IC50 = 25 μM. The central phenylethyl moiety of compound **7** is filling the S1 pocket of the BACE active site effectively and its terminal 3-methoxy-phenyl group is penetrating deep into the adjacent S3 pocket (Fig. 5.6c). Further optimization of this lead is likely to focus on substitution of the biaryl moiety as well as exploration of additional vectors for further potency improvement.

The fragment hits **4** and **5** identified by X-ray crystallography screening were not only used for direct optimization but also to generate focused libraries for virtual fragment screening [12]. This approach resulted in the identification of the 3-substituted 2-aminopyridine BACE inhibitor **8** (IC50 = 310 μM). Compared to compounds **4–7**, the binding mode of the virtual screening hit **8** is flipped. Its primary

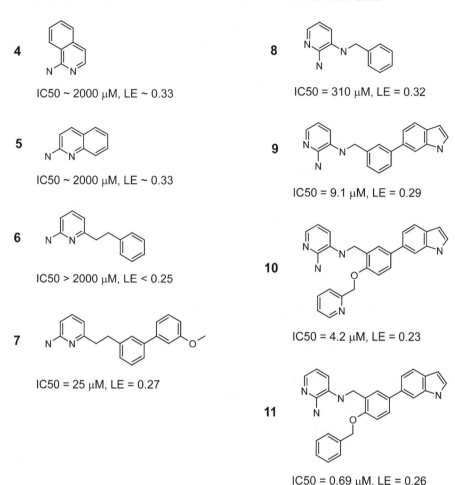

4

IC50 ~ 2000 µM, LE ~ 0.33

5

IC50 ~ 2000 µM, LE ~ 0.33

6

IC50 > 2000 µM, LE < 0.25

7

IC50 = 25 µM, LE = 0.27

8

IC50 = 310 µM, LE = 0.32

9

IC50 = 9.1 µM, LE = 0.29

10

IC50 = 4.2 µM, LE = 0.23

11

IC50 = 0.69 µM, LE = 0.26

Figure 5.5   Fragments and fragment-derived BACE inhibitors reported by Astex.

amine is still positioned between the side chain of the catalytic residues Asp32 and Asp228, but the protonated pyridine nitrogen is now forming a hydrogen bond with the carboxy side chain of Asp228 (Fig. 5.6d). The 3-amino group of **8** is donating an additional hydrogen bond to the Asp32 side chain. Similar as observed for the 6-substituted 2-aminopyridine **7**, the benzyl group of the 3-substituted 2-aminopyridine **8** is occupying the S1 pocket.

The significantly higher ligand efficiency of the 3-substituted 2-aminopyridine **8** (LE = 0.32) over its 6-substituted 2-aminopyridine analog **6** made it a promising starting point for further optimization. Addition of a 6-indolyl to **8** resulted in compound **9** which inhibits BACE with IC50 = 9.1 µM. The indole ring of the 3-substituted 2-aminopyridine **9** is penetrating the S3 pocket in a similar fashion as observed for the 6-substituted 2-aminopyridine **7**. This modification leads to an ~1.5 Å shift of almost the entire ligand toward the prime side of the substrate binding pocket

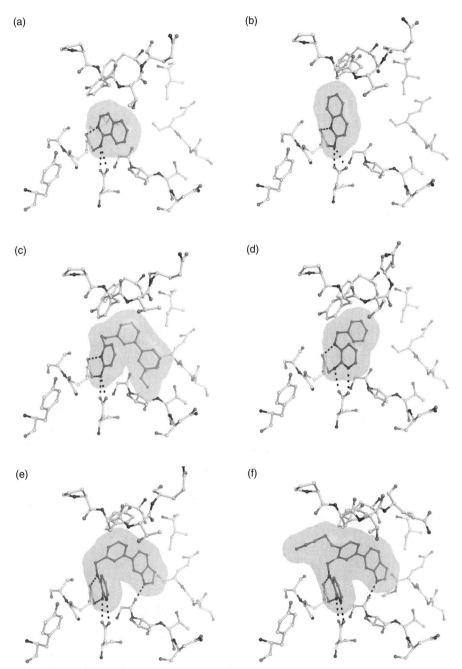

Figure 5.6 X-ray crystal structures of BACE protease domain in complex with the compounds (a) **4**, PDB accession number 2OHK, (b) **5**, 2OHL, (c) **7**, 2OHQ, (d) **8**, 2OHM, (e) **9**, 2OHT, and (f) **10**, 2OHU. (See color insert.)

while keeping its primary amino group in place between the side chains of the catalytic residues Asp32 and Asp228 (Fig. 5.6e). The indole NH of **9** is forming a hydrogen bond with the backbone carbonyl of Gly230. To further increase ligand potency, aryl-ethyl substituents were inserted at the 2-position of the central benzyl ring. The pyridin-2-ylmethoxy analog **10** inhibits BACE with IC50 = 4.2 µM. Its additional pyridine ring is occupying the S2′ pocket (Fig. 5.6f). Finally, the benzyloxy analog **11** was the first sub-micromolecular fragment-based BACE inhibitor reported in the literature with IC50 = 0.69 µM. This was a remarkable achievement considering the low chemical tractability of this enzyme.

5.3.4 Tyramines

Tyramine analogs have been discovered to bind to the BACE active site by a fragment screening approach that included surface plasmon resonance measurements with immobilized BACE, computational chemistry, and X-ray crystallography [10]. One of the hits that were identified from a library of fragments with molecular weight 100–150 Da and confirmed with a BACE crystal structure was the tyrosine metabolite tyramine **12** (Fig. 5.7). It binds to the S1 pocket of the BACE active site (Fig. 5.8a) with KD = 2 mM. Unlike most other BACE inhibitors reported so far, tyramine **12** does not displace the catalytic water molecule, which in the apo structure is positioned between the two carboxy side chains of Asp32 and Asp228 [17]. Instead, the protonated primary amine of tyramine **12** form a hydrogen bond with the catalytic water molecule [10]. In addition, the tyramine **12** amine is forming a direct hydrogen bond with a carboxylate oxygen of Asp32 and a water-mediated one with the side chain of the flap residue Tyr71. The hydroxyl group of tyramine **12** is forming a hydrogen bond with the backbone carbonyl of Phe108.

Hit expansion was performed by soaking of tyramine **12** analogs from the Roche compound collection into BACE crystals and subsequent structure determination by X-ray crystallography. Two *ortho*-substituted tyramine derivatives were identified to bind to BACE with increased binding affinity: the ethyl analog **13** (KD = 660 µM) and the cyclohexyl analog **14** (KD = 220 µM). The additional ethyl

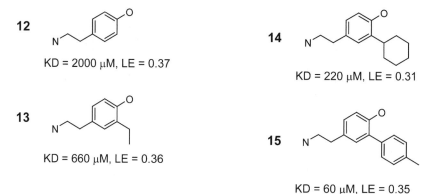

12

KD = 2000 µM, LE = 0.37

13

KD = 660 µM, LE = 0.36

14

KD = 220 µM, LE = 0.31

15

KD = 60 µM, LE = 0.35

Figure 5.7 Fragments and fragment-derived BACE inhibitors reported by Roche.

(a)   (b)

(c)

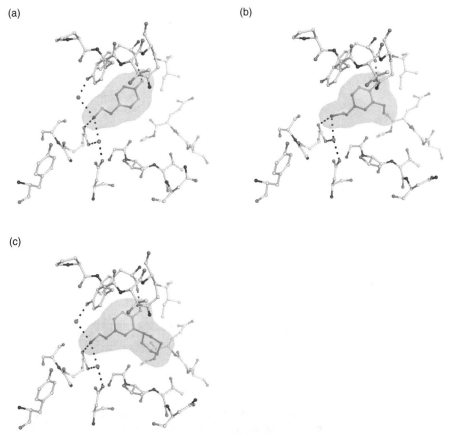

Figure 5.8   X-ray crystal structures of BACE protease domain in complex with the compounds (a) **12**, PDB accession number 2BRA, (b) **13**, 3BUG, and (c) **14**, 3BUH. (See color insert.)

moiety of compound **13** is pointing into the adjacent S3 pocket (Fig. 5.8b), and the cyclohexyl moiety of compound **14** is filling this pocket even further (Fig. 5.8c). Finally, the tyramine derivative **15** was synthesized with a goal to further optimize interactions with the BACE S3 pocket, resulting in a compound with a dissociation constant of 60 μM.

The identified tyramine analogs are of low molecular weight and high ligand efficiency, which makes them a suitable starting point for optimization of BACE inhibitors with central nervous system (CNS) pharmacological activity.

5.3.5   From Isocytosines to Dihydroisocysteines

A 2000-compound fragment library was screened for binding to the BACE active site with 1D NMR, and the identified hits were subsequently analyzed and character-ized by surface plasmon resonance competition measurements using an immobilized substrate peptide analog [14]. One of the discovered fragments was the 6-substituted

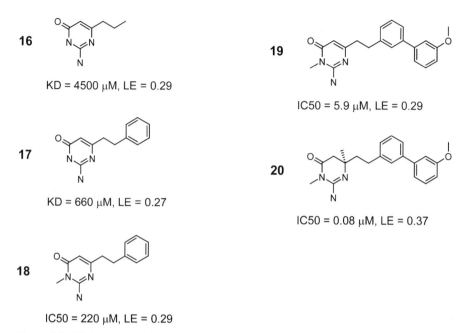

16

KD = 4500 μM, LE = 0.29

17

KD = 660 μM, LE = 0.27

18

IC50 = 220 μM, LE = 0.29

19

IC50 = 5.9 μM, LE = 0.29

20

IC50 = 0.08 μM, LE = 0.37

Figure 5.9   Fragments and fragment-derived BACE inhibitors reported by AstraZeneca.

isocytosine **16** (Fig. 5.9) which binds to BACE with KD = 4.5 mM as determined by surface plasmon resonance.

Hit expansion, the search for potent analogs of screening hits in proprietary and public compound libraries, showed that the isocytosine derivative **17** binds to BACE with KD = 0.66 mM. Compound **17** binds to endothiapepsin, used as a structural surrogate for BACE, in a way similar to the 6-substituted 2-aminopyridine **7** (Fig. 5.6c). The primary amine of **17** is positioned in between the side chains of the catalytic residues Asp35 and Asp219 of endothiapepsin forming hydrogen bonds to both carboxy groups (Fig. 5.10a). The nitrogen at the isocytosine 1-position of compound **17** is accepting a hydrogen bond from the presumably protonated Asp35 side chain, and the isocytosine carbonyl group is accepting a hydrogen bond from the backbone NH of Asp81. The phenylethyl moiety of **17** is occupying the S1 pocket of the endothiapepsin substrate binding site.

The fragment-based isocytosines served then as a starting point for further optimization [13]. N-methylation at the isocytosine 3-position resulted in more potent BACE inhibitors like compound **18** (IC50 = 220 μM). Further improvement of the ligand potency to IC50 = 5.9 μM was achieved with the isocytosine analog **19** where the benzyl ring is replaced with a 3-methoxy-biphenyl group. The critical breakthrough was achieved by replacing the isocytosine with dihydroisocytosine, resulting in compound **20** which inhibits BACE not only in an enzyme assay with IC50 = 0.08 μM but also in a cell-based assay with IC50 = 0.47 μM. Examination of the crystal structure of BACE complexed with compound **20** (Fig. 5.10b) shows that compared to the isocytosine, the dihydroisocytosine core is rotated toward the

(a)   (b)

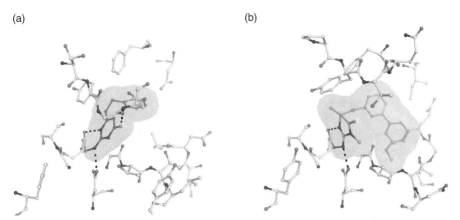

Figure 5.10   X-ray crystal structures of BACE protease domain in complex with the compounds (a) **17**, PDB accession number 2V00 and (b) **20**, 2VA7. (See color insert.)

prime side of the substrate binding site while maintaining critical interaction with the catalytic residues Asp32 and Asp228. The 3-methoxy-biphenyl moiety of **20** is filling the joint S1-S3 subpocket region in essentially the same way as observed for the 6-substituted 2-aminopyridine **7** (Fig. 5.6c).

To our knowledge, the dihydroisocytosine **20** is the only fragment-derived BACE inhibitor with submicromolar cellular potency reported so far.

5.4 FINAL REMARKS

In the early days of fragment-based drug discovery, organic solvent molecules were screened by X-ray crystallography for binding to the surface of a target protein with the goal to identify potential small molecule binding sites [18]. In the same way, analyzing the binding modes of a diverse set of fragment molecules on a target protein can indicate which sections of a binding pocket are more tractable and what interactions a small molecule can or should make with the protein to maximize the free energy of binding. For BACE, the identified fragments with experimentally confirmed binding modes clearly indicate two binding hot spots in the substrate binding site: the side chains of the catalytic residues Asp32 and Asp228, and the S1 pocket (Fig. 5.11a). The Asp carboxy groups seem to prefer to interact with a basic or primary amino group. The S1 pocket is consistently filled with a benzyl ring, even though the exact position and orientation varies. In addition, lipophilic extensions of the ligand from the S1 pocket directly into the adjacent S3 pocket are a recurring theme for potency improvement while maintaining ligand efficiency (Fig. 5.11b). Interestingly, vectors that explore the prime side of the peptide-binding pocket appear to be less frequently explored or reported. The common amine-aryl-hydrophobic pharmacophore derived from the published crystal structures of BACE complexed with fragment molecules can serve as guidance for the design of BACE inhibitors with novel chemotypes. Overall, the fragment screening

(a)   (b)

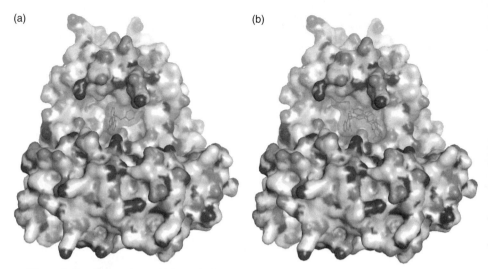

Figure 5.11   Composite volumes filled by experimentally identified fragments and fragment-derived BACE inhibitors. The volume filled by (a) the originally identified fragments **4, 5,** and **12** compared with (b) the fragment-derived inhibitors **10, 14,** and **20.** Ligands and composite molecular surfaces are drawn in green. The molecular surface of BACE protease is colored by atom types. Flap residues 70–75 have been omitted for clarity. (See color insert.)

efforts have been remarkably successful in identifying truly novel chemotypes for BACE inhibitors, a target that is generally considered to be of low chemical tractability. The future will show how these molecules are further optimized to fulfill all the requirements for a clinical candidate aiming for the inhibition of amyloid cleavage in patients. Several molecules that are in clinical research today claim its origin from fragment-based drug discovery [19–22]. However, BACE would provide the first example for a success in targeting the CNS with this approach. Given the urgent need for a treatment of Alzheimer's disease, such a breakthrough would be more than welcome.

REFERENCES

1. Boehm, H.J., Boehringer, M., Bur, D., Gmuender, H., Huber, W., Klaus, W., Kostrewa, D., Kuehne, H., Luebbers, T., Meunier-Keller, N., and Mueller, F. 2000. Novel inhibitors of DNA gyrase: 3D structure-based biased needle screening, hit validation by biophysical methods, and 3D-guided optimization: a promising alternative to random screening. *J Med Chem* **43**:2664–2674.
2. Erlanson, D.A., McDowell, R.S., and O'Brien, T. 2004. Fragment-based drug discovery. *J Med Chem* **47**:3463–3482.
3. Hubbard, R.E., Davis, B., Chen, I., and Drysdale, M.J. 2007. The SeeDs approach: integrating fragments into drug discovery. *Curr Top Med Chem* **7**:1568–1581.
4. Rees, D.C., Congreve, M., Murray, C.W., and Carr, R. 2004. Fragment-based lead discovery. *Nat Rev Drug Discov* **3**:660–672.
5. Hopkins, A.L., Groom, C.R., and Alex, A. 2004. Ligand efficiency: a useful metric for lead selection. *Drug Discov Today* **9**:430–431.

6. Kuntz, I.D., Chen, K., Sharp, K.A., and Kollman, P.A. 1999. The maximal affinity of ligands. *Proc Natl Acad Sci U S A* **96**:9997–10002.

7. Hong, L., Koelsch, G., Lin, X., Wu, S., Terzyan, S., Ghosh, A.K., Zhang, X.C., and Tang, J. 2000. Structure of the protease domain of memapsin 2 (beta-secretase) complexed with inhibitor. *Science* **290**:150–153.

8. Lullau, E., Kanttinen, A., Hassel, J., Berg, M., Haag-Alvarsson, A., Cederbrant, K., Greenberg, B., Fenge, C., and Schweikart, F. 2003. Comparison of batch and perfusion culture in combination with pilot-scale expanded bed purification for the production of soluble recombinant beta-secretase. *Biotechnol Prog* **19**:37–44.

9. Gruninger-Leitch, F., Schlatter, D., Kung, E., Nelbock, P., and Dobeli, H. 2002. Substrate and inhibitor profile of BACE (beta-secretase) and comparison with other mammalian aspartic proteases. *J Biol Chem* **277**:4687–4693.

10. Kuglstatter, A., Stahl, M., Peters, J.U., Huber, W., Stihle, M., Schlatter, D., Benz, J., Ruf, A., Roth, D., Enderle, T., and Hennig, M. 2008. Tyramine fragment binding to BACE-1. *Bioorg Med Chem Lett* **18**:1304–1307.

11. Congreve, M, Aharony, D., Albert, J., Callaghan, O., Campbell, J., Carr, R.A., Chessari, G., Cowan, S., Edwards, P.D., Frederickson, M., McMenamin, R., Murray, C.W., Patel, S., and Wallis, N. 2007. Application of fragment screening by X-ray crystallography to the discovery of aminopyridines as inhibitors of beta-secretase. *J Med Chem* **50**:1124–1132.

12. Murray, C.W., Callaghan, O., Chessari, G., Cleasby, A., Congreve, M., Frederickson, M., Hartshorn, M.J., McMenamin, R., Patel, S., and Wallis, N. 2007. Application of fragment screening by X-ray crystallography to beta-secretase. *J Med Chem* **50**:1116–1123.

13. Edwards, P.D., Albert, J.S., Sylvester, M., Aharony, D., Andisik, D., Callaghan, O., Campbell, J.B., Carr, R.A., Chessari, G., Congreve, M., Frederickson, M., Folmer, R.H., Geschwindner, S., Koether, G., Kolmodin, K., Krumrine, J., Mauger, R.C., Murray, C.W., Olsson, L.L., Patel, S., Spear, N., and Tian, G. 2007. Application of fragment-based lead generation to the discovery of novel, cyclic amidine beta-secretase inhibitors with nanomolar potency, cellular activity, and high ligand efficiency. *J Med Chem* **50**:5912–5925.

14. Geschwindner, S., Olsson, L.L., Albert, J.S., Deinum, J., Edwards, P.D., de Beer, T., and Folmer, R.H. 2007. Discovery of a novel warhead against beta-secretase through fragment-based lead generation. *J Med Chem* **50**:5903–5911.

15. Huang, D., Luthi, U., Kolb, P., Edler, K., Cecchini, M., Audetat, S., Barberis, A., and Caflisch, A. 2005. Discovery of cell-permeable non-peptide inhibitors of beta-secretase by high-throughput docking and continuum electrostatics calculations. *J Med Chem* **48**:5108–5111.

16. Huang, D., Luthi, U., Kolb, P., Cecchini, M., Barberis, A., and Caflisch, A. 2006. In silico discovery of beta-secretase inhibitors. *J Am Chem Soc* **128**:5436–5443.

17. Patel, S., Vuillard, L., Cleasby, A., Murray, C.W., and Yon, J. 2004. Apo and inhibitor complex structures of BACE (beta-secretase). *J Mol Biol* **343**:407–416.

18. Ringe, D. 1995. What makes a binding site a binding site? *Curr Opin Struct Biol* **5**:825–829.

19. Barril, X., Brough, P., Drysdale, M., Hubbard, R.E., Massey, A., Surgenor, A., and Wright, L. 2005. Structure-based discovery of a new class of Hsp90 inhibitors. *Bioorg Med Chem Lett* **15**:5187–5191.

20. Card, G.L., Blasdel, L., England, B.P., Zhang, C., Suzuki, Y., Gillette, S., Fong, D., Ibrahim, P.N., Artis, D.R., Bollag, G., Milburn, M.V., Kim, S.H., Schlessinger, J., and Zhang, K.Y. 2005. A family of phosphodiesterase inhibitors discovered by cocrystallography and scaffold-based drug design. *Nat Biotechnol* **23**:201–207.

21. Gill, A.L., Frederickson, M., Cleasby, A., Woodhead, S.J., Carr, M.G., Woodhead, A.J., Walker, M.T., Congreve, M.S., Devine, L.A., Tisi, D., O'Reilly, M., Seavers, L.C., Davis, D.J., Curry, J., Anthony, R., Padova, A., Murray, C.W., Carr, R.A., and Jhoti, H. 2005. Identification of novel p38alpha MAP kinase inhibitors using fragment-based lead generation. *J Med Chem* **48**:414–426.

22. Petros, A.M., Dinges, J., Augeri, D.J., Baumeister, S.A., Betebenner, D.A., Bures, M.G., Elmore, S.W., Hajduk, P.J., Joseph, M.K., Landis, S.K., Nettesheim, D.G., Rosenberg, S.H., Shen, W., Thomas, S., Wang, X., Zanze, I., Zhang, H., and Fesik, S.W. 2006. Discovery of a potent inhibitor of the antiapoptotic protein Bcl-xL from NMR and parallel synthesis. *J Med Chem* **49**:656–663.

STRUCTURE-BASED DESIGN OF BACE INHIBITORS: TECHNICAL AND PRACTICAL ASPECTS OF PREPARATION, 3-DIMENSIONAL STRUCTURE, AND COMPUTATIONAL ANALYSIS

Felix F. Vajdos,[1] *Veerabahu Shanmugasundaram,*[1] *and Alfredo G. Tomasselli*[2]

[1]Pfizer Global Research and Development, Groton, CT and [2]Pfizer Global Research and Development, Chesterfield, MO

6.1 INTRODUCTION

According to the widely accepted "amyloid hypothesis," the increased production of toxic amyloid beta (Aβ) peptides in the brain and/or decreased removal from it are the triggers of the series of pathogenic events leading to Alzheimer's disease (AD) [1]. Aβ peptides are generated from the amyloid precursor protein (APP) by the action of two enzymes referred to as β- and γ-secretase, a fact that makes them attractive targets for AD treatment [2, 3]. β-secretase is a Type I membrane anchored aspartyl protease that catalyzes the first mandatory step in APP processing [4–7], while γ-secretase, which catalyzes the second step, is a complex of at least four membrane-bound proteins [8]: presenilin, nicastrin, Aph1, and Pen2. Presenilin, also an aspartyl protease, constitutes the catalytic core of the complex [9, 10]. Aspartic proteases (AP) are the smallest class of proteases in the human genome with only 15 members. β-secretase, also named BACE (β-site APP Cleaving Enzyme), Asp-2, and memapsin 2, is a so-called classical AP because it has the catalytic triads $D^{32}S/TG \ldots D^{228}S/TG$ (BACE-1 numbering, Fig. 6.1) typical of renin, cathepsin D, pepsin, and HIV protease. In contrast, presenilin is a membrane AP with the catalytic

BACE: Lead Target for Orchestrated Therapy of Alzheimer's Disease, Edited by Varghese John

M^{-21L}*AQALPWLLLWMGAGVLPAHG***T^{1P}QHGIRLPLRSG**
LGGAPLGLRLPR^{24P}↓E^{25P}PTDEEP^{30P}EEPGRRGSFV^{40P}E^1
MVDNLRGKSGQGYYVEMTV^{20}GSPPQTLNILV**DTG**SS
NFAV^{40}GAAPHPFLHRYYQRQLSSTY^{60}RDLRKGVYVP
YTQGKWEGEL^{80}GTDLVSIPHGPNVTVRANIA^{100}AITES
DKFFINGSNWEGILG^{120}LAYAEIARPDDSLEPFFDSL^{140}
VKQTHVPCNLFSLQLCGAGFP^{160}LNQSEVLASVGGSM
IIGGID^{180}HSLYTGSLWYTPIRREWYYE^{200}VIIVRVEING
QDLKMDCKEY^{220}NYDKSIV**DSG**TTNLRLPKKV^{240}FEA
AVKSIKAASSTEKFPDG^{260}FWLGEQLVCWQAGTTPW
NIF^{280}PVISLYLMGEVTNQSFRITI^{300}LPQQYLRPVEDVA
TSQDDCY^{320}KFAISQSSTGTVMGAVIMEG^{340}FYVVFDR
ARKRIGFAVSACH^{360}VHDEFRTAAVEGPFVTLDME^{380}
DCGYNIPQTDESTLMTIAYV^{400}MAAICALFMLPLCLM
VCQWR^{420}CLRCLRQQHDDFADDISLLK^{440}

Figure 6.1 The primary structure of BACE. Prominent features of BACE amino acid sequence are highlighted: a 21-aa leader sequence (M^{-21L} ... G^{-1L}) and a 24-aa prosegment (T^{1P} ... R^{24P}) precedes the mature enzyme sequence starting at the E^{25P} and extending to K^{440} (according to the sequence of the enzyme isolated from human brain). BACE contains the classic catalytic triad D^{32}TG ... D^{228}SG, six cysteine residues paired to form three disulfide bridges: Cys^{155}–Cys^{359}, Cys^{217}–Cys^{382}, and Cys^{269}–Cys^{319}, and four glycosylated asparagines, 92, 111, 162, and 293. Residue S^{392} precedes the BACE transmembrane domain of 27-aa (T^{393} ... R^{420}), and a cytoplasmic tail of 21 residues (R^{420} ... K^{440}) completes the primary structure. (See color insert.)

signature YD^{257} ... GxGD^{385} (presenilin 1 numbering) typical of peptidyl peptidases [11].

6.1.1 β- and γ-Secretase as AD Targets

Aspartyl proteases have generated successful drugs. Prominent examples are inhibitors of the HIV protease and renin to treat AIDS and high blood pressure, respectively [12]. With regard to AD therapies, targeting BACE might offer some advantages over γ-secretase inhibition or modulation due to the fact that γ-secretase cleaves a myriad of substrates [13] including Notch, a protein involved in animal development and in immune system processes, such as B- and T-cell differentiation [14, 15]. In addition, a presenilin –/– genotype is lethal in mice, supporting a mechanism-based toxicity. In fact, the most advanced γ-secretase inhibitor, LY-450139 now in Phase 3, has shown gastrointestinal problems in clinical tests [2]. The γ-secretase modulation approach has recently suffered some setbacks since *R*-Flurbiprofen, a compound that apparently spares Notch, has failed in Phase 3 clinical trials because of a lack of efficacy [16]. On the other hand, there are compelling reasons to target BACE in AD [3]; for example, because of its role as the first obligatory step in Aβ formation and its elevated level in AD, BACE inhibition would dampen Aβ production and its associated toxic effects on neuron and role in plaques formation. In addition, the BACE knockout mouse has demonstrated the validity of BACE as a therapeutic target in AD and, together with its relatively clean phenotype, would suggest BACE inhibition is a safer strategy than γ-secretase inhibition. Contrary to γ-secretase, BACE can be prepared in highly purified forms and, as described in the following narrative, dozens of three-dimensional (3D) structures in complexation with a variety of inhibitors have been solved to support vigorous efforts in rational drug design.

6.1.2   Challenges in Drug Design: The Role of Crystallography and Computational Chemistry

It is now well appreciated that compounds that are effective in a patient generally possess certain physical characteristics, often referred to as drug-like properties. Among these properties are low molecular weight, a balance between polarity and lipophilicity, and a reasonable number of hydrogen bond donors and acceptors. Often referred to as the "rule of five," owing to the observation by Lipinski et al. that these properties are typically exemplified in marketed drugs as multiples of the number five (i.e., MW < 500, ClogP < 5, sum of hydrogen bond donors < 5, sum of hydrogen bond acceptors < 10) [17], these are not hard and fast rules, but rather serve as general rubrics to guide the drug discovery process. Consequently, although it is necessary to have an inhibitor with potency in the low nanomolar to picomolar range, this is not sufficient. In view of chronic use, specificity for the intended molecular target is of paramount importance, as even a modest inhibition of other biological targets might lead to some level of toxicity. The drug has to reach therapeutic levels in the areas where it needs to exercise its effect, and to be bioavailable to fulfill its task. The drug may need to show synergy with other drugs, and must not interfere with other medicines that the patient is taking. Considering the length of the treatment in the case of AD, the drug must also be inexpensive.

To inhibit BACE in the brain, then, it is mandatory that the inhibitor be sufficiently small in order to cross the blood–brain barrier (BBB); in addition, the inhibitor must not be ejected from the brain by the P-glycoprotein (P-gp) drug efflux pump expressed in the luminal surface of cerebral endothelial cells forming the BBB [18]. In addition, a BACE inhibitor must also be permeable to cell membranes, as there is good evidence that BACE performs most of its APP cleavage intracellularly, in acidic compartments such as the endosome and the trans-golgi network (TGN) [19].

Hence the need of an effective alliance of disparate yet synergistic disciplines encompassing molecular biology, protein chemistry, high-throughput screening (HTS), enzymology, medicinal chemistry, crystallography, computational chemistry, drug delivery, pharmacokinetics, and drug safety to endow a BACE inhibitor with the desirable properties of an AD drug. Modern drug design strives to exploit crystallography and the closely related discipline of computational chemistry in the earlier stages of lead discovery to offer the medicinal chemist a wide chemistry space at the beginning of the lead optimization process. Over the last several decades in the pharmaceutical and biotherapeutic industries, this process, known as structure-based drug design (SBDD), has emerged as its own subdiscipline of drug discovery. Once dominated by physicists and enzymologists, X-ray crystallography has now become a vital tool for medicinal and computational chemists, and the ability to map structure–activity relationships (SAR) and binding interactions directly to protein structure has informed and accelerated the process of lead development. Although still requiring sophisticated technical training, the end result of the experiment (a set of validated 3D coordinates describing the relative placement of each non-hydrogen atom in a protein–ligand complex) has been made much more accessible through the use of sophisticated interactive modeling and visualization software, often at the chemist's desktop.

The challenge is to obtain 3D structures of lead inhibitors complexed to the enzyme and start the iterative process of lead optimization. Leads are obtained from various sources, which include HTS, fragment screening, *de novo* design, from inhibitors of enzymes homologous to the target of interest, or from other activities. A thorough understanding of the network of interactions between the subsites of the enzyme and the various parts of the lead compound allow us to make informed predictions on the moieties that have the best possibilities to maximize the contact at that site and produce important opportunities for further optimization. It is important to remember that this optimization is not limited solely to increasing the potency of the inhibitor for BACE. Rather, all of the above-mentioned properties must be balanced in order to increase the probability of successful modulation of BACE activity in a clinical setting.

6.2 PREPARATION OF BACE FOR STRUCTURAL STUDIES

Protein expression, purification, and crystallization are fundamental steps in X-ray crystallography, a discipline that normally requires large quantities of proteins, and demands certain high standards regarding protein purity, activity, and refolding status. Membrane proteins and multiple domain proteins have been proven rather difficult to express, purify, and crystallize. These difficulties increase when heterogeneity are present because of posttranslational modifications such as glycosylation and phosphorylation. When dealing with such complex proteins, multiple options are explored to obtain products suitable for crystallography and other activities, for example, HTS and inhibitor validation, needed for drug development. Of course, it is always desirable to express and purify the authentic full-length protein; mammalian cells are the systems of choice when production of a protein close to the human form is desirable, and insect cell systems are the reasonable next choices. Both systems yield proteins that are refolded and active, but are in general relatively low producers, and the culture media are expensive to support the gram amounts of protein often needed. When the protein from these systems is not crystallizable, enzymatic removal of posttranslational modifications are performed along with proteolytic excision of protein fragments that might be fastidious to crystallization. To facilitate the latter task, proteolytically cleavable sequences can be inserted at specific sites in the protein sequence. Alternatively, various differently truncated constructs can be engineered, and/or glycosylation sites can be mutated to prevent them from being glycosylated. In many cases, posttranslational modifications are dispensable for both proper protein refolding and functionality. In these cases, *Escherichia coli* expression offers many advantages since these bacteria are easy to grow, are relatively inexpensive, and do not carry out posttranslational modifications.

BACE is a rather complex enzyme; the primary structure of the protein as synthesized in the endoplasmatic reticulum is given in Fig. 6.1. We would like to point out that given the literature inconsistency with regard to BACE amino acid numbering, we have numbered, in this and in Chapter 3 [20], BACE leader sequence M^{-21L} ... G^{-1L}, its prosegment T^{1P} ... V^{40P}, though the prosegment ends at R^{24P} in the mature form isolated from brain [6]. The residue V^{40P} is followed by E^1 to agree with the majority of the reports on BACE 3D structure and kinetics. A more detailed description of BACE primary structure is given in Chapter 3 [20]. Many of the previously mentioned options have been used to obtain diffraction quality crystals of BACE. In fact, in the beginning, it was not possible to predict whether removal of any domains and/or posttranslational modifications would still preserve sound catalytic and structural features. It was likewise unpredictable which constructs and expression systems would yield reasonable expression and a facile purification. These uncertainties fostered a multipronged expression approach for both construct design and cell system selection.

The general approach for BACE expression and purification for crystallography has been consistently to make constructs lacking BACE membrane and cytosolic domains; these constructs were then further truncated at various points in the N-terminal portion of the enzyme.

Various groups have reported the expression and purification of glycosylated BACE from mammalian [21–24] and insect [25–28] cells. Notwithstanding, only two groups have published the accomplishment of diffracting crystals for glycosylated enzyme from these sources: specifically, Emmons et al. [24] from mammalian cells, and Wang et al. [28] from insect cells. Two other groups have published the expression and purification of crystallizable recombinant BACE from insect [25] and mammalian cells [21], respectively, but in both instances, the glycosylation sites were modified to avoid glycosylation. Yet, both the most successful preparations and the highest resolution structures of BACE have been obtained for the enzyme expressed in *E. coli* cells [29–33].

6.2.1 Preparation of Soluble BACE Derivatives in Insect and Mammalian Cells

Wang et al. [28] successfully expressed BACE-M^{-21L} ... Leu^{394}-c-myc-His$_6$ (this chapter's nomenclature, Fig. 6.1) in High Five cells and purified it by a two-step procedure on Ni-NTA and Superdex 200 columns. This procedure allowed the obtainment of about 2.5 mg enzyme, containing its prosegment T^{1P}QHGIR ... , per liter of cell culture. Single orthorhombic crystals with two BACE molecules in the asymmetric unit were obtained in the absence of a bound inhibitor, and a complete 3.4 Å data set was collected. Interestingly, characterization of the crystalline enzyme showed equal mixtures of two sequences P^{23P}RETD ... and E^{25P}TDEEP ... lacking both c-myc and hexa-His tags; the authors ascribed the processing of the tags to autocleavage.

Bruinzeel et al. [25] also reported the purification of crystallizable BACE expressed in High Five insect cells, but in this instance, the glycosylation sites were mutated. In addition, these investigators designed their construct to replace the leader sequence (21 aa) by the viral gp67 signal sequence to increase expression level; also, they inserted a FLAG tag between the gp67 signal and the prodomain sequences, and a $(His)_6$ tag at the enzyme C-terminus. They co-expressed BACE with Furin and obtained properly processed enzyme to the extent of 0.5 mg/L cell culture. A four-step purification resulted in pure enzyme to the extent of 0.1 mg/L cell culture that produced crystal structures in the presence of inhibitors.

Clarke et al. [21] engineered the mutation asparagine to glutamine at the positions 92, 111, 162, 293 fused to Fc and introduced a thrombin cleavage site after residues R24P and L439. This construct, referred to as pro/thr/Asp2-QQQQ/thr/Fc, was expressed in a Chinese hamster ovary (CHO) secretion system. After capturing by ProSep-A High Capacity resin and elution, the Pro/thr/Asp2-QQQQ/thr/Fc was neutralized and dialyzed into 25 mM Hepes, 0.25 M NaCl, pH 7.4. Bovine alpha thrombin was used to cleave the BACE construct and liberate Asp2-QQQQ. The thrombin digest that did not bind to ProSep A was further cleaved by pepsin to yield V^{40P}-E^{431} form of Asp2-QQQQ, which was then purified by MonoQ at pH 7.4. The enzyme yielded high-resolution crystals, which aided in the discovery of potent inhibitors.

Our general strategy for recombinant expression was to express BACE constructs such as Met^{-21L} … $Ser^{392}(His)_6$, in insect and mammalian cell lines, such as CHO-K1, human embryonic kidney (HEK), and CHO-Lec-1 [24] that would yield catalytically active enzyme and would possess different patterns of N-linked glycosylation. The goal was to be able to select among these expression systems the one with both the best crystallographic and kinetic properties for inhibitor identification and development. Although we were able to obtain reasonable expressions in all these systems, preliminary crystallography experiments led to the selection of CHO-K1 cells as the expression system to carry forward.

BACE was expressed in stable CHO-K1 cells to the extent of 4.5 mg/L of conditioned media and was about 40% pure at this stage. It was further purified by a two-step procedure: the first step consisted of a Ni^{2+}NTA resin from which BACE was highly purified by elution with an imidazole gradient. The second step utilized a BACE inhibitor bound to matrix to ensure that only protein that was properly folded was captured and eluted. A total of 293 mg of BACE of more than 99% final purity was obtained from 150 L of conditioned media. This heavily glycosylated enzyme yielded crystals that allowed 3.2 Å resolution 3D structures in the presence of inhibitors, but was a mixture of pro-BACE T^{1P}QHGIRLPL … and processed BACE E^{25P}TDEEPEEP. … Treatment of this BACE mixture with HIV protease allowed us to produce a catalytically competent enzyme $V^{40P}E^1MV$ … $Ser^{392}(His)_6$ that was purified by affinity column on a peptido-mimetic inhibitor. Crystals typically diffracted between 2.8 to 2.6 Å resolution and allowed to solve structures with a variety of inhibitors. This is an example that demonstrates improvement of crystal diffraction by proteolytic cleavage of a protein.

6.2.2   Preparation of Soluble BACE Derivatives in *E. coli*

The first purification procedure leading to crystal structure was reported by Lin et al. [29, 30]. These investigators expressed a BACE construct containing residues A^{-8L} (Leader) to A^{359} in *E. coli* as inclusion bodies (IB). They dissolved the IB in 0.1 M Tris, 1 mM ethylenediaminetetraacetic acid (EDTA), 1 mM glycine, 8 M urea, and 0.1 M β-mercaptoethanol, and then refolded by rapid dilution in buffer. Purification was accomplished in a two-step procedure by gel filtration on Sepharose S-300 and fast protein liquid chromatography (FPLC) on Resource-Q column. Subsequently, Hong et al. [29] reported the expression and purification of BACE (A^{-8L} ... T^{393}). The final product had Leu^{20P} with a minor component starting at Leu^{30P} as its N-terminus generated by the removal of 28 and 30 residues, respectively, from their original construct in the course of refolding and purification. Good activity and purity was obtained, and crystals yielding a 1.9 Å resolution were generated.

Patel et al. [31] used the same construct (from Ala^{-8} to T^{393}, our numbering) used by Hong et al. [29]. In the attempt to remove the prosegment with clostripain, they observed cleavages after R^{35P} and R^{36P} and were not able to generate crystals from these samples. They mutated the two Arg residues to Lys to obtain a protein that gave a robust expression and that was subjected to refolding. IBs were dissolved in 8 M urea, 50 mM Tris, 0.1 M β-mercaptoethanol, 10 mM dithiothreitol (DTT) to the extent of 22.5 mL of buffer per gram of inclusion body preparation. They diluted the supernatant 10-fold with 8 M urea, 0.2 mM oxidized glutathione, 1.0 mM reduced glutathione, and refolded by a 20-fold dilution into 20 mM Tris, 10 mM 3-(benzyldi-methylammonio)propanesulfonate (NDSB256). After a step consisting of overnight incubation at 4°C, they adjusted the pH to 9.0 and left the mixture at 4°C for 2 to 3 weeks. The refolding mixture was then concentrated by ultrafiltration, and the concentrated and refolded BACE was subjected to purification by Sephacryl 300 column equilibrated in 0.4 M urea, 20 mM Tris (pH 8.2). Refolded BACE was treated with clostripain to remove the prosegment portion preceeding Leu^{22P}, and the sample was loaded onto a Mono Q HR5-5 column equilibrated in 0.4 M urea, 20 mM Tris (pH 8.2), followed by washing and elution with a NaCl gradient. Yields of the final purified product were up to 10 mg/L cell culture; this protein started at residue L^{22} and yielded crystals with apoenzyme that allowed soaking of a hydroxyethylamine (HEA) inhibitor to produce a 1.75 Å structure.

Sardana et al. expressed a series of BACE constructs with various N-terminal truncations in *E. coli* IB [32]. IB solubilization was carried out in 50 mM Tris–HCl, pH 9.0, 8 M urea, and 10 mM β-mercaptoethanol to a concentration of ~1.5 mg/mL. Refolding was initiated by a 20-fold dilution at ambient temperature in a refolding buffer composed of 20 mM Tris–HCl, pH 9.0, 0.5 mM oxidized glutathione, and 1.25 mM reduced glutathione. After storage of the refolding solution at 4°C for 4 h, its pH was then lowered to 8.0. The sample was de-gassed, and β-mercaptoethanol and reduced and oxidized glutathione were added. After about 48 h, the pH was lowered to 6.8 and was left at 4°C for another 48 h. A Q-Sepharose fast flow column in 20 mM Tris–HCl buffer, pH 7.5, 0.4 M urea served to concentrate the protein and remove the majority of aggregated forms of BACE. The refolded BACE bound to the column was eluted with the same buffer indicated above in the presence of 0.5 M

NaCl. After concentration, a HiPrep Sephacryl 26/60 S-300 sizing column was used to separate residual aggregates from monomers. Purification was completed by using a HiTrap Q-Sepharose HP column.

Final yields depended on the construct used and ranged from 0.4–0.6 mg/mL for BACE 35–433 to 2.5–3.5 mg/mL for BACE 22–433. Crystals yielding 3D structure to 1.8 Å resolutions were obtained.

BACE refolding and purification of constructs expressed in *E. coli* as IBs by a procedure developed in our group [33] were even simpler than those reported above. Major steps in our process were: (a) the ability to reproducibly express large quantities of several BACE constructs, for example, (1) pET11a-T7.Tag-GSM-(A^{-8L}GV......QTDES^{392}), (2) pQE80L-Met-RGS-(His)$_6$-GSIETD-(T^{1P}QH... QTDES^{392}), and (3) pQE70-Met-BACE (R^{36P}GSFVEMG....PQTDES^{392}(His)$_6$ as IBs using *E. coli* strain such as BL21 CodonPlus (DE3) and BL21 (pREP4); (b) a simple, and robust refolding method; and (c) a two-step purification procedure.

Our refolding process is preceded by dissolution of washed IBs in 7.5 M urea, 100 mM AMPSO buffer, and 100 mM BME, to have a pH = 10.8. This solution is further diluted with the same buffer, not including BME, to obtain an A$_{280}$ = 1.5, and the BME concentration is adjusted to 10 mM. Refolding is started by diluting 20-fold with cold water (4–8°C) and allowing the resulting solution to rest in the cold room. Usually, constructs including the prodomain, (1) and (2), take 3–4 days to reach maximal activity, while the construct missing the prodomain, (3), takes about 21 days. It has been shown that the prosegment is not needed for refolding [33]. Our studies confirm this finding; in addition, they show that under the conditions used, the prosegment accelerates refolding. Once the sample has reached the desirable activity, it is brought to pH 8.5 and delivered to a Q-Sepharose column. After elution with a salt gradient, the BACE activity containing fractions are dialyzed against 20 mM Hepes buffer pH 8.0, which allows removing urea and salt. The pH of the sample is dropped to 5.0, and this acidic solution is delivered to the affinity column with attached the BACE inhibitor used to prepare CHO cell expressed BACE [24]. A highly purified and properly refolded sample is eluted from this column with a yield of 7–10 mg (depending on the construct) of BACE/ liter cell culture. This process is scalable up to at least to 60-L cell culture with yields of up to 500 mg and provides large quantities of enzyme that can be easily stored and employed for consistently reproducible crystallographic studies. Both apoenzyme and enzyme complexed to inhibitor yield crystals diffracting up to 1.4 Å resolution [33].

6.3 CRYSTALLOGRAPHIC STUDIES OF BACE

Crystallization of macromolecules is an inexact science, often requiring large amounts of exquisitely pure and homogeneous protein at high concentration. Since it is not possible to predict a priori the solution conditions that will promote crystallization (as opposed to random precipitation), a battery of solution conditions (hundreds to thousands) are typically screened in order to find a lead condition which can then be further optimized to yield reproducible, single, and well-diffracting crystals of the target protein. Generally, crystallization solutions contain a precipitant (polyalcohols, chaotropic salts), a buffer, and may include one or more salts to act as counterions. Following the identification of a lead condition, the various components may be systematically varied, as well as the concentrations (of both the components and the protein itself) and temperature. A typical experimental setup involves the incubation of a mixture of protein and crystallization solution in a 1:1 ratio, with a larger volume of the undiluted crystallization solution in a sealed vessel. This setup, known as a vapor diffusion experiment, allows for the rapid and parallel evaluation of many crystallization conditions. Once the optimal crystallization conditions have been identified, crystals may be harvested into a solution closely mimicking the solution from which they are grown (the "mother liquor"), and soaked with inhibitor compounds prior to data collection. It should be noted that in some cases, the inhibitor induces a conformation of the protein which is more amenable to crystallization, and in these cases the protein–inhibitor complex itself must be crystallized. As protein crystals are typically 30–70% solvent, they accurately recapitulate the solution structure of the component protein; consequently, the active site of the protein is typically in its bioactive form, and is capable of forming most, if not all, of the relevant protein–ligand interactions. X-ray diffraction data may then be collected on the resultant protein–ligand complex, and through the use of algorithms ultimately converted to a 3D crystal structure that reveals the exact interactions between the protein active site and the bound inhibitor (for an excellent review of the technical and applied aspects of X-ray crystallography in SBDD, the reader is referred to Qiu et al. [34]). At the time this chapter was being written, a total of 79 BACE crystal structures were available from the Research Collaboratory for Structural Bioinformatics [35]. It should be noted that while there are many examples of BACE–ligand complexes that have been disclosed in the patent literature, we have elected to omit these examples due to the non-refereed nature of patent applications as well as the difficulty of analysis in their current form. BACE lends itself to many different crystallization strategies, and this is reflected in the wide variety of well-diffracting crystal forms crystallized from many different precipitant mixtures (Table 6.1). The 79 publicly available crystal structures of BACE represent 11 unique crystal forms. Most of these protein data bank (PDB) entries report high-resolution data ($d_{min} \leq 2.50 \text{Å}$). The vast majority utilizes refolded BACE protein produced in *E. coli*, although three groups have produced BACE crystal structures utilizing protein expressed in a native form from CHO and insect cells. Specifically, Clarke et al. (Glaxo-SmithKline [GSK]) [21] and Emmons et al. (Pfizer [PFE]) [24] used CHO-cell expressed protein, while Baxter et al. (Johnson & Johnson [J&J]) [36] employed protein from insect cells. The crystal forms include two face-centered monoclinic (C2_A and C2_B, Table 6.1), a face-centered orthorhombic (C222₁), four primitive monoclinic (P2₁ A-D), two primitive orthorhombic (P2₁2₁2₁_A and _B), hexagonal (P6₁22), and trigonal (H3) lattices. While some forms are associated with a single crystallography group (e.g., P2₁2₁2₁ with the GSK effort) several seem to have been independently discovered by multiple groups (e.g., P6₁22 by researchers from Astex, J&J, Roche, and Riken).

Despite the wide variety of sources, crystallization protocols, and structures, the overall fold and topology of BACE is extremely well preserved in each of these structures. BACE possesses a now familiar aspartyl protease fold [12, 29, 37, 38],

TABLE 6.1 BACE Crystal Forms and PDB Entry Codes

C2_A	C2_B	C222₁	H3	P2₁_A	P2₁_B	P2₁_C	P2₁_D	P2₁2₁2₁_A	P2₁2₁2₁_B	P6₁22
2QU3	1YM4	2QZK	2EWY	1FKN	2FDP	1XS7	1SGZ	2VIE	3CID	2OHR
2QU2	3CKP	3E3W			2P83		1XN3	2VNM	2ZHR	2OHM
2HM1	3CKR	2PH6			2HIZ		1XN2	2VIJ	3CIC	2OHS
2IQG	2Q11	2PH8			2F3E		2G94	2VJ7	2QP8	2VA5
		2NTR			2F3F		2P4J	2VNN	1M4H	2OHU
		2IRZ			1YM2			2VJ6	2QMD	2ZHV
		2P8H						2VIZ	2QK5	2Q15
		2IS0						2VIY	2QMG	1W51
		2B8L						2VJ9	2QMF	2OHN
		2OAH							3CIB	2OF0
		2B8V								3BUH
		1TQF								2OHP
		2QZL								2ZHT
										2VA7
										2OHQ
										2OHL
										3BUF
										2OHK
										2ZHU
										3BRA
										2VA6
										2ZHS
										2OHT
										1W50
										3BUG

with N-terminal and C-terminal domains which each follow the same topology identified early on as a common supersecondary structure of all aspartic acid proteinases [38]. This similar topology generates a pseudo two-fold symmetry in the enzyme, analogous to the exact symmetry observed for the retroviral HIV protease, which is an exact dimer of a monomeric subunit. This close similarity between the N- and C-terminal domains suggests a common evolutionary origin in a gene duplication event [39]. The two domains can be described as highly twisted, eight-stranded beta sheet structures that are anchored to a six-stranded beta sheet platform (Fig. 6.2). The primary feature of the BACE active site is the disposition of two catalytic aspartic acid residues (Asp32/Asp228), which are in turn contributed by each lobe of the protease. These two aspartic acids are directed symmetrically at each other with an extremely well-ordered catalytic water molecule coordinated between them. At the pH maximum of 4.5–5.0, a proton is abstracted from this water by one of the catalytic Asp residues, thereby generating the nucleophile which attacks the scissile peptide bond in a substrate polypeptide [12, 20, 40]. As do all sequence-specific proteases [41–43], BACE achieves sequence-specific proteolysis of substrate peptides via specificity pockets which are situated N-terminal (denoted Sn, where n is the number of residues N-terminal to the site of cleavage) and C-terminal (denoted similarly by Sn′, where n is the number of residues removed from the scissile bond). BACE appears to have at least eight specificity pockets (S4-S1 and S1′-S4′) that are required for reasonable binding of substrate to the active site [29]. In addition, three additional N-terminal specificity pockets (S5, S6, and S7) have been identified [44], although the contribution of these sites to the high

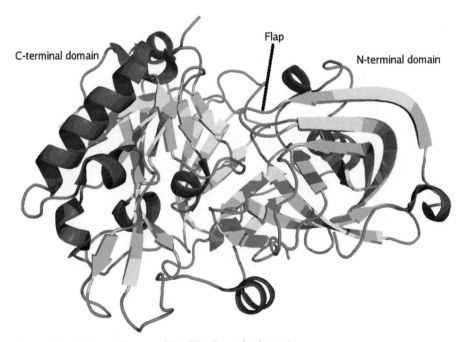

Figure 6.2   Ribbon diagram of BACE. (See color insert.)

affinity binding of inhibitors is probably less than the central eight specificity pockets. In general, the active site of BACE is dominated by hydrophobic residues (S1, S3, S1′, and S2′) matching the preference at these respective positions in substrate sequences for hydrophobic residues [45]. S4, S2, and S3′ are notably more hydrophilic and solvent exposed, and furthermore, S2 differs from the corresponding specificity pocket in the related human protease cat-D, suggesting that this may offer a potential route for gaining selectivity in inhibitor design [29].

All of the crystal forms described in Table 6.1 appear to be compatible with various ligands, suggesting that crystal packing plays a minor role in affecting protein–ligand interactions. Among the published structures, two key areas exhibit dramatic conformational changes depending on the ligand that is bound. The first, a beta hairpin structure known simply as the "flap" region, spans residues 70–76 in BACE (Fig. 6.3). This structure exhibits typically high B-factors (thermal factors) and consequently is sometimes disordered. Upon binding a substrate or peptidomimetic inhibitor the flap closes down, covering the catalytic machinery and sequestering the enzyme substrate complex from solvent. In their discussion of the apo forms of BACE, Hong and Tang [46] observed that a key residue in the flap, Tyr71, adopts an alternate rotamer, forming a hydrogen bond with the carbonyl oxygen of Lys107. They also observed two additional interactions that are unique to free BACE: a hydrogen bond between the backbone atoms of Tyr71 (O) and Gly74 (N), as well as a salt bridge between the side chains of Lys75 (NZ) and Glu77 (OE2). Together, these three interactions may serve to lock the enzyme active site in an "open" configuration to allow substrate access. The authors note, however, that a similar conformation for a conserved tyrosine residue in the eukaryotic aspartyl proteases chymosin and proteinase A serve to lock the flap in those enzymes in a closed, or

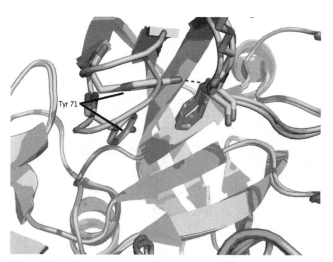

Figure 6.3   Close-up view of flap region (residues 70–75) of BACE, showing open (apo) form in cyan, and the closed (ligand bound) form in green. Note the alternate rotamer for Tyr71. (See color insert.)

autoinhibited, conformation. The open form observed by these authors suggests a role for substrate selection on the surface of the cell membrane, as opposed to an autoinhibited form. In contrast, Shimizu et al. [47] observed no altered conformation of Tyr71 in several structures of apo BACE; instead they argue that the flap undergoes a pH-dependent closing, resulting in a fully "closed" inactive structure at pH 7.0. Conversely, at lower pH, the flap opens up, allowing substrate access to the catalytic machinery. Since both of these structures were determined from crystals grown under similar conditions (1SG7 : 13–15% PEG8000, 0.1 M Na Cacodylate pH 6.2–7.4, 2ZHV, 1W50 : 10–18.5% PEG5000, 200 mM sodium citrate pH 7.0, 6.6, 0.2 M ammonium iodide), the primary difference may be due to the crystal packing environment. 1SGZ is a P2$_1$ crystal form with four molecules of BACE per asymmetric unit, while 2ZHV and 1W50 are a P6$_1$22 crystal form with one molecule of BACE per asymmetric unit. On the basis of these two structures, the biological relevance of the altered side chain rotamer seen for Tyr71 in 1SGZ is unclear.

The second region in BACE that undergoes significant conformational change is a deep cleft immediately adjacent to the S3 specificity pocket, often termed the S3 subpocket. This region, bordered on one side by residues 10–20 (the "tens" loop) and on the other by the 230's loop, can adopt an open and closed configuration depending on the nature of the ligand that is bound. Several groups have independently discovered the propensity of this region to collapse in response to ligand binding [29, 48, 49]. In the "open" or "up" conformation, the main chain carbonyl oxygen (O) atom of Ser10 is 10 Å from the side chain hydroxyl (OH) of Thr232, creating the large hydrophobic S3 subpocket. In contrast, the "closed" or "down" conformation places the Ser10 carbonyl O atom 2.7 Å from Thr232 OH, forcing a collapse of the S3 subpocket around the ligand R group at this site (Fig. 6.4). This collapse appears to be facilitated by the introduction of a lipophilic group (methyl-cyclopropyl, methoxyphenyl, valine) at the S3 position. However, McGaughey et al. [50] have shown that a key prerequisite lies in the nature of the interaction with the side chain OH of Thr232. In the case of a small P3 substituent, the preferred configuration would be for the S3 subpocket to close down to sequester the lipophilic component. However, in the case where a hydrogen bond acceptor on the ligand is in close proximity to the sidechain OH of Thr232, an alternate interaction is established between these two atoms, precluding the preferred hydrogen bond between Thr232 (OH) and Ser10 (O) [50]. The remainder of the BACE active site is remarkably well conserved among all of these structures. Certain residues do appear to undergo modest rearrangement in response to specific inhibitor interactions (e.g., Arg228, Leu30), but these rearrangements are relatively minor in light of the preceding discussion.

6.4 STRUCTURAL STUDIES WITH BACE INHIBITORS: PEPTIDOMIMETICS AND NONPEPTIDOMIMETICS

We now turn our attention to the interactions between specific classes of inhibitors and the BACE active site.

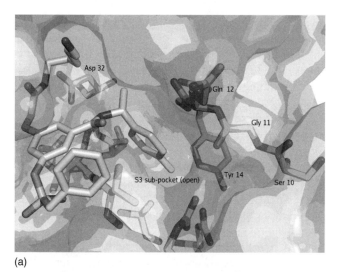

(a)

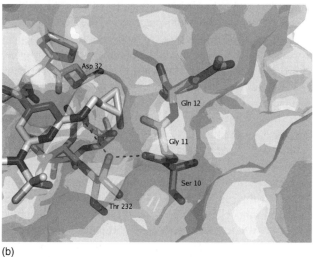

(b)

Figure 6.4 Surface representations of the S3 subpocket and 10s loop interactions: (a) the open form of the S3sp and (b) the closed form of the S3sp, with the H-bond formed between Ser10 and Thr232. (See color insert.)

6.4.1 Peptidomimetic BACE Inhibitors

The first of these, the peptidomimetics, are essentially short peptides in which the (usually central) scissile peptide bond is replaced with a non-cleavable transition-state isostere (TSI). Typical TSIs for peptidomimetics are the hydroxyethylene (HE), HEA, statine, and aminoethylenes (Fig. 6.5). The choice of TSI is often dictated by the desired pharmacokinetic properties, as certain TSIs are more brain- and/or cell-penetrant than others. In the HE and HEA class of inhibitors, the TSI hydroxyl mimics the gem-diol transition state of the activated peptide bond [20]. In the case

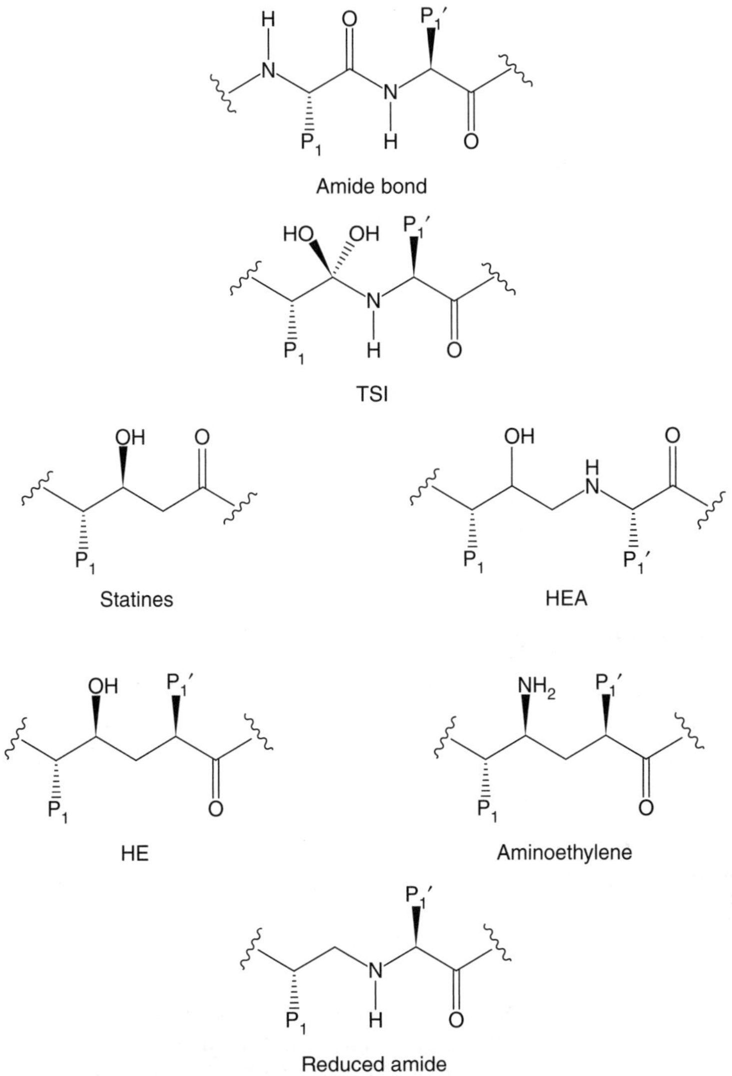

Amide bond

TSI

Statines

HEA

HE

Aminoethylene

Reduced amide

Figure 6.5   Typical transition-state isosteres for aspartyl proteases.

of a peptide bond, the amino terminal half of the substrate serves as a leaving group, resulting in cleavage of the scissile bond. However, in the case of the HE and HEA inhibitors, the ethylene moiety cannot function as a leaving group, resulting in a competitive inhibitor. The HEAs possess a distinct advantage over the HEs in that they are much more cell-penetrant, resulting in higher whole cell and *in vivo* efficacy [51]. Structurally, the additional hydrogen bond donor in the HEAs adds some potency due to a hydrogen bond established between the NH and the carbonyl oxygen of Gly34, as well as to the catalytic aspartic acid, Asp228. Perhaps because of this additional interaction, the stereochemical preference at the HEA hydroxyl is opposite from that seen for the HE TSI [51].

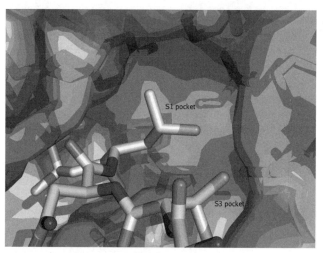

Figure 6.6   BACE S1 specificity pocket, shown bound to a hydroxyethylene peptidomimetic inhibitor OM99-2 (PDB entry 1FKN [29]). (See color insert.)

6.4.2   The S1 Specificity Pocket

Outside the TSI interactions with the catalytic aspartic acid dyad, the S1 specificity pocket is probably the most important contributor to both potency and specificity. The "normal" APP sequence that is recognized by BACE (SEVKM↓DAEFR, where the arrow indicates the cleavage site), with a Met as the P1 residue, is poorly hydrolyzed ($k_{cat}/K_m = 40$ s^{-1}M^{-1}), while the equivalent sequence from a mutated form of APP (SEVNL↓DAEFR), with an Asn and Leu as the P2 and P1 residues, respectively (the so-called "Swedish mutation," APPswe), is a robust substrate for BACE ($k_{cat}/K_m = 2450$ s^{-1}M^{-1}) [52]. S1 is a large hydrophobic cleft formed by the side chains of Tyr71, Phe108, Trp115, Ile118, and Leu30 (Fig. 6.6). The presence of the aromatic residues Tyr71 and Phe108, as well as the continuity with S3, suggests that a significant boost in potency may be achieved through engineering a series of aromatic stacking interactions [51]. Not surprisingly, most inhibitors in this class contain some sort of aromatic residue at P1 [21, 51, 53–65]. The large size of S1 clearly accommodates the added bulk of the aromatic moiety, and additional potency appears to come from the addition of highly electronegative fluorine (F) atoms at the 3- and 5-positions [51, 58–61, 63].

6.4.3   The S3 Specificity Pocket

Like S1, S3 is largely hydrophobic, being formed by side chain atoms from Leu30, Trp115, and Ile110, as well as main chain atoms from Gln12, Gly11, Gly230, Thr231, and Thr232 (Fig. 6.7). As mentioned previously, the S3 pocket extends into a deep cleft, the conformationally variable S3 subpocket. Impressive potency gains have been achieved by exploiting this region of the BACE active site, and a similar approach has also been utilized in the design of inhibitors to renin [66]. However,

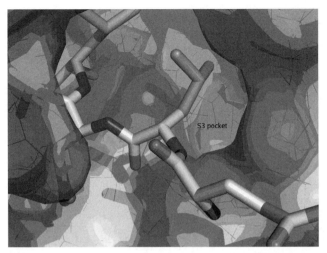

Figure 6.7   BACE S3 specificity pocket, shown bound to OM99-2 (PDB entry 1FK [29]). (See color insert.)

the potency to be gained in this pocket must be balanced against the physical properties in the resulting molecule. Most of the SAR in this area has focused on simple aliphatic chains (which exploit the hydrophobic character of S3) although Osterman and colleagues at Novartis recently published the crystal structure (PDB entry 2EWY) of a HEA inhibitor bound to the peripherally expressed BACE2 enzyme (43% sequence identity to BACE1), which places an intriguing tricyclic aromatic group in S3, suggesting that this pocket may be receptive to aromatics as well [67].

6.4.4   The S2 and S4 Binding Pockets

Unlike the S1/S3 cleft, both S2 and S4 are more polar and solvent exposed. Besides residues Tyr71, Thr72, and Glu73 from the flap, which fold over in the flap-"closed" conformation to interact with this pocket, the key feature of the S2 pocket is the side chain of Arg235, which provides much of the polar character (Fig. 6.8). Consequently, much of the SAR in this region has revealed a preference for negatively charged groups, which complement the positive charge of Arg235. Examples of P2 groups that have been exemplified in the literature are benzyl carbamates (2HIZ), pyridyl (2HM1), isophthalate (2IQG), sulfones (2VIY), pyrrolidinones (2VIZ), sultams (2VIJ), and aromatics (2EWY). While this pocket has been suggested to be a potential area to gain selectivity against other cellular aspartyl proteases such as pepsin gastricsin, and cathepsins D and E, which do not share this hydrophilic character [29], the requirement for a BACE inhibitor to be brain-penetrant places limits on the polarity that may be introduced here.

The S4 specificity pocket, likewise, is highly polar and is solvent exposed, but in the structure of the OM99-2 HE inhibitor, the P4 Glu residue is observed to be interacting primarily with the P2 Asn residue, along with Arg235 and Arg307. While gains in potency with peptidomimetics by introducing interactions at the S4 site have

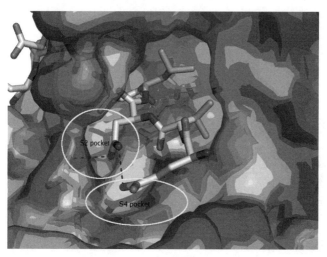

Figure 6.8   BACE S2 and S4 specificity pockets, showing the hydrogen bond between the polar P2 Asn side chain and the BACE specific Arg235. In OM99-2 (shown), there is an additional intramolecular interaction between the P2 (Asn) and P4 (Glu) side chains. (See color insert.)

been reported, the need to minimize molecular weight in order to improve physical properties has resulted in this position usually being left unoccupied.

6.4.5   The Prime Side – S1′, S2′, S3′, and S4′

The prime side of the BACE active site constitutes the S1′ S4′ specificity pockets, which interact with the four-substrate residues on the C-terminal side of the scissile peptide bond (Fig 6.9). Turner et al. [45] have shown that the prime side specificity pockets are far less stringent than the non-prime pockets. The S1′ pocket, while being large enough to accommodate a cyclohexyl group, as in 2VJ9 [55], is often unoccupied, or at best is occupied by a small substituent such as a methyl group, as in 1FKN [29]. Hong and Tang [46] have postulated that the preference for small groups at the P1′ position in substrates may be the result of a bottleneck created in part by closure of the flap, especially Thr72. Although molecules with small P1′ substituents may not be able to fully capitalize on the range of interactions available in S1′, the influence of the bottleneck residues on the kinetics of binding may allow for an overall enhancement in potency. This model is called into question, however, given the clear preference for large side chain residues in their earlier work [45].

In contrast to S1′, the S2′ pocket has been extensively explored by several independent groups. The preferred amino acid at this position is clearly Val, with Ile a close second. However, like all of the prime-side specificity pockets, the stringency at S2′ is fairly poor, and a wide array of large, mostly hydrophobic side chains is accommodated here [45]. Clarke et al. have explored this pocket in the context of an HEA TSI, with large bulky ring structures ranging in size from cyclopentyl to

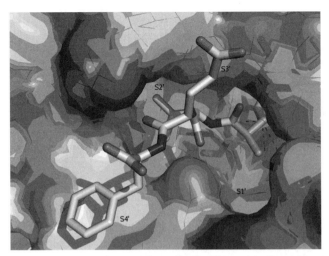

Figure 6.9 BACE prime side specificity pockets (S1'-S4'), shown bound to hydroxyethylene inhibitor OM-003 (PDB entry 1M4H [68]). (See color insert.)

azepine as well as branched aliphatics effectively filling the pocket [21, 55]. They also showed that meta-substituted aromatic groups provide reasonable potency despite lacking both interactions with S1' and the H-bonding capacity of an amide linker between P1' and P2'. Ostermann et al. [67] have also used a meta-substituated phenyl substituent at S2' in their studies of inhibitors of the closely related BACE2 enzyme. Similarly, Iserloh et al. [60, 61] and later Cumming et al. [57] have developed constrained peptidomimetics (pyrrolidine, piperidine, and piperazinone/imidazodinone) that exploit the S2' pocket via a naked phenyl ring. It will be interesting to observe whether the SAR in this region of the BACE active site is modular, which may allow for grafting of optimized substituents from one series to another.

The remainder of the prime side (S3' and S4') does not show much of a preference for specific interactions [45]. Early work by Hong et al. [68] suggested that occupation of these sites formed by Pro70, Tyr71, Arg128, and Tyr198 (S3'), and Gly125, Ile126, Trp197, and Tyr198 (S4') is crucial to achieving high potency inhibitors. However, the resulting compounds tend to be very large (e.g., 917 Da for inhibitor OM-003), a property not likely to be beneficial for brain penetration. Perhaps due to this, most inhibitors with cellular and *in vivo* potency tend to not rely on these sites.

6.4.6 Nonpeptidomimetic BACE Inhibitors

Owing to their typically large size, large numbers of hydrogen bonding groups, and dependence on lipophilicity to derive potency, peptidomimetics are notoriously difficult to optimize into safe and effective drugs. Consequently, many groups are now pursuing nonpeptidomimetic molecules. For BACE, which has at the center of its enzymatic mechanism a pair of catalytic aspartates, most of the disclosed nonpeptidomimetic inhibitors utilize a charged amino group, which may present other difficulties in optimization late in development. A distinctive feature of all of these compounds is the fact that since they do not explicitly mimic a substrate peptide, they are not limited to a linear set of interactions with the BACE active site. Consequently, a variety of binding modes have been observed, including indirect (water-mediated) interactions with the catalytic aspartates and dramatic conformational changes, especially in the flap residues. At the time of this writing, there were three examples of nonpeptidomimetic BACE inhibitors reported in the scholarly literature: the carbenimines (Merck), acylguanadines (Wyeth), and dihydroquinolines (J&J).

6.4.7 The Carbenimines

One of the first nonpeptidomimetics to be described in the literature is the carbenimine series (PDB entry 1TQF) [69]. Intriguingly, the lead compound, an aminopentyl oxyacetamide, was identified using a solution phase binding assay, and later was confirmed as a *bona fide* BACE inhibitor (BACE IC_{50} = 25 μM). This compound occupies sites from S4 to S1, making no prime side interactions, and interacts only indirectly with the catalytic machinery via a hydrogen bond between the oxyacetamide NH and the catalytic water, a heretofore unprecedented binding mode (Fig. 6.10). Besides this unusual water-mediated interaction, this structure revealed several novel interactions. The S3 pocket, which normally prefers small hydrophobic residues [45], opens up dramatically to accommodate the aromatic fluorophenyl of the inhibitor. S2 is occupied, as expected, by a polar benzyl-sulfonate, which also partially occupies S4. Finally, the amino pentyl side chain coils back into the S1 pocket, reminiscent of aliphatic side chains such as the Leu residue present in this position in 1FKN [29]. Following on this initial work, McGaughey et al. went on to further

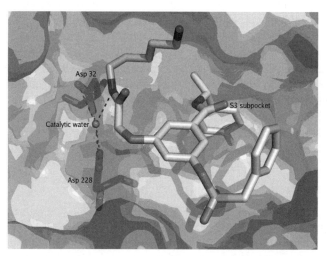

Figure 6.10 Nonpeptidomimetic carbenimine BACE inhibitor (PDB entry 1TQF [69]). (See color insert.)

elucidate the mechanism by which the ligand interactions modulate the conformation of S3, as discussed earlier [50]. The absence of a hydrogen bond donor proximal to Thr232 allows for a productive hydrogen bond between Thr232 and Ser10, thereby closing the S3 pocket down, and restricting the access of this pocket only to small, usually aliphatic, substituents [50]. Indeed, Stauffer et al. showed that the amide usually present at this position could be replaced with a highly constrained cis-olefin linker, constraining a small cyclopropyl P3 substituent within the S3 pocket, while allowing for a 10s loop "down" conformation via a productive Thr232-Ser10 hydrogen bond [49]. During the course of optimizing this series of inhibitors, the original oxyacetamide, which forms a water-mediated interaction with the catalytic aspartates, was replaced with a primary amine, which displaces the catalytic water and forms a direct interaction with the catalytic machinery [49, 50, 70]. Recognition of the close spatial relationship between the P1 and P3 substituents within this series led to the design of macrocyclic derivatives, with an aliphatic linker stabilizing the bioactive conformation of the inhibitor [71, 72], with a concomitant enhancement of potency. However, further exploration will be required to balance the usual requirements for inhibitor potency with brain penetration and Pgp-efflux properties [72].

6.4.8   The Acylguanidines

The acylguanidine class of BACE inhibitors was first disclosed by researchers at Wyeth [73, 74], and was discovered via a traditional HTS strategy. An X-ray crystal structure of the complex between BACE and the symmetric tri-substituted pyrrole (PDB entry 2QU2) led to the discovery that, while the charged guanidinium "warhead" interacted as predicted with the catalytic aspartic dyad, the substituted pyrrole was directed upward toward the flap, resulting in a disposition of Tyr71 in which the side chain of Tyr71 is rotated by 120 degrees and forms a hydrogen bond between the side chain hydroxyl and the main chain carbonyl of Asp105 (Asp168 according the authors' numbering scheme) [73] (Fig. 6.11). This interaction is reminiscent of the altered apo structure (PDB entry 1SGZ) [46] in which the corresponding interaction is between Tyr71 and the carbonyl O of Lys107. This placed the pendant aryl groups symmetrically in S1 and S2′, with the authors quickly recognizing the potential for further potency gains by engineering a halogen bond [74] between an ortho Cl P2′ aryl group and the indole NH of Trp76 [74]. This is an exquisite example of an induced pocket interaction, which has not been demonstrated in the peptidomimetic inhibitors. Elaboration on the non-prime side aryl group has led to a modest (six-fold) improvement in potency over the original lead compound, with both aryl and small alkyl groups directed toward the S3 pocket giving similar results [73]. While these results suggest that modification of these inhibitors in this region may be leading to modulation of the S3 pocket, as seen in the carbenimines, the available structural data (PDB entries 2QU2, 2QU3, 2ZDZ, 2ZE1) involve only aryl P3 substituents, with the S3 pocket in a unique conformation which does not fully recapitulate the features of the carbenimine 10s loop model [50]. Whether this discrepancy reflects inaccuracies in the model or is the result of different crystal forms remains to be seen.

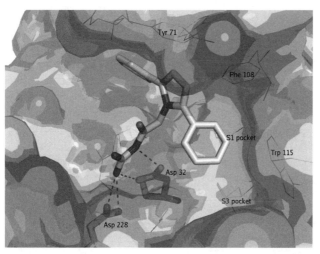

Figure 6.11 Nonpeptidomimetic acylguanidine BACE inhibitor (PDB entry 2QU2 [73]). (See color insert.)

6.4.9 The Dihydroaminoquinazolines

A third class of nonpeptidomimetic BACE inhibitor has recently been disclosed that exemplifies yet another novel, induced fit binding mode: the dihydroaminoquinazolines. This chemotype utilizes a charged amino group as the primary warhead to engage the catalytic aspartic acids as seen in the acylguanidines, but in this series, the NH_2 group is fused to a novel dihydroquinazoline scaffold [36] (Fig. 6.12). This series was discovered as part of a traditional inhibitor screen by J&J, with subsequent X-ray crystallographic analysis conducted in collaboration with Astex Therapeutics [36]. The quinazoline 2-amino group engages the cataylic aspartates, while the N1 atom is well positioned to accept a hydrogen bond from the outer side chain oxygen atom of Asp32, contradicting the computational result, which suggested that the monoprotonated form of the BACE catalytic aspartates prefers to place the proton on the inner oxygen of Asp228 [75]. It is not clear if this result is due to perturbed electrostatics in the active site as a result of ligand binding, or due to the fact that the aminoheterocycle TSI does not recapitulate the features of the tetrahedral transition state of the intermediate formed during proteolysis. As in the acylguanidines, the flap residues of BACE adopt an open structure, and the side chain of Tyr71 adopts yet a third rotamer conformation, now oriented outward with the side chain hydroxyl directed toward the S1′ pocket, but failing to form a productive hydrogen bond with either inhibitor or protein atoms. The quinazoline 6 position bears an aryl substituent, which fills the void left by Tyr71, making what appear to be predominantly hydrophobic interactions with the flap. The S1 pocket is filled by a cyclohexyl moiety, consistent with the broad specificity in this region for large aromatic or branched alkyl groups. The original lead compound exhibited reasonable potency (0.9 μM Ki), presumably from the extensive network of hydrogen bonds, as well as from the hydrophobic interactions conferred by the quinazoline and 6-aryl groups.

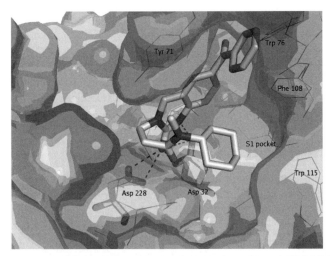

Figure 6.12   Nonpeptidomimetic dihydroquinazoline BACE inhibitor (PDB entry 2Q11 [36]). (See color insert.)

It is not clear whether this scaffold will allow for a better balance of central nervous system (CNS) properties and enzyme potency.

6.5   COMPUTATIONAL APPROACHES

The advantages of using computational methods include their high-throughput nature, the ability to work with large amounts of virtual structures and virtual testing of hypotheses before carrying out experiments in the lab, thereby reducing both design cycle times and costs in drug discovery. Computational methods continue to play a critical role in drug discovery research, and this is certainly the case in the discovery and development of novel BACE inhibitors.

6.5.1   Protein Flexibility

As discussed earlier, several BACE crystal structures solved to date provide information on the flexibility of BACE. Both the flap and 10s loop are present in both open/closed and up/down conformational states, respectively, depending on the ligands that bind to the enzyme. As is expected for a protein of flexible nature, there is significant variation in the location of crystallographic waters among various crystal structures. Furthermore, the flap and 10s loop can change up to 10 Å in orientation. Three molecular dynamic studies with BACE have been reported thus far. Gorfe and Caflisch [76] ran molecular dynamic simulations of BACE in explicit water bath for a long simulation time (0.3 μs). During this simulation they noted motions of the flap as well as orientations of two conserved water molecules – one that interacts with Ser35 and Asp32 that is hypothesized to be involved in proton transfer and a second one that is located between Tyr71, the flap and the catalytic residues. In a shorter simulation study (1200 ps), Park and Lee [77] found that the hydrogen bonding interactions between inhibitor OM99-2 and Asp228 can only exist when Asp32 is protonated and Asp228 is negatively charged. Xiong et al. [78] ran simulations in explicit water (1.2–4.5 ns) using unliganded BACE and observed that motions corresponded to low-frequency and large-amplitude fluctuations of the enzyme.

6.5.2   Binding Affinity Predictions

One of the most challenging and difficult problems in computational chemistry is the accurate computation of absolute free energies of binding. Current computational methods use several approximations to model the underlying physics of protein–ligand interactions to varying degrees of accuracy and speed. Absolute and relative ligand-binding free energies are best computed using rigorous statistical mechanics methods. These include the free-energy perturbation (FEP) and thermodynamic integration (TI) in conjunction with molecular dynamics (MD) or Monte Carlo (MC) simulations using a thermodynamic cycle. The computational demand of adequately sampling the intermediate states of the ligand along the pathway makes the absolute calculations very expensive and sometimes difficult to converge. The linear interaction energy (LIE) approximation is a way of combining molecular mechanics calculations with experimental data to build a model scoring function for evaluation of protein–ligand binding energies. In contrast to FEP, where a large number of intermediate windows must be evaluated, the LIE method only requires simulations of the two ending windows. Tounge and Reynolds [79] derived a LIE model for BACE. Rajamani and Reynolds [80] reported an improved model using a slightly different functional form of the computed interaction energies and predicted binding affinities of a series of HE-based BACE inhibitors. This model was in good agreement with experimental results and was used to study subsite specificity (P_2-P_2') and relative inhibitor activities of a series of C-terminal analogs. Scoring functions are the most widely used methods in evaluating protein–ligand interaction energies as they are very fast and are easy to compute. But in terms of accuracy of predicting rank ordering of compounds (relative free energies of binding), scoring function performance varies greatly from system to system. In a recent publication [81], Holloway et al. examined several simple scoring methods for two series of substrate-based BACE inhibitors to identify a docking/scoring protocol that could be used to design BACE inhibitors. They observed that both PLP1 score and Merck molecular force field (MMFF) interaction energy (E_{inter}) performed as well or better than other methods and recommended the use of MMFF E_{inter} for rank ordering potential inhibitors in a high-throughput mode prior to synthesis.

6.5.3   Selectivity Assessment

BACE selectivity is important since the target is localized in the brain where other related aspartyl proteases such as cathepsin D (cat-D) and renin are also present. Inhibitors of BACE that have poor selectivity against these enzymes are likely to cause undesirable side effects. Most of the selectivity design for BACE inhibitors involves a structure-based approach, as crystal structures of both cat-D and renin are also available. Through a systematic analysis of the several crystal structures and binding sites, it has been noted that significant differences in both the length and sequence of loop defining the S1′/S3′ subsites between BACE, renin, and cat-D can be differentially utilized to engender selectivity toward BACE. BACE is primarily hydrophilic whereas renin and cat-D are hydrophobic. In addition, there is a specific residue Arg235 in BACE that is distinctly different in cat-D (Val233) and renin (Ser222).

6.5.4 Brain Penetration Modeling

The human BBB consists of an intricate network of capillaries estimated to be ~600 km in length and ~ 12 m^2 in surface area [82, 83]. These capillaries are lined with endothelial cells that are distinguished by a number of important features – (1) paracellular transport is highly restricted, (2) active transport, both uptake and efflux, is prevalent, (3) metabolizing enzymes are also prevalent, and (4) the efflux transporters lining the BBB recognize a wide variety of substrates. In combination, these present a formidable and complex biological barrier to both large and small molecule entry into the brain. Computational models for predicting brain penetration can be divided into three categories [84–86]: (1) "rules-of-thumb" based on favorable physicochemical property space; (2) classification models that categorize compounds into CNS-penetrant or CNS-non-penetrant; and (3) continuous models that predict the extent of BBB permeability over a range of values. The benefits of predictive models include their high-throughput nature and the ability to work with virtual structures. The limitations include the amount of *in vivo* data that is typically available to generate hypotheses and construct models. Therefore, extensive use of *in vitro* permeability data is necessary to derive large data sets for computational modeling. However, in many cases, these large *in vitro* data sets are not entirely predictive of *in vivo* permeability [87]. In designing potent BACE inhibitors, optimal placement of hydrogen bond donors and acceptors are generally required for tight binding to the active site of the aspartyl protease. In addition, there appears to be a general requirement to span at least three to four subsites for effective inhibition. BACE inhibitors often possess a combination of high molecular weight, large polar surface area (PSA), and several freely rotatable bonds, relative to well-established CNS drugs that act on other target classes such as G protein-coupled receptors (GPCRs) and ion channels. This creates significant challenges in developing CNS-active BACE inhibitors due to the BBB, specifically P-gp susceptibility (*vide supra*). Several reports in the literature have implicitly either utilized either "rules of thumb" or *in-silico* BBB model to take into account the design principles necessary to effectively develop a CNS-active BACE inhibitor [88]. However, explicit use of *in-silico* BBB model to effectively design BACE inhibitors has not yet been heavily reported in the literature perhaps because this remains to be a hot area of research. Rishton et al. have recently taken a set of BACE inhibitors from literature and computed logBB using the ACD/Labs BBB permeability model [89]. All logBB values were <0, indicating that these inhibitors will not be CNS permeable. The ACD/Labs BBB model was developed from a training set gathered from examining literature data. This model is a linear QSAR model that contains a hydrophobicity term (logP) and a PSA term. Other parameters such as molecular weight, rotatable bonds, and pKa were not strong predictors of the training set logBB.

6.5.5 Protonation States and Impact on Structure-Based Virtual Screening

There are several possible conformational states of the catalytic residues, Asp32 and Asp228, resulting in at least eight different hydrogen bonding patterns based on four protonation states and three overall net charge (−2, −1, or 0). The two aspartic acid residues exist in a variety of configurations from coplanar to conformations that are orthogonal to each other in a variety of reported X-ray crystal structures. Based on a full linear-scaling quantum mechanical study, Rajamani and Reynolds [75] have suggested that in the presence of a ligand, a monoprotonated state is preferred where the inner oxygen of Asp228 is protonated. A more recent study by Yu et al. [90] suggests that the inner oxygen of Asp32 is protonated in the presence of a ligand. It appears that the absence of a correction for solubility is the reason for the different conclusions drawn by these two studies. The protonated state of Asp32 is in alignment with an experimental work performed on HIV-1 protease and a molecular dynamics study of BACE [77]). It is important that the protonation states of the active site residues are accurately represented during lead identification as demonstrated by Polgar and Keserue [91]. This can have a significant effect on the retrieval of actives in a virtual screening study. In a comparative study with OM99-2 crystal structure and docking with FlexX and FlexX-Pharm (BioSolveIT GmbH, Sankt Augustin, Germany) and scoring using Dock, Gold, Chem, PMF, and FlexX, they observed that the enrichment factor can vary anywhere from 0 to 36 depending on the protonation state of the aspartic acids. Adding pharmacophoric constraints to docking, as one would expect, further increased the enrichment factor to 41. It was noted that Dock and Gold performed better than other scoring functions as they explicitly use polar interaction terms. The choice of the crystal structure and/or the conformational state of the protein used to dock ligands will also have a significant effect on the virtual screening results. Cross-docking studies with ligands on different conformational protein states have given varying results depending on the nature of the docking protocol – rigid versus induced fit.

6.5.6 Ligand-Based Virtual Screening

A 3D pharmacophore model has sometimes been used in combination with a structure-based virtual screening approach either as a pre-filtering or a post-processing tool to reduce the massive amount of culling or selection work that needs to be performed in identifying virtual hit-lists. The FlexX-Pharm pharmacophore constraints used in the study by Polgar and Keserue [92] (*vide supra*) were retrieved from a Vertex patent [93] in which a congeneric series of BACE inhibitors were presented. The Vertex pharmacophore is a seven-point pharmacophore that contains four hydrophobic features and three hydrogen-bonding features. Specifically, a hydrogen bonding feature that interacts with one or both catalytic aspartic acids, two hydrogen bond donors with G34 and/or G230, hydrophobic groups in flap/S1 pocket, S2, and/or S2′ sites, and stacking interactions with Trp71, Phe108, and/or Trp76. In another approach [94], a set of most active and selective compounds for each class of BACE inhibitors was selected and subjected to an ensemble molecular docking process into five BACE X-ray structures. The superimposition of the calculated bioactive conformations of these inhibitors was then used to generate a common feature pharmacophore. The differences found between this pharmacophore and the Vertex pharmacophore model can be assigned to the different compounds used in the model generation. The Vertex pharmacophore was derived from a congeneric series based on a piperazine scaffold that was thought to stabilize the flap in an open conformation. Consequently, in that pharmacophoric model, an additional hydrophobic point is involved in the interactions with the flap pocket (Trp76, Phe108, Phe109, Trp115, and Ile102). In the Limongelli model, with the flap in a closed conformation, this hydrophobic pocket is no longer present [94]. In this nine-point pharmacophore model, five points are essential features for ligand recognition, and the remaining four points are accessory points of interaction.

6.5.7 Fragment-Based Virtual Screening

Screening campaigns against novel protein families are often disappointing due to the lack of quality chemical leads possessing overall characteristics of a compound class that make them an attractive starting point for lead optimization. This is particularly the case with BACE where not only does one have to identify potent compounds that bind and inhibit a large binding site but the compounds have to provide avenues for developing brain-penetrant molecules. Large molecule hits are often difficult to optimize for affinity and pharmacological properties without further increasing the molecular weight to a point that is unfavorable for pharmacological properties. Fragment-hits, on the other hand, provide good ligand-efficient starting points, exhibit a higher probability of making sufficient interactions with proteins through better complementarity of shapes and electrostatic properties, further increasing the likelihood of finding chemical leads and improving the value of fragment screens. Based on Astex Therapeutics Library of Available Substances (ATLAS), Murray and colleagues, using a proprietary version of the GOLD docking algorithm and a scoring protocol using GoldScore & ChemScore identified fragment-hits that were later optimized to increase potency using fragment-bound BACE crystal structure. Please refer to Chapter 5 for more details on this topic and other successful fragment-based virtual screening campaigns.

6.5.8 Combination Virtual Screening Approaches

In virtual screening (VS) approaches, due to the approximations used in the methods and the inherent orthogonal nature/bias of each VS methodology, there are severe shortcomings in both rank ordering the individual virtual screening hit-lists and/or combining hit-lists that arrive from different VS methods. It is now well-known that nearest neighbor relationships will not be preserved in different chemistry spaces

[95]. This leads to different chemistry-space representations, leading to different distributions of compounds that will significantly violate the similarity principle. Several researchers in the field have, hence, developed and applied a variety of novel computational tools to mitigate some of these representation-dependent and similarity-biased views of chemistry space [96–99]. Data-fusion approaches are used to provide the highest enrichment factor in a given system [100]. Successful data fusion approaches could reduce the uncertainty involved in selecting the appropriate VS method. The rationale behind this is to perform better than the worst individual VS method in the chosen subset of methods. Similarly, one can combine several diverse and alike VS approaches in selecting the final list. These types of data-aggregation approaches could potentially result in a merged result that is superior to any of the individual input method results and thus is able to extract useful information from all input lists, including inferior methods [98, 101]. In BACE, although we can be quite sure that a variety of combination approaches have been attempted within the research community, the challenges in developing efficacious BACE inhibitors have perhaps obviated any public announcement of successful VS campaigns. In a sequential VS workflow reported recently [102], a large database of compounds was screened for potential inhibitors of BACE using a sequential workflow approach that contained a substructural searching (2D Unity pharmacophore using a hydroxyl functionality and a benzene ring), structure-based coarse docking using HTVS-Glide (High-Throughput Virtual Screen setup) against four BACE crystal structures to approximate protein flexibility, refined Standard Precision-Glide docking and molecular mechanics Poisson-Boltzmann surface area (MM/PBSA) binding free-energy calculation to score the top hits, and finally a partial interaction energy analysis using a computational alanine scanning study to further cull down the VS hit-lists. By using this VS workflow, the authors reported identifying five compounds as VS hits (two of which were known BACE inhibitors) from a database of 3.5 million compounds.

6.6   FINAL REMARKS

The prevalence of AD in modern society presents a health-care challenge of enormous magnitude. According to the Alzheimer's Association, over 5 million Americans suffer from this debilitating disorder, with nearly 10 million more expected to develop AD over the coming decades [103]. Since its identification as one of the primary enzymes involved in the formation of beta amyloid, BACE has been the subject of an intense drug discovery effort by many different groups. An enormous amount of work over the last decade resulted in the rapid identification, cloning, expression, and structural characterization of BACE. Despite the breadth of technologies brought to bear on this enzyme, BACE remains a particularly difficult drug target. Brain penetration and P-gp efflux continue to be critical issues for most of the BACE inhibitors that have been disclosed in the literature, especially the peptidomimetic inhibitors. Safety and selectivity risks will continue to be major concerns, owing to the existence of important, closely related aspartyl proteases. The relatively recent evolution of more chemically tractable nonpeptidomimetic inhibitors suggests that the pharmaceutical industry is moving beyond substrate mimetics into more novel modes of enzyme inhibition. This shift in inhibitor design, combined with the wealth of enzymological, structural, and computational data offers hope that a safe, efficacious BACE inhibitor may soon be forthcoming.

ACKNOWLEDGMENT

We would like to thank Thomas L. Emmons for his invaluable help and insightful discussions.

REFERENCES

1. Hardy, J. and Selkoe, D.J. 2002. The amyloid hypothesis of Alzheimer's disease: progress and problems on the road to therapeutics. *Science* **297**(5580):353–356.
2. Imbimbo, B.P. 2008. Therapeutic potential of γ-secretase inhibitors and modulators. *Current Topics in Medicinal Chemistry* **1**:54–61.
3. Vassar, R. 2004. BACE1: the beta-secretase enzyme in Alzheimer's disease. *Journal of Molecular Neuroscience* **23**:105–114.
4. Hussain, I., Powell, D., Howlett, D.R., Tew, D.G., Meek, T.D., Chapman, C., Gloger, I.S., Murphy, K.E., Southan, C.D., Ryan, D.M., Smith, T.S., Simmons, D.L., Walsh, F.S., Dingwall, C., and Christie, G. 1999. Identification of a novel aspartic protease (Asp 2) as β-secretase. *Molecular and Cellular Neuroscience* **14**(6):419–427.
5. Sinha, S., Anderson, J.P., Barbour, R., Basi, G.S., Caccavello, R., Davis, D., Doan, M., Dovey, H.F., Frigon, N., Hong, J., Jacobson-Croak, K., Jewett, N., Keim, P., Knops, J., Lieberburg, I., Power, M., Tan, H., Tatsuno, G., Tung, J., Schenk, D., Seubert, P., Suomensaari, S.M., Wang, S., Walker, D., Zhao, J., McConlogue, L., and John, V. 1999. Purification and cloning of amyloid precursor protein β-secretase from human brain. *Nature* **402**(6761):537–540.
6. Vassar, R., Bennett, B.D., Babu-Khan, S., Kahn, S., Mendiaz, E.A., Denis, P., Teplow, D.B., Ross, S., Amarante, P., Loeloff, R., Luo, Y., Fisher, S., Fuller, J., Edenson, S., Lile, J., Jarosinski, M.A., Biere, A.L., Curran, E., Burgess, T., Louis, J.-C., Collins, F., Treanor, J., Rogers, G., and Citron, M. 1999. β-secretase cleavage of Alzheimer's amyloid precursor protein by the transmembrane aspartic protease BACE. *Science* **286**(5440):735–741.
7. Yan, R., Bienkowski, M.J., Shuck, M.E., Miao, H., Tory, M.C., Pauley, A.M., Brashler, J.R., Stratman, N.C., Mathews, W.R., Buhl, A.E., Carter, D.B., Tomasselli, A.G., Parodi, L.A., Heinrikson, R.L., and Gurney, M.E. 1999. Membrane-anchored aspartyl protease with Alzheimer's disease β-secretase activity. *Nature* **402**(6761):533–537.
8. Wolfe, M.S. 2006. The γ-secretase complex: membrane-embedded proteolytic ensemble. *Biochemistry* **45**(26):7931–7939.
9. Esler, W.P., Kimberly, W.T., Ostaszewski, B.L., Diehl, T.S., Moore, C.L., Tsai, J.-Y., Rahmati, T., Xia, W., Selkoe, D.J., and Wolfe, M.S. 2000. Transition-state analogue inhibitors of γ-secretase bind directly to presenilin-1. *Nature Cell Biology* **2**(7):428–434.
10. Li, Y.-M., Xu, M., Lai, M.-T., Huang, Q., Castro, J.L., DiMuzio-Mower, J., Harrison, T., Lellis, C., Nadin, A., Neduvelil, J.G., Register, R.B., Sardana, M.K., Shearman, M.S., Smith, A.L., Shi, X.-P., Yin, K.-C., Shafer, J.A., and Gardell, S.J. 2000. Photoactivated γ-secretase inhibitors directed to the active site covalently label presenilin 1. *Nature* **405**(6787):689–694.
11. Steiner, H. and Haass, C. 2007. GXGD-type intramembrane proteases – a family of novel aspartate proteases. In *Intramembrane-Cleaving Proteases (I-CLiPs)* (N.M. Hooper and U. Lendeckel, eds.). New York: Springer, pp. 31–49.
12. Eder, J., Hommel, U., Cumin, F., Martoglio, B., and Gerhartz, B. 2007. Aspartic proteases in drug discovery. *Current Pharmaceutical Design* **13**:271–285.

13. Lleó, A. 2008. Activity of γ-secretase on substrates other than APP. *Current Topics in Medicinal Chemistry* **8**:9–16.

14. Maillard, I., Adler, S.H., and Pear, W.S. 2003. Notch and the immune system. *Immunity*, **19**(6):781–791.

15. Stanger, B.Z., Datar, R., Murtaugh, L.C., and Melton, D.A. 2005. Direct regulation of intestinal fate by Notch. *Proceedings of the National Academy of Sciences of the United States of America* **102**(35):12443–12448.

16. *Myriad Genetics Reports Results of U.S. Phase 3 Trial of Flurizan™ in Alzheimer's Disease* [cited June 1, 2009]. Available at http://www.myriad.com/news/release/1170283.

17. Lipinski, C.A., Lombardo, F., Dominy, B.W., and Feeney, P.J. 2001. Experimental and computational approaches to estimate solubility and permeability in drug discovery and development settings. *Advanced Drug Delivery Reviews* **46**(1–3):3–26.

18. Löscher, W. and Potschka, H. 2005. Blood–brain barrier active efflux transporters: ATP-binding cassette gene family. *Neurotherapeutics: The Journal of the American Society for Experimental NeuroTherapeutics* **2**(1):86–98.

19. Huse, J.T., Liu, K., Pijak, D.S., Carlin, D., Lee, V.M.Y., and Doms, R.W. 2002. β-secretase processing in the trans-golgi network preferentially generates truncated amyloid species that accumulate in Alzheimer's disease brain. *The Journal of Biological Chemistry* **277**(18):16278–16284.

20. See Chapter 3 of this book.

21. Clarke, B., Demont, E., Dingwall, C., Dunsdon, R., Faller, A., Hawkins, J., Hussain, I., MacPherson, D., Maile, G., Matico, R., Milner, P., Mosley, J., Naylor, A., O'Brien, A., Redshaw, S., Riddell, D., Rowland, P., Soleil, V., Smith, K.J., Stanway, S., Stemp, G., Sweitzer, S., Theobald, P., Vesey, D., Walter, D.S., Ward, J., and Wayne, G. 2008. BACE-1 inhibitors part 1: Identification of novel hydroxy ethylamines (HEAs). *Bioorganic & Medicinal Chemistry Letters* **18**(3):1011–1016.

22. Lüllau, E., Kanttinen, A., Hassel, J., Berg, M., Haag-Alvarsson, A., Cederbrant, K., Greenberg, B., Fenge, C., and Schweikart, F. 2003. Comparison of batch and perfusion culture in combination with pilot-scale expanded bed purification for the production of soluble recombinant beta-secretase. *Biotechnology Progress* **19**(1):37–44.

23. Sidera, C., Liu, C., and Austen, B. 2002. Pro-domain removal in ASP-2 and the cleavage of the amyloid precursor are influenced by pH. *BMC Biochemistry* **3**(1):25.

24. Emmons, T.L., Shuck, M.E., Babcock, M.S., Holloway, J.S., Leone, J.W., Durbin, J.D., Paddock, D.J., Prince, D.B., Heinrikson, R.L., Fischer, H.D., Bienkowski, M.J., Benson, T.E., and Tomasselli, A.G. 2008. Large-scale purification of human BACE expressed in mammalian cells and removal of the prosegment with HIV-1 protease to improve crystal diffraction. *Protein and Peptide Letters* **15**(2):119–130.

25. Bruinzeel, W., Yon, J., Giovannelli, S., and Masure, S. 2002. Recombinant insect cell expression and purification of human β-secretase (BACE-1) for X-ray crystallography. *Protein Expression and Purification* **26**(1):139–148.

26. Chang, K.H., Baek, N.I., Yang, J.M., Lee, J.M., Bo, J.H., and Chung, I.S. 2005. Expression and characterization of recombinant β-secretase from *Trichoplusia ni* BTI Tn5B1-4 cells transformed with cDNAs encoding human β1,4-galactosyltransferase and Gal β1,4-GlcNAc α 2,6-sialyltransferase. *Protein Expression and Purification* **44**(2):87–93.

27. Mallender, W.D., Yager, D., Onstead, L., Nichols, M.R., Eckman, C., Sambamurti, K., Kopcho, L.M., Marcinkeviciene, J., Copeland, R.A., and Rosenberry, T.L. 2001. Characterization of recombinant, soluble β-secretase from an insect cell expression system. *Molecular Pharmacology* **59**(3):619–626.

28. Wang, W., Reichert, P., Beyer, B.M., Liu, J., Lee, J., Zhang, L., Liu, Y.-H., Taremi, S.S., Le, H.V., and Strickland, C. 2004. Crystallization of glycosylated human BACE protease domain expressed in *Trichoplusia ni*. *Biochimica et Biophysica Acta (BBA) – Proteins & Proteomics* **1698**(2):255–259.

29. Hong, L., Koelsch, G., Lin, X., Wu, S., Terzyan, S., Ghosh, A.K., Zhang, X.C., and Tang, J. 2000. Structure of the protease domain of memapsin 2 (β-secretase) complexed with inhibitor. *Science* **290**(5489):150–153.

30. Lin, X., Koelsch, G., Wu, S., Downs, D., Dashti, A., and Tang, J. 2000. Human aspartic protease memapsin 2 cleaves the β-secretase site of β-amyloid precursor protein. *Proceedings of the National Academy of Sciences of the United States of America* **97**(4):1456–1460.
31. Patel, S., Vuillard, L., Cleasby, A., Murray, C.W., and Yon, J. 2004. Apo and inhibitor complex structures of BACE (β-secretase). *Journal of Molecular Biology* **343**(2):407–416.
32. Sardana, V., Xu, B., Zugay-Murphy, J., Chen, Z., Sardana, M., Darke, P.L., Munshi, S., and Kuo, L.C. 2004. A general procedure for the purification of human β-secretase expressed in *Escherichia coli. Protein Expression and Purification* **34**(2):190–196.
33. Tomasselli, A.G., Paddock, D.J., Emmons, T.L., Mildner, A.M., Leone, J.W., Lull, J.M., Cialdella, J.I., Prince, D.B., Fischer, H.D., Heinrikson, R.L., and Benson, T.E. 2008. High yield expression of human BACE constructs in *Eschericia coli* for refolding, purification, and high resolution diffracting crystal forms. *Protein and Peptide Letters* **15**(2):131–143.
34. Qiu, X. and Abdel-Meguid, S.S. 2004. Protein crystallography in structure-based drug design. In *Drug Discovery Strategies and Methods* (A. Makriyannis and D. Biegel, eds.). New York: Marcel Dekker, pp. 1–21.
35. Berman, H.M., Westbrook, J., Feng, Z., Gilliland, G., Bhat, T.N., Weissig, H., Shindyalov, I.N., and Bourne, P.E. 2000. The protein data bank. *Nucleic Acids Research* **28**(1):235–242.
36. Baxter, E.W., Conway, K.A., Kennis, L., Bischoff, F., Mercken, M.H., De Winter, H.L., Reynolds, C.H., Tounge, B.A., Luo, C., Scott, M.K., Huang, Y., Braeken, M., Pieters, S.M.A., Berthelot, D.J.C., Masure, S., Bruinzeel, W.D., Jordan, A.D., Parker, M.H., Boyd, R.E., Qu, J., Alexander, R.S., Brenneman, D.E., and Reitz, A.B. 2007. 2-amino-3,4-dihydroquinazolines as inhibitors of BACE-1 (β-site APP cleaving enzyme): use of structure-based design to convert a micromolar hit into a nanomolar lead. *Journal of Medicinal Chemistry* **50**(18):4261–4264.
37. Dunn, B.M. 2002. Structure and mechanism of the pepsin-like family of aspartic peptidases. *Chemical Reviews* **102**(12):4431–4458.
38. Blundell, T.L., Cooper, J.B., Sali, A., and Zhu, Z.-Y. 1991. Comparisons of the sequences, 3-D structures and mechanisms of pepsin-like and retroviral aspartic proteinases. In *Structure and Function of the Aspartic Proteinases* (B.M. Dunn, ed.). New York: Plenum Press, pp. 443–453.
39. Tang, J., James, M.N.G., Hsu, I.N., Jenkins, J.A., and Blundell, T.L. 1978. Structural evidence for gene duplication in the evolution of the acid proteases. *Nature* **271**(5646):618–621.
40. Coates, L., Erskine, P.T., Mall, S., Gill, R., Wood, S.P., Myles, D.A.A., and Cooper, J.B. 2006. X-ray, neutron and NMR studies of the catalytic mechanism of aspartic proteinases. *European Biophysics Journal: EBJ* **35**:559–566.
41. Abramowitz, N., Schechter, I., and Berger, A. 1967. On the size of the active site in proteases. II: Carboxypeptidase-A. *Biochemical and Biophysical Research Communications* **29**(6):862–867.
42. Schechter, I. and Berger, A. 1967. On the size of the active site in proteases. I: Papain. *Biochemical and Biophysical Research Communications* **27**(2):157–162.
43. Schechter, I. and Berger, A. 1968. On the active site of proteases. III: Mapping the active site of papain; specific peptide inhibitors of papain. *Biochemical and Biophysical Research Communications* **32**(5):898–902.
44. Turner, R.T., Hong, L., Koelsch, G., Ghosh, A.K., and Tang, J. 2005. Structural locations and functional roles of new subsites S5, S6, and S7 in memapsin 2 (β-secretase). *Biochemistry* **44**(1):105–112.
45. Turner, R.T., Koelsch, G., Hong, L., Castenheira, P., Ghosh, A., and Tang, J. 2001. Subsite specificity of memapsin 2 (β-secretase): implications for inhibitor design. *Biochemistry* **40**(34):10001–10006.
46. Hong, L. and Tang, J. 2004. Flap position of free memapsin 2 (β-secretase), a model for flap opening in aspartic protease catalysis. *Biochemistry* **43**(16):4689–4695.
47. Shimizu, H., Tosaki, A., Kaneko, K., Hisano, T., Sakurai, T., and Nukina, N. 2008. Crystal structure of an active form of BACE1, an enzyme responsible for amyloid β protein production. *Molecular and Cellular Biology* **28**(11):3663–3671.
48. Edwards, P.D., Albert, J.S., Sylvester, M., Aharony, D., Andisik, D., Callaghan, O., Campbell, J.B., Carr, R.A., Chessari, G., Congreve, M., Frederickson, M., Folmer, R.H.A., Geschwindner, S., Koether, G., Kolmodin, K., Krumrine, J., Mauger, R.C., Murray, C.W., Olsson, L.-L., Patel, S., Spear, N., and Tian, G. 2007. Application of fragment-based lead generation to the discovery of

novel, cyclic amidine β-secretase inhibitors with nanomolar potency, cellular activity, and high ligand efficiency. *Journal of Medicinal Chemistry* **50**(24):5912–5925.

49. Stauffer, S.R., Stanton, M.G., Gregro, A.R., Steinbeiser, M.A., Shaffer, J.R., Nantermet, P.G., Barrow, J.C., Rittle, K.E., Collusi, D., Espeseth, A.S., Lai, M.-T., Pietrak, B.L., Holloway, M.K., McGaughey, G.B., Munshi, S.K., Hochman, J.H., Simon, A.J., Selnick, H.G., Graham, S.L., and Vacca, J.P. 2007. Discovery and SAR of isonicotinamide BACE-1 inhibitors that bind β-secretase in an N-terminal 10s-loop down conformation. *Bioorganic & Medicinal Chemistry Letters* **17**(6):1788–1792.

50. McGaughey, G.B., Colussi, D., Graham, S.L., Lai, M.-T., Munshi, S.K., Nantermet, P.G., Pietrak, B., Rajapakse, H.A., Selnick, H.G., Stauffer, S.R., and Holloway, M.K. 2007. β-secretase (BACE-1) inhibitors: accounting for 10s loop flexibility using rigid active sites. *Bioorganic & Medicinal Chemistry Letters* **17**(4):1117–1121.

51. Maillard, M.C., Hom, R.K., Benson, T.E., Moon, J.B., Mamo, S., Bienkowski, M., Tomasselli, A.G., Woods, D.D., Prince, D.B., Paddock, D.J., Emmons, T.L., Tucker, J.A., Dappen, M.S., Brogley, L., Thorsett, E.D., Jewett, N., Sinha, S., and John, V. 2007. Design, synthesis, and crystal structure of hydroxyethyl secondary amine-based peptidomimetic inhibitors of human β-secretase. *Journal of Medicinal Chemistry* **50**(4):776–781.

52. Ghosh, A.K., Shin, D., Koelsch, G., Lin, X., Ermolieff, J., and Tang, J. 2000. Design of potent inhibitors for human brain memapsin 2 (β-secretase). *Journal of the American Chemical Society* **122**(14):3522–3523.

53. Bridges, K.G., Chopra, R., Lin, L., Svenson, K., Tam, A., Jin, G., Cowling, R., Lovering, F., Akopian, T.N., DiBlasio-Smith, E., Annis-Freeman, B., Marvell, T.H., LaVallie, E.R., Zollner, R.S., Bard, J., Somers, W.S., Stahl, M.L., and Kriz, R.W. 2006. A novel approach to identifying β-secretase inhibitors: bis-statine peptide mimetics discovered using structure and spot synthesis. *Peptides* **27**(7):1877–1885.

54. Beswick, P., Charrier, N., Clarke, B., Demont, E., Dingwall, C., Dunsdon, R., Faller, A., Gleave, R., Hawkins, J., Hussain, I., Johnson, C.N., MacPherson, D., Maile, G., Matico, R., Milner, P., Mosley, J., Naylor, A., O'Brien, A., Redshaw, S., Riddell, D., Rowland, P., Skidmore, J., Soleil, V., Smith, K.J., Stanway, S., Stemp, G., Stuart, A., Sweitzer, S., Theobald, P., Vesey, D., Walter, D.S., Ward, J., and Wayne, G. 2008. BACE-1 inhibitors part 3: Identification of hydroxy ethyl-amines (HEAs) with nanomolar potency in cells. *Bioorganic & Medicinal Chemistry Letters* **18**(3):1022–1026.

55. Clarke, B., Demont, E., Dingwall, C., Dunsdon, R., Faller, A., Hawkins, J., Hussain, I., MacPherson, D., Maile, G., Matico, R., Milner, P., Mosley, J., Naylor, A., O'Brien, A., Redshaw, S., Riddell, D., Rowland, P., Soleil, V., Smith, K.J., Stanway, S., Stemp, G., Sweitzer, S., Theobald, P., Vesey, D., Walter, D.S., Ward, J., and Wayne, G. 2008. BACE-1 inhibitors part 2: Identification of hydroxy ethylamines (HEAs) with reduced peptidic character. *Bioorganic & Medicinal Chemistry Letters* **18**(3):1017–1021.

56. Coburn, C.A., Stachel, S.J., Jones, K.G., Steele, T.G., Rush, D.M., DiMuzio, J., Pietrak, B.L., Lai, M.-T., Huang, Q., Lineberger, J., Jin, L., Munshi, S., Katharine Holloway, M., Espeseth, A., Simon, A., Hazuda, D., Graham, S.L., and Vacca, J.P. 2006. BACE-1 inhibition by a series of ψ[CH2NH] reduced amide isosteres. *Bioorganic & Medicinal Chemistry Letters* **16**(14):3635–3638.

57. Cumming, J.N., Le, T.X., Babu, S., Carroll, C., Chen, X., Favreau, L., Gaspari, P., Guo, T., Hobbs, D.W., Huang, Y., Iserloh, U., Kennedy, M.E., Kuvelkar, R., Li, G., Lowrie, J., McHugh, N.A., Ozgur, L., Pan, J., Parker, E.M., Saionz, K., Stamford, A.W., Strickland, C., Tadesse, D., Voigt, J., Wang, L., Wu, Y., Zhang, L., and Zhang, Q. 2008. Rational design of novel, potent piperazinone and imidazolidinone BACE1 inhibitors. *Bioorganic & Medicinal Chemistry Letters* **18**(11):3236–3241.

58. Freskos, J.N., Fobian, Y.M., Benson, T.E., Bienkowski, M.J., Brown, D.L., Emmons, T.L., Heintz, R., Laborde, A., McDonald, J.J., Mischke, B.V., Molyneaux, J.M., Moon, J.B., Mullins, P.B., Bryan Prince, D., Paddock, D.J., Tomasselli, A.G., and Winterrowd, G. 2007. Design of potent inhibitors of human β-secretase. Part 1. *Bioorganic & Medicinal Chemistry Letters* **17**(1):73–77.

59. Freskos, J.N., Fobian, Y.M., Benson, T.E., Moon, J.B., Bienkowski, M.J., Brown, D.L., Emmons, T.L., Heintz, R., Laborde, A., McDonald, J.J., Mischke, B.V., Molyneaux, J.M., Mullins, P.B., Bryan Prince, D., Paddock, D.J., Tomasselli, A.G., and Winterrowd, G. 2007. Design of potent

inhibitors of human β-secretase. Part 2. *Bioorganic & Medicinal Chemistry Letters* **17**(1):78–81.

60. Iserloh, U., Pan, J., Stamford, A.W., Kennedy, M.E., Zhang, Q., Zhang, L., Parker, E.M., McHugh, N.A., Favreau, L., Strickland, C., and Voigt, J. 2008. Discovery of an orally efficaceous 4-phenoxy-pyrrolidine-based BACE-1 inhibitor. *Bioorganic & Medicinal Chemistry Letters* **18**(1):418–422.

61. Iserloh, U., Wu, Y., Cumming, J.N., Pan, J., Wang, L.Y., Stamford, A.W., Kennedy, M.E., Kuvelkar, R., Chen, X., Parker, E.M., Strickland, C., and Voigt, J. 2008. Potent pyrrolidine- and piperidine-based BACE-1 inhibitors. *Bioorganic & Medicinal Chemistry Letters* **18**(1):414–417.

62. Kortum, S.W., Benson, T.E., Bienkowski, M.J., Emmons, T.L., Prince, D.B., Paddock, D.J., Tomaselli, A.G., Moon, J.B., LaBorde, A., and TenBrink, R.E. 2007. Potent and selective isoph-thalamide S2 hydroxyethylamine inhibitors of BACE1. *Bioorganic & Medicinal Chemistry Letters* **17**(12):3378–3383.

63. Park, H., Min, K., Kwak, H.-S., Koo, K.D., Lim, D., Seo, S.-W., Choi, J.-U., Platt, B., and Choi, D.-Y. 2008. Synthesis, SAR, and X-ray structure of human BACE-1 inhibitors with cyclic urea derivatives. *Bioorganic & Medicinal Chemistry Letters* **18**(9):2900–2904.

64. Stachel, S.J., Coburn, C.A., Steele, T.G., Crouthamel, M.-C., Pietrak, B.L., Lai, M.-T., Holloway, M.K., Munshi, S.K., Graham, S.L., and Vacca, J.P. 2006. Conformationally biased P3 amide replacements of β-secretase inhibitors. *Bioorganic & Medicinal Chemistry Letters* **16**(3):641–644.

65. Yang, W., Lu, W., Lu, Y., Zhong, M., Sun, J., Thomas, A.E., Wilkinson, J.M., Fucini, R.V., Lam, M., Randal, M., Shi, X.-P., Jacobs, J.W., McDowell, R.S., Gordon, E.M., and Ballinger, M.D. 2006. Aminoethylenes: a tetrahedral intermediate isostere yielding potent inhibitors of the aspartyl pro-tease BACE-1. *Journal of Medicinal Chemistry* **49**(3):839–842.

66. Rahuel, J., Rasetti, V., Maibaum, J., Rüeger, H., Göschke, R., Cohen, N.C., Stutz, S., Cumin, F., Fuhrer, W., Wood, J.M., and Grütter, M.G. 2000. Structure-based drug design: the discovery of novel nonpeptide orally active inhibitors of human renin. *Chemistry & Biology* **7**(7):493–504.

67. Ostermann, N., Eder, J., Eidhoff, U., Zink, F., Hassiepen, U., Worpenberg, S., Maibaum, J., Simic, O., Hommel, U., and Gerhartz, B. 2006. Crystal structure of human BACE2 in complex with a hydroxyethylamine transition-state inhibitor. *Journal of Molecular Biology* **355**(2):249–261.

68. Hong, L., Turner, R.T., Koelsch, G., Shin, D., Ghosh, A.K., and Tang, J. 2002. Crystal structure of memapsin 2 (β-secretase) in complex with an inhibitor OM00-3. *Biochemistry* **41**(36): 10963–10967.

69. Coburn, C.A., Stachel, S.J., Li, Y.-M., Rush, D.M., Steele, T.G., Chen-Dodson, E., Holloway, M.K., Xu, M., Huang, Q., Lai, M.-T., DiMuzio, J., Crouthamel, M.-C., Shi, X.-P., Sardana, V., Chen, Z., Munshi, S., Kuo, L., Makara, G.M., Annis, D.A., Tadikonda, P.K., Nash, H.M., Vacca, J.P., and Wang, T. 2004. Identification of a small molecule nonpeptide active site β-secretase inhibitor that displays a nontraditional binding mode for aspartyl proteases. *Journal of Medicinal Chemistry* **47**(25):6117–6119.

70. Rajapakse, H.A., Nantermet, P.G., Selnick, H.G., Munshi, S., McGaughey, G.B., Lindsley, S.R., Young, M.B., Lai, M.-T., Espeseth, A.S., Shi, X.-P., Colussi, D., Pietrak, B., Crouthamel, M.-C., Tugusheva, K., Huang, Q., Xu, M., Simon, A.J., Kuo, L., Hazuda, D.J., Graham, S., and Vacca, J.P. 2006. Discovery of oxadiazoyl tertiary carbinamine inhibitors of β-secretase (BACE-1). *Journal of Medicinal Chemistry* **49**(25):7270–7273.

71. Lindsley, S.R., Moore, K.P., Rajapakse, H.A., Selnick, H.G., Young, M.B., Zhu, H., Munshi, S., Kuo, L., McGaughey, G.B., Colussi, D., Crouthamel, M.-C., Lai, M.-T., Pietrak, B., Price, E.A., Sankaranarayanan, S., Simon, A.J., Seabrook, G.R., Hazuda, D.J., Pudvah, N.T., Hochman, J.H., Graham, S.L., Vacca, J.P., and Nantermet, P.G. 2007. Design, synthesis, and SAR of macrocyclic tertiary carbinamine BACE-1 inhibitors. *Bioorganic & Medicinal Chemistry Letters* **17**(14): 4057–4061.

72. Moore, K.P., Zhu, H., Rajapakse, H.A., McGaughey, G.B., Colussi, D., Price, E.A., Sankaranarayanan, S., Simon, A.J., Pudvah, N.T., Hochman, J.H., Allison, T., Munshi, S.K., Graham, S.L., Vacca, J.P., and Nantermet, P.G. 2007. Strategies toward improving the brain penetration of macrocyclic tertiary carbinamine BACE-1 inhibitors. *Bioorganic & Medicinal Chemistry Letters* **17**(21):5831–5835.

73. Cole, D.C., Stock, J.R., Chopra, R., Cowling, R., Ellingboe, J.W., Fan, K.Y., Harrison, B.L., Hu, Y., Jacobsen, S., Jennings, L.D., Jin, G., Lohse, P.A., Malamas, M.S., Manas, E.S., Moore, W.J., O'Donnell, M.-M., Olland, A.M., Robichaud, A.J., Svenson, K., Wu, J., Wagner, E., and Bard, J. 2008. Acylguanidine inhibitors of β-secretase: optimization of the pyrrole ring substituents extending into the S1 and S3 substrate binding pockets. *Bioorganic & Medicinal Chemistry Letters* **18**(3):1063–1066.

74. Fobare, W.F., Solvibile, W.R., Robichaud, A.J., Malamas, M.S., Manas, E., Turner, J., Hu, Y., Wagner, E., Chopra, R., Cowling, R., Jin, G., and Bard, J. 2007. Thiophene substituted acylguanidines as BACE1 inhibitors. *Bioorganic & Medicinal Chemistry Letters* **17**(19):5353–5356.

75. Rajamani, R. and Reynolds, C.H. 2004. Modeling the protonation states of the catalytic aspartates in β-secretase. *Journal of Medicinal Chemistry* **47**(21):5159–5166.

76. Gorfe, A.A. and Caflisch, A. 2005. Functional plasticity in the substrate binding site of β-secretase. *Structure* **13**(10):1487–1498.

77. Park, H. and Lee, S. 2003. Determination of the active site protonation state of β-secretase from molecular dynamics simulation and docking experiment: implications for structure-based inhibitor design. *Journal of the American Chemical Society* **125**(52):16416–16422.

78. Xiong, B., Huang, X.-Q., Shen, L.-L., Shen, J.-H., Luo, X.-M., Shen, X., Jiang, H.-L., and Chen, K.-X. 2004. Conformational flexibility of β-secretase: molecular dynamics simulation and essential dynamics analysis. *Acta Pharmacologica Sinica* **25**(6):705–713.

79. Tounge, B.A. and Reynolds, C.H. 2003. Calculation of the binding affinity of β-secretase inhibitors using the linear interaction energy method. *Journal of Medicinal Chemistry* **46**(11): 2074–2082.

80. Rajamani, R. and Reynolds, C.H. 2004. Modeling the binding affinities of β-secretase inhibitors: application to subsite specificity. *Bioorganic & Medicinal Chemistry Letters* **14**(19):4843–4846.

81. Holloway, M.K., McGaughey, G.B., Coburn, C.A., Stachel, S.J., Jones, K.G., Stanton, E.L., Gregro, A.R., Lai, M.-T., Crouthamel, M.-C., Pietrak, B.L., and Munshi, S.K. 2007. Evaluating scoring functions for docking and designing β-secretase inhibitors. *Bioorganic & Medicinal Chemistry Letters* **17**(3):823–827.

82. Pardridge, W.M. 1995. Transport of small molecules through the blood–brain barrier: biology and methodology. *Advanced Drug Delivery Reviews* **15**(1–3):5–36.

83. Pardridge, W.M. 2003. Blood–brain barrier drug targeting: the future of brain drug development. *Molecular Interventions* **3**(2):90–105.

84. Clark, D.E. 2003. In silico prediction of blood–brain barrier permeation. *Drug Discovery Today* **8**(20):927–933.

85. Clark, D.E. 2005. Computational prediction of blood–brain barrier permeation. *Annual Reports in Medicinal Chemistry* **40**:403–415.

86. Goodwin, J.T. and Clark, D.E. 2005. In silico predictions of blood–brain barrier penetration: considerations to "keep in mind." *The Journal of Pharmacology and Experimental Therepeutics* **315**(2):477–483.

87. Faassen, F., Vogel, G., Spanings, H., and Vromans, H. 2003. Caco-2 permeability, P-glycoprotein transport ratios and brain penetration of heterocyclic drugs. *International Journal of Pharmaceutics* **263**(1–2):113–122.

88. Norinder, U. and Haeberlein, M. 2002. Computational approaches to the prediction of the blood–brain distribution. *Advanced Drug Delivery Reviews* **54**(3):291–313.

89. Rishton, G.M., LaBonte, K., Williams, A.J., Kassam, K., and Kolovanov, E. 2006. Computational approaches to the prediction of blood–brain barrier permeability: a comparative analysis of central nervous system drugs versus secretase inhibitors for Alzheimer's disease. *Current Opinion in Drug Discovery & Development* **9**(3):303–313.

90. Yu, N., Hayik, S.A., Wang, B., Liao, N., Reynolds, C.H., and Merz, K.M. Jr. 2006. Assigning the protonation states of the key aspartates in β-secretase using QM/MM X-ray structure refinement. *Journal of Chemical Theory and Computation* **2**(4):1057–1069.

91. Polgar, T. and Keserue, G.M. 2006. Ensemble docking into flexible active sites: critical evaluation of FlexE against JNK-3 and β-secretase. *Journal of Chemical Information and Modeling* **46**(4):1795–1805.

92. Polgar, T. and Keserue, G.M. 2005. Virtual screening for β-secretase (BACE1) inhibitors reveals the importance of protonation states at Asp32 and Asp228. *Journal of Medicinal Chemistry* **48**(11):3749–3755.

93. Bhisetti, G.R., Saunders, J.O., Murcko, M.A., Lepre, C.A., Britt, S.D., Come, J.H., Deninger, D.D., and Wang, T. 2002. Preparation of β-carbolines and other inhibitors of BACE-1 aspartic proteinase useful against Alzheimer's and other BACE-mediated diseases. *Vertex Pharmaceuticals Incorporated*, WO-2002088101, p. 208.

94. Limongelli, V., Marinelli, L., Cosconati, S., Braun, H.A., Schmidt, B., and Novellino, E. 2007. Ensemble-docking approach on BACE-1: pharmacophore perception and guidelines for drug design. *ChemMedChem* **2**(5):667–678.

95. Maggiora, G.M. and Shanmugasundaram, V. 2005. An information-theoretic characterization of partitioned property spaces. *Journal of Mathematical Chemistry* **38**(1):1–20.

96. Bajorath, J. 2002. Integration of virtual and high-throughput screening. *Nature Reviews: Drug Discovery* **1**:882–894.

97. Maggiora, G.M. and Shanmugasundaram, V. 2004. Molecular similarity measures. In Bajorath, J, ed., *Chemoinformatics: Concepts, Methods and Tools for Drug Discovery*. Clifton, NJ: Humana Press, pp. 1–50.

98. Shanmugasundaram, V., Maggiora, G.M., and Lajiness, M.S. 2005. Hit-directed nearest-neighbor searching. *Journal of Medicinal Chemistry* **48**(1):240–248.

99. Willett, P. 2003. Similarity-based approaches to virtual screening. *Biochemical Society Transactions* **31**:603–606.

100. Raymond, J.W., Jalaie, M., and Bradley, M.P. 2004. Conditional probability: a new fusion method for merging disparate virtual screening results. *Journal of Chemical Information and Computer Sciences* **44**(2):601–609.

101. Sheridan Robert, P. and Kearsley Simon, K. 2002. Why do we need so many chemical similarity search methods? *Drug Discovery Today* **7**(17):903–911.

102. Fujimoto, T., Matsushita, Y., Gouda, H., Yamaotsu, N., and Hirono, S. 2008. In silico multi-filter screening approaches for developing novel β-secretase inhibitors. *Bioorganic and Medicinal Chemistry Letters* **18**(9):2771–2775.

103. Maslow, K. 2008. 2008 Alzheimer's disease facts and figures. *Alzheimer's and Dementia* **4**(2):110–133.

PHARMACOLOGICAL MODELS FOR PRECLINICAL TESTING: FROM MOUSE TO DOG TO NONHUMAN PRIMATES

Jason L. Eriksen,[1] *Michael Paul Murphy,*[2] *and Elizabeth Head*[2]

[1]Department of Pharmacological and Pharmaceutical Sciences, University of Houston, Houston, TX and [2]Department of Molecular and Cellular Biochemistry and the Sanders-Brown Center on Aging, University of Kentucky, Lexington, KY

7.1 INTRODUCTION

Postmortem studies of the brains of patients with Alzheimer's disease (AD) demonstrate a progressive accumulation of senile plaques and neurofibrillary tangles, and a significant loss of synapses and neurons [1, 2]. Convincing evidence suggests that there is a strong mechanistic link between the accumulation of a protein found in senile plaques, beta-amyloid (Aβ), and altered processing of its precursor protein, amyloid precursor protein (APP) in AD [3]. Aβ protein is produced from the larger APP molecule through β- and γ-secretase cleavage, two sequential enzymatic activities. APP is an integral membrane protein containing a single transmembrane domain and first undergoes cleavage by β-secretase APP-cleaving enzyme 1 (BACE is also known as BACE1 – the isoform that is predominately localized in the brain), resulting in production of an N-terminal secreted fragment of APP and a membrane anchored C-terminal fragment (C99) [4]. The C99 fragment is cleaved by γ-secretase within a small but variable region of its transmembrane domain, resulting in the production of Aβ peptides of varying lengths. The majority of Aβ species produced is 40 amino acids long (Aβ_{40}), but a small proportion (<10%) is slightly longer (Aβ_{42}) [5]. The minor Aβ_{42} species is extremely amyloidogenic, and accumulation of aggregated Aβ_{42} results in the formation of senile plaques [6]. In familial forms of AD, mutations in APP favor production of the longest forms of the protein, enhancing the production of aggregation-prone and neurotoxic Aβ_{42} peptides. APP can also be alternatively processed through the non-amyloidogenic α-secretase pathway, resulting in a shorter P3 peptide fragment and a longer form of the secreted peptide (sAPPα) [5].

BACE: Lead Target for Orchestrated Therapy of Alzheimer's Disease, Edited by Varghese John
Copyright © 2010 John Wiley & Sons, Inc.

The steady accumulation of $A\beta_{42}$ peptide fosters the assembly of $A\beta$ into progressively higher-order structures, from dimers all the way up to the insoluble plaques that accumulate in the brain. Soluble assembled forms of the peptide are also directly toxic, and as the amount of $A\beta$ increases, neurons start to suffer deleterious consequences. Affected neurons develop neurofibrillary tangles composed of the cytoskeletal protein tau, ultimately leading to widespread neuronal dysfunction and loss [7]. It is the loss of neurons that causes the severe memory deficit that eventually leads to the inability of patients to sustain normal daily cognitive function. Thus, a steady accumulation of $A\beta$ levels results in downstream pathological events in the brain and researchers have developed the amyloid cascade hypothesis, which posits that $A\beta$ is an initial causative factor in the development of AD [6].

Although the range of data supporting the amyloid cascade hypothesis is compelling, the strongest evidence for the amyloid cascade is genetic. Autosomal dominant mutations that cause familial AD are predominantly within two proteins: APP, the substrate from which $A\beta$ originates, and in presenilins, part of the γ-secretase enzyme complex in the pathway that produces $A\beta$. Many familial mutations have now been identified (an up to date list is maintained at http://www.alzforum.org/res/com/mut/). Mutations in the presenilins lead to a shift in the production of $A\beta$ toward the long, more amyloidogenic forms, generally seen as an increase in the ratio of $A\beta_{42}:A\beta_{40}$; although there is some debate on the issue. This phenomenon is usually thought to reflect a loss rather than a gain of function [8, 9]. Disease causing mutations in APP are clustered either within the $A\beta$ region or in close proximity to the β- or γ-secretase cleavage sites (outlined in Chapter 1).

Given the well-defined enzymatic pathways that have been identified in human AD, both γ-secretase and β-secretase have been targeted for lowering $A\beta$ production *in vivo*. Early efforts to target γ-secretase were successful with the development of extremely potent, selective, blood–brain permeable compounds. Unfortunately, extended preclinical dosing studies with γ-secretase inhibitors demonstrated these compounds had adverse effects in mouse models and were unsuitable for clinical use. Although these compounds displayed excellent $A\beta$ lowering ability, it became clear that γ-secretase enzyme is an important but promiscuous enzyme that cleaves multiple substrates. In addition to blocking $A\beta$ production, the inhibition of γ-secretase also inhibited the production of other key molecules, such as Notch, an important regulatory component of the immune system function, leading to significant adverse side effects [10–12].

BACE1 is also considered to be a very promising target for the lowering of $A\beta$, as this enzyme activity is also an essential step in the generation of the potentially neurotoxic $A\beta_{42}$ peptides in AD. In preclinical studies of BACE1 inhibitors, transgenic mouse models of AD demonstrated brain $A\beta$ lowering after inhibition of the enzyme. The development of a robust, potent, and active BACE1 inhibitor *in vivo* has been quite difficult because of the open catalytic structure of this enzyme, coupled with the presence of numerous charged residues. BACE1 is an aspartic protease with a wide catalytic cleft, similar to HIV protease and renin [13], requiring multiple binding sites in order to achieve adequate affinities. As a consequence, inhibitors of these enzymes tend to be quite large in size [14]. Small molecules are typically favored in blood–brain barrier permeability; however, the development of

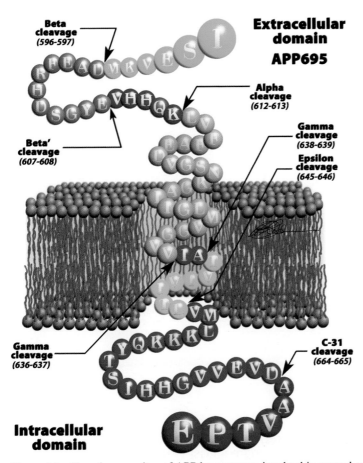

Figure 1.1   Key cleavage sites of APP by proteases involved in normal and aberrant processing.

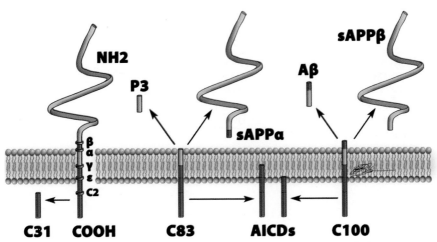

Figure 1.2   Alternative cleavage patterns of APP generate distinct extracellular, transmembrane, and intracytoplasmic fragments.

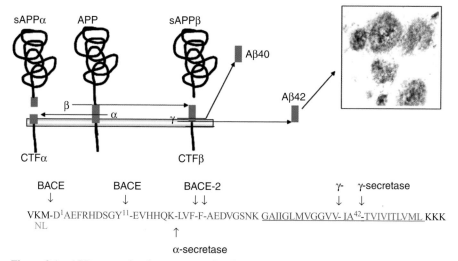

Figure 3.1 APP processing by secretases leading to the formation of APP fragments of which $A\beta_{1-42}$ and $A\beta_{11-42}$ are toxic forms.

$M^{-21L}AQALPWLLLWMGAGVLPAHG$T^{1P}QHGIRLPLRSG
LGGAPLGLRLPR^{24P}↓E^{25P}TDEEP^{30P}EEPGRRGSFV^{40P}E^1
MVDNLRGKSGQGYYVEMTV^{20}GSPPQTLNILV**DTG**SS
NFAV^{40}GAAPHPFLHRYYQRQLSSTY^{60}RDLRKGVYVP
YTQGKWEGEL^{80}GTDLVSIPHGP∧VTVRANIA^{100}AITES
DKFFI∧GSNWEGILG^{120}LAYAEIARPDDSLEPFFDSL^{140}
VKQTHVPCNLFSLQLCGAGFP^{160}L∧QSEVLASVGGSM
IIGGID^{180}HSLYTGSLWYTPIRREWYYE^{200}VIIVRVEING
QDLKMDCKEY^{220}NYDKSIV**DSG**TTNLRLPKKV^{240}FEA
AVKSIKAASSTEKFPDG^{260}FWLGEQLVCWQAGTTPW
NIF^{280}PVISLYLMGEVT∧QSFRITI^{300}LPQQYLRPVEDVA
TSQDDCY^{320}KFAISQSSTGTVMGAVIMEG^{340}FYVVFDR
ARKRIGFAVSACH^{360}VHDEFRTAAVEGPFVTLDME^{380}
DCGYNIPQTDESTLMTIAYV^{400}MAAICALFMLPLCLM
VCQWR^{420}CLRCLRQQHDDFADDISLLK^{440}

Figure 3.2 The primary structure of BACE with features relevant to the enzyme cellular trafficking and functions.

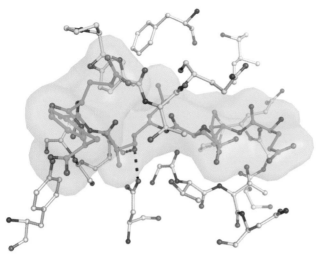

Figure 5.2   X-ray crystal structure of BACE protease domain in complex with **OM99-2** (PDB accession number 1FKN). **OM99-2** and its molecular surface are indicated in green. BACE flap residues are drawn in yellow, all other residues in the proximity of the ligand are drawn in grey.

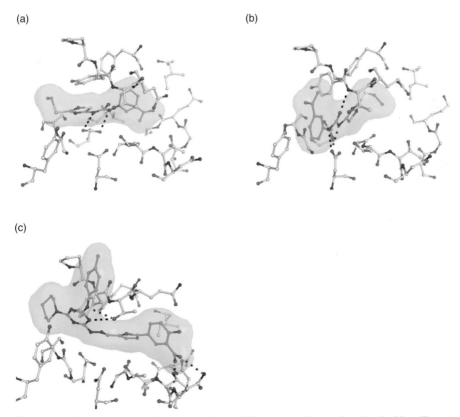

(a)

(b)

(c)

Figure 5.4   Binding modes of compounds **1** and **3** as derived by molecular docking. Two preferred docking modes have been reported for compound **1** (a, b) and one for compound **2** (c).

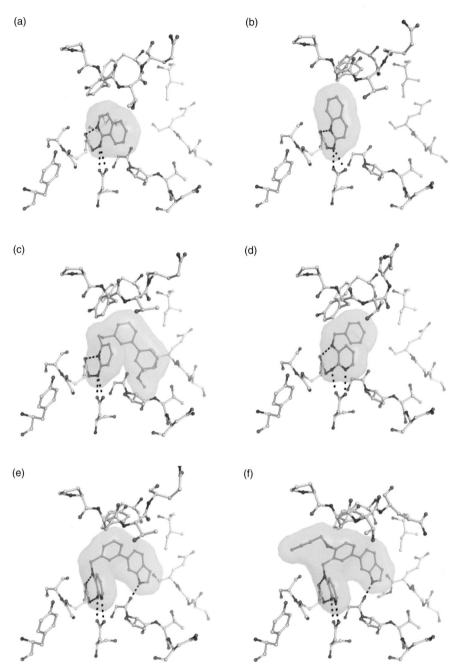

Figure 5.6   X-ray crystal structures of BACE protease domain in complex with the compounds (a) **4**, PDB accession number 2OHK, (b) **5**, 2OHL, (c) **7**, 2OHQ, (d) **8**, 2OHM, (e) **9**, 2OHT, and (f) **10**, 2OHU.

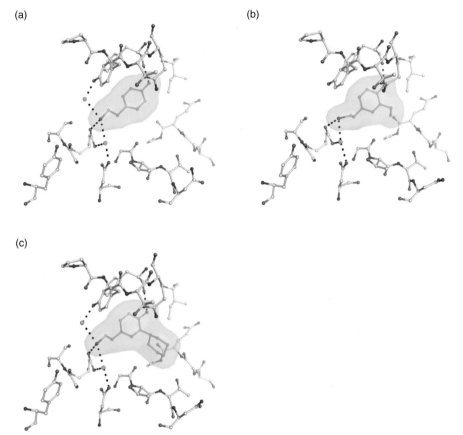

Figure 5.8 X-ray crystal structures of BACE protease domain in complex with the compounds (a) **12**, PDB accession number 2BRA, (b) **13**, 3BUG, and (c) **14**, 3BUH.

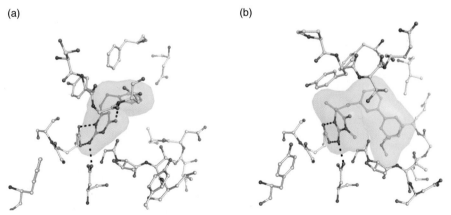

Figure 5.10 X-ray crystal structures of BACE protease domain in complex with the compounds (a) **17**, PDB accession number 2V00 and (b) **20**, 2VA7.

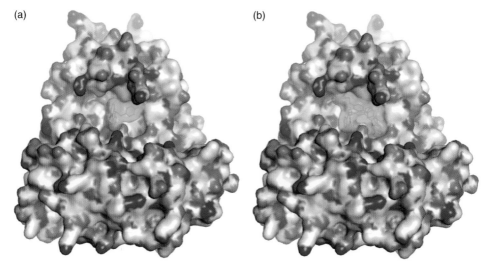

Figure 5.11 Composite volumes filled by experimentally identified fragments and fragment-derived BACE inhibitors. The volume filled by (a) the originally identified fragments **4, 5,** and **12** compared with (b) the fragment-derived inhibitors **10, 14,** and **20.** Ligands and composite molecular surfaces are drawn in green. The molecular surface of BACE protease is colored by atom types. Flap residues 70–75 have been omitted for clarity.

*M^{-21L}AQALPWLLLWMGAGVLPAHG*T^{1P}QHGIRLPLRSG
LGGAPLGLRLPR^{24P}↓E^{25P}TDEEP^{30P}EEPGRRGSFV^{40P}E^{1}
MVDNLRGKSGQGYYVEMTV^{20}GSPPQTLNILV**DTG**SS
NFAV^{40}GAAPHPFLHRYYQRQLSSTY^{60}RDLRKGVYVP
YTQGKWEGEL^{80}GTDLVSIPHGPNVTVRANIA^{100}AITES
DKFFINGSNWEGILG^{120}LAYAEIARPDDSLEPFFDSL^{140}
VKQTHVPCNLFSLQLCGAGFP^{160}LNQSEVLASVGGSM
IIGGID^{180}HSLYTGSLWYTPIRREWYYE^{200}VIIVRVEING
QDLKMDCKEY^{220}NYDKSIV**DSG**TTNLRLPKKV^{240}FEA
AVKSIKAASSTEKFPDG^{260}FWLGEQLVCWQAGTTPW
NIF^{280}PVISLYLMGEVTNQSFRITI^{300}LPQQYLRPVEDVA
TSQDDCY^{320}KFAISQSSTGTVMGAVIMEG^{340}FYVVFDR
ARKRIGFAVSACH^{360}VHDEFRTAAVEGPFVTLDME^{380}
DCGYNIPQTDESTLMTIAYV^{400}MAAICALFMLPLCLM
VCQWR^{420}CLRCLRQQHDDFADDISLLK^{440}

Figure 6.1 The primary structure of BACE. Prominent features of BACE amino acid sequence are highlighted: a 21-aa leader sequence (M^{-21L} ... G^{-1L}) and a 24-aa prosegment (T^{1P} ... R^{24P}) precedes the mature enzyme sequence starting at the E^{25P} and extending to K^{440} (according to the sequence of the enzyme isolated from human brain). BACE contains the classic catalytic triad D^{32}TG ... D^{228}SG, six cysteine residues paired to form three disulfide bridges: Cys^{155}–Cys^{359}, Cys^{217}–Cys^{382}, and Cys^{269}–Cys^{319}, and four glycosylated asparagines, 92, 111, 162, and 293. Residue S^{392} precedes the BACE transmembrane domain of 27-aa (T^{393} ... R^{420}), and a cytoplasmic tail of 21 residues (R^{420} ... K^{440}) completes the primary structure.

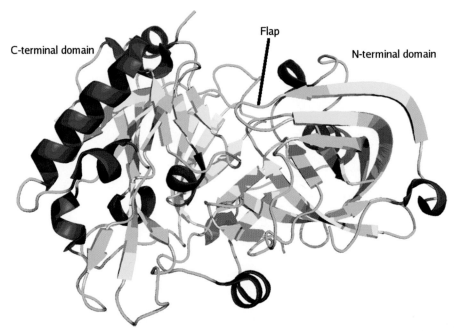

Figure 6.2   Ribbon diagram of BACE.

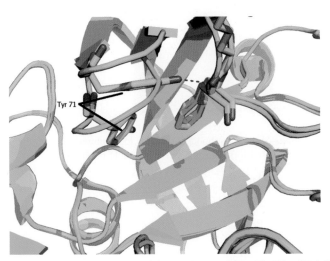

Figure 6.3   Close-up view of flap region (residues 70–75) of BACE, showing open (apo) form in cyan, and the closed (ligand bound) form in green. Note the alternate rotamer for Tyr71.

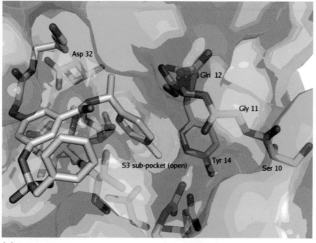

(a)

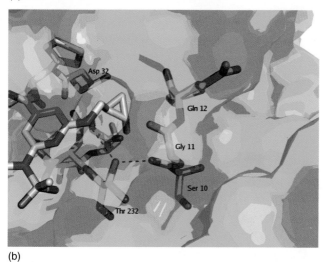

(b)

Figure 6.4   Surface representations of the S3 subpocket and 10s loop interactions: (a) the open form of the S3sp and (b) the closed form of the S3sp, with the H-bond formed between Ser10 and Thr232.

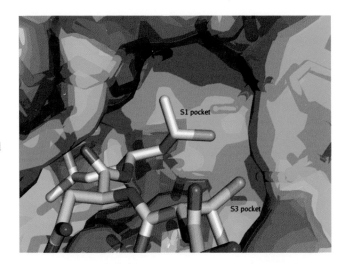

Figure 6.6   BACE S1 specificity pocket, shown bound to a hydroxyethylene peptidomimetic inhibitor OM99-2 (PDB entry 1FKN [29]).

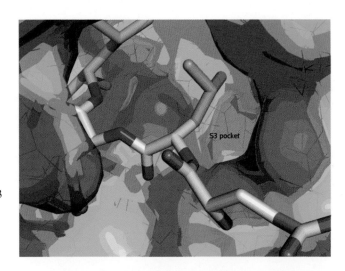

Figure 6.7   BACE S3 specificity pocket, shown bound to OM99-2 (PDB entry 1FK [29]).

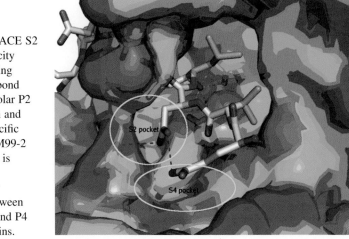

Figure 6.8   BACE S2 and S4 specificity pockets, showing the hydrogen bond between the polar P2 Asn side chain and the BACE specific Arg235. In OM99-2 (shown), there is an additional intramolecular interaction between the P2 (Asn) and P4 (Glu) side chains.

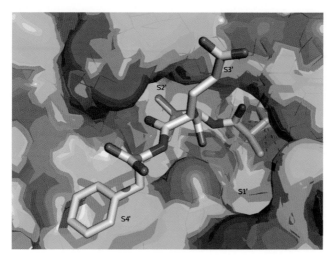

Figure 6.9 BACE prime side specificity pockets (S1′-S4′), shown bound to hydroxyethylene inhibitor OM-003 (PDB entry 1M4H [68]).

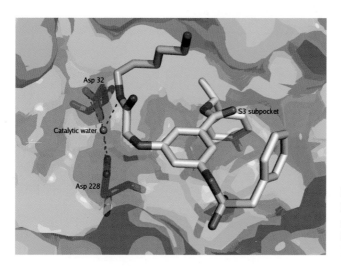

Figure 6.10 Nonpeptidomimetic carbenimine BACE inhibitor (PDB entry 1TQF [69]).

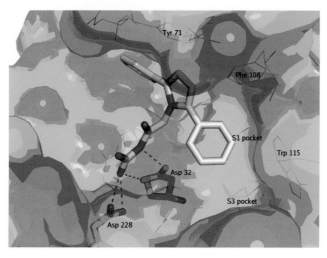

Figure 6.11 Nonpeptidomimetic acylguanidine BACE inhibitor (PDB entry 2QU2 [73]).

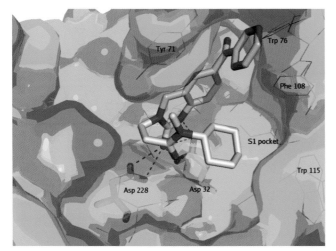

Figure 6.12 Nonpeptidomimetic dihydroquinazoline BACE inhibitor (PDB entry 2Q11 [36]).

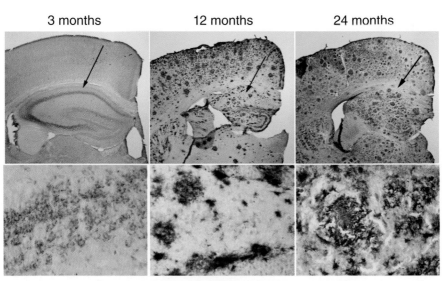

Figure 7.1 Neuropathology in a transgenic mouse with age. Cortical and hippocampal immunostaining for $A\beta_{1-16}$ in the APP/PS1 transgenic mouse shows that at 3 months of age, $A\beta$ can be seen within neurons in the hippocampus (arrow) although no plaques are present. As animals age (12 months and 24 months), the extent of $A\beta$ increases dramatically with plaques becoming more compact with time (arrow). Brain tissue kindly provided by Dr. Karen Duff (Columbia University Medical Center, NY, NY).

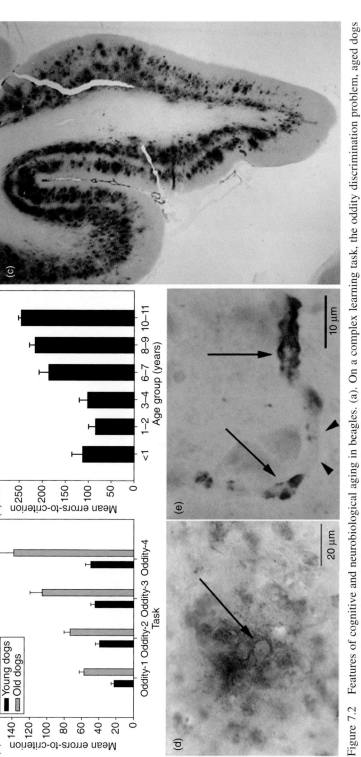

Figure 7.2 Features of cognitive and neurobiological aging in beagles. (a). On a complex learning task, the oddity discrimination problem, aged dogs commit more errors when reaching criterion levels of responding relative to young animals. In addition, progressive increases in error scores for each oddity problem suggest that aged dogs solve each successive problem individually whereas young dogs learn the concept of the task. (b). Acquisition of a spatial memory task is age-dependent in dogs and deficits first appear in middle age (6–7 years). (c). Significant Aβ neuropathology can be observed using antibodies against $Aβ_{1-16}$ and immunohistochemistry in the prefrontal cortex of aged dogs and can accumulate across all cortical layers. (d). A higher magnification photograph showing that intact neurons (arrow) may be surrounded by clouds of diffuse Aβ (brown – $Aβ_{1-16}$ immunostaining) in the aged canine brain (counterstained with cresyl violet). (e). In addition to Aβ in diffuse plaques, subsets of blood vessels also accumulate Aβ (brown – $Aβ_{1-40}$ immunostaining – arrows) whereas other regions of the same vessel may be free of Aβ (arrowheads). Bars in (a) and (b) represent means, and error bars represent standard errors of the mean and reproduced or modified with permission from Elsevier Limited [17, 92].

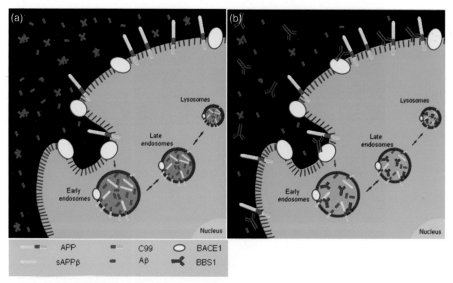

	APP		C99	○	BACE1
	sAPPβ		Aβ		BBS1

Figure 10.1   Illustration of anti β-site antibody mediating the inhibition of Aβ production via the endocytic pathway. (a) Aβ peptides are generated by two pathways: the secretory and the endocytic pathways, after which the generated peptides are either secreted or degraded in the cell. For simplicity purposes, only the endocytic pathway of Aβ production is illustrated. Accordingly, cell surface APP molecules, which are in close interaction with BACE1 molecules, are internalized into the early endosomes where the acidic pH favors BACE1 cleavage. The immediate product of BACE1 cleavage, C99, is further cleaved by γ-secretase to release Aβ peptides, which in turn can be either secreted or degraded in the cell. (b) The addition of BBS1, anti-APP β-site antibody, results in APP binding on the surface, flowing co-internalization of both APP and the antibody into the early endosomes. Within the endosomes, antibody binding is speculated to interfere with BACE1 cleavage and thus restrict Aβ production. In such a scenario, both the immediate products of BACE1 cleavage, soluble APPβ and C99, and Aβ levels are reduced. Since Aβ peptides are generated inside the cell, inhibition of its generation will be reflected in both the intra- and extracellular Aβ pools. The production of Aβ through the secretory pathway is not illustrated for simplicity purposes.

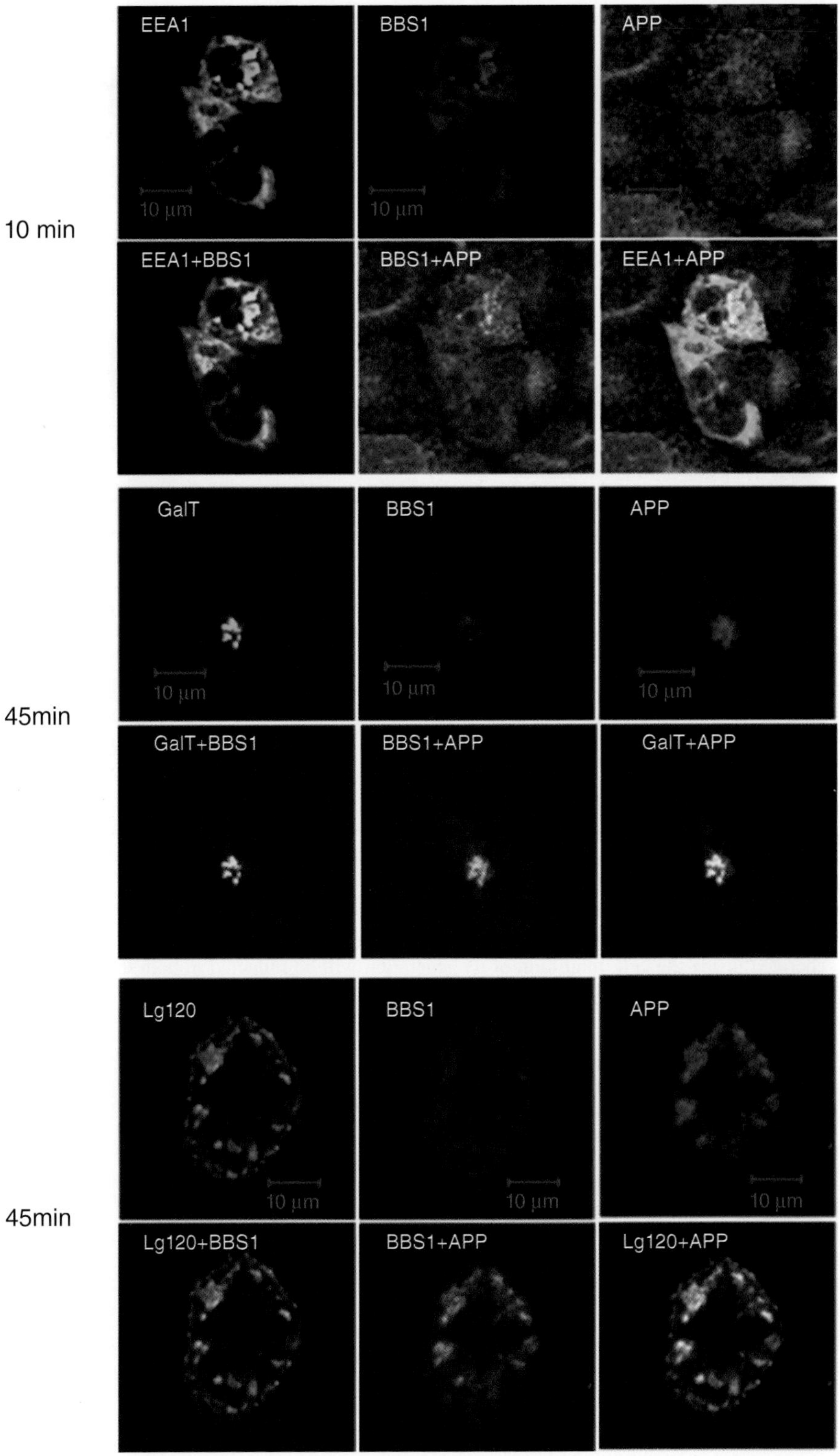

10 min

EEA1 | BBS1 | APP
10 μm | 10 μm |

EEA1+BBS1 | BBS1+APP | EEA1+APP

45min

GalT | BBS1 | APP
10 μm | 10 μm | 10 μm

GalT+BBS1 | BBS1+APP | GalT+APP

45min

Lg120 | BBS1 | APP
10 μm | 10 μm | 10 μm

Lg120+BBS1 | BBS1+APP | Lg120+APP

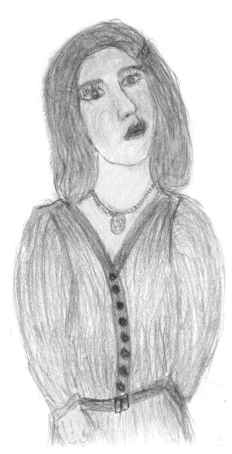

Image 1   Sheila used sharp pointed pencil crayons to create many pictures of women. The small repetitive hatched lines with which she painstakingly filled areas of the dress, skin, and hair, were a means to calm her compulsive tendencies and agitated state (mild cognitive impairment).

Figure 10.2   BBS1 internalization and trafficking in CHO cells overexpressing APP. Mammalian expression vectors consisting of either EEA1, Lg120, or GalT fused to eGFP, were used to label the early endosomes, lysosomes, and Golgi apparatus, respectively. Twenty-four hours post transfection, BBS1 antibody was administered to the growing media and incubated at 37°C for different intervals. Cells were then fixed and permeabilized and anti-mouse secondary antibody conjugated to Cy3 (red) was added to follow BBS1 localization. Anti-APP carboxy terminal antibody followed by secondary antibody conjugated to Cy5 (purple) was used to detect APP localization. Cell labeling was visualized using LSM-510 Zeiss confocal microscope and a co-localization software. The bottom panels at each time point represent merged images as indicated. Bars = 10μm.

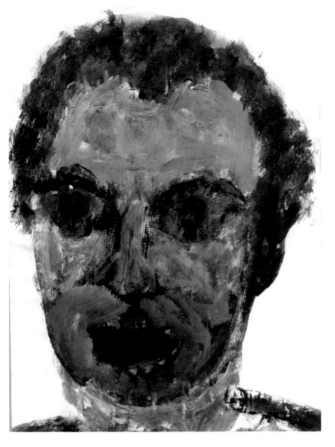

Image 3   Joe was struggling with severe paranoia which he portrayed in the glaring eyes of this portrait. A mild mannered man, he repeatedly used the art to express anger and fear that lay hidden behind his unemotional facade. The rich layering of liquid paint (gouache) and dramatic use of color lends expressive power to the work (moderate stage dementia).

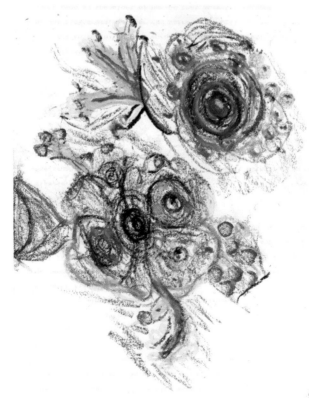

Image 5   This is Alice's attempt to copy a still life. It was a great achievement, given that her perception of figure and ground was already seriously impaired. She made joyful use of oil pastel to create many colorful works (late stage dementia).

potent BACE1 inhibitors that can cross the blood–brain barrier with acceptable pharmacokinetic properties has proven to be challenging.

Since the structure of aspartic protease inhibitors predisposes them to undergo rapid metabolism, resulting to poor systemic exposure, the early development of BACE1 inhibitors that were active *in* vivo was problematic. Additionally, the structural requirements for inhibitors that bind and inhibit aspartic proteases typically impart strong susceptibility to p-glycoprotein transporters associated with the blood–brain barrier, additionally reducing the concentrations of compounds such as BACE1 inhibitors *in vivo*. To overcome these challenges, much of the early work on BACE1 inhibitors *in vivo* used intracranial administration of compounds [15–17], or peripheral administration of very high doses of compound in mouse models of AD [18–21], but it became evident that the use of these compounds would be difficult to translate beyond the initial preclinical evaluation for these reasons. The lack of potent inhibitors also possessing acceptable pharmacokinetics and brain penetration properties has prevented the further validation of BACE1 inhibitors in other animals such as canines and nonhuman primates, which naturally develop similar types of human cognitive decline and neuropathology. In contrast, recent BACE1 inhibitors that have been used *in vivo* utilize non-hydroxyethylamine and tertiary carbinamine backbones similar to that of HIV protease inhibitors [21–25]. These compounds have shown promise in overcoming many of the previous problems and display generally good passive membrane permeability and limited p-glycoprotein susceptibility.

7.2   BACE1 AND MOUSE MODELS OF AD

Transgenic mouse models of AD have been critically important in developing BACE1 inhibitors. Indeed, it was research using mouse model systems that led to the discovery that BACE1 may be considered to be one of the most promising enzymatic targets for slowing AD. Much of the early momentum for the development of BACE1 inhibitors came from observations that few phenotypic abnormalities have been identified in BACE1 knockout mice ($Bace1^{-/-}$) [26, 27], and these lines also have very low Aβ levels in brain tissue, a lack of amyloid plaques, and increased α-secretase processing of APP [28–30].

To address the role of BACE1 in AD, $Bace1^{-/-}$ mice have been crossed with transgenic mouse models that recapitulate the key features of human AD pathology. Over the past decade, a large number of transgenic mouse models that develop amyloid plaque pathology have been developed, typically by overexpressing human APP containing mutations associated with early onset AD [31]. Commonly used lines include PDAPP mice, containing a minigene construct encoding APPV717F[32], the Tg 2576 mouse model, expressing a human APP cDNA transgene with the K670M/N671NL double mutation (APPswe) [33], and mouse crosses of mutant APP mice with mice expressing mutant presenilin transgenes (APP/PS1) [34–36] (Fig. 7.1). The pathology of the vast majority of APP mice includes diffuse amyloid deposits and dense cored amyloid plaques resembling the senile plaques in AD; the cored plaques in transgenic mice are typically surrounded by dystrophic neurites

3 months   12 months   24 months

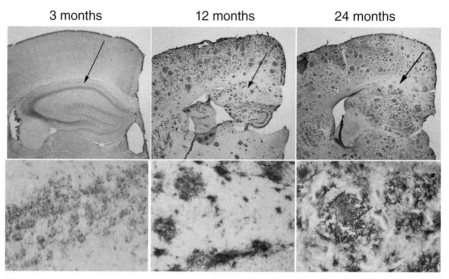

Figure 7.1   Neuropathology in a transgenic mouse with age. Cortical and hippocampal immunostaining for $A\beta_{1-16}$ in the APP/PS1 transgenic mouse shows that at 3 months of age, $A\beta$ can be seen within neurons in the hippocampus (arrow) although no plaques are present. As animals age (12 months and 24 months), the extent of $A\beta$ increases dramatically with plaques becoming more compact with time (arrow). Brain tissue kindly provided by Dr. Karen Duff (Columbia University Medical Center, NY, NY). (See color insert.)

associated with increased amyloid deposits. However, it should be emphasized that despite the robust amyloid accumulation observed in these mouse models, they do not fully recapitulate the AD phenotype; none of these models develop widespread neuronal loss or the intracellular neuronal tangles found in AD [37–39].

Using transgenic mouse models, BACE1 was unequivocally shown to be essential for amyloid formation on the AD phenotype, and this enzyme was shown to be the primary β-secretase that is responsible for Aβ generation in the brain. In one experiment, Tg2576 were crossed with $Bace1^{-/-}$ line. In comparison with $Bace1^{+/-}$·Tg2576 or $Bace1^{+/+}$·Tg2576 mice, bigenic $Bace1^{-/-}$·Tg2576 lacked brain Aβ, APPsβ, and C99 fragments, and failed to develop amyloid plaques [29]. Similar findings were reported in another APP overexpressing BACE1-deficient mouse line [40]. Manipulation of BACE1 has also been used to test the impact of Aβ expression on memory function. Although reports varied by the degree of impairment, the Tg2576 and APP/PS1 crosses develop robust memory defects. In studies of young, pre-plaque Tg2576 mice with high levels of soluble Aβ, they were shown to have significant memory dysfunction compared with their wild-type counterparts. When the Tg2576 line was crossed with $Bace1^{-/-}$, memory deficits failed to develop in the $Bace1^{-/-}$·Tg2576 bigenic line [30]. Similarly, ablation of BACE1 in APP/PS1 rescues both the aggressive Aβ accumulation and Aβ-associated memory deficits normally observed in these animals [40–43]. These results showed that the accumulation of Aβ peptides was responsible, at least in part, for age-associated cognitive impairments that develop in these transgenic mouse lines.

While the loss of BACE1 does not appear to have gross phenotypic effects, the loss of this enzymatic activity is not inconsequential. Although the initial reports of *Bace1$^{-/-}$* mice showed these animals to be relatively normal [26, 27], follow-up reports of *Bace1$^{-/-}$* lines have demonstrated enhanced early lethality [44], increased evidence of cognitive deficits [40], and effects upon early developmental processes [45, 46]. Recent studies have identified neuregulin-1 and the sodium channel β-subunit as BACE1 substrates, implicating this enzyme in myelination and neuronal activity, two pathways that are implicated in cognitive function. BACE1 is required for specific hippocampal memory processes, and complete *Bace1* suppression results in mechanism-based toxicities [30, 40, 42], and these *Bace1$^{-/-}$* animals also exhibit hyperactivity and enhanced locomotion [40, 44]. The studies suggest that complete inhibition of BACE1 is likely to be therapeutically undesirable, but a further understanding of partial BACE1 inactivation is critically important. From a clinical viewpoint, partial suppression of BACE1 is likely to have little effect on normal learning or memory processes, but may be sufficient to target Aβ-associated pathology and cognitive deficits.

Although the methods of administration vary widely, pharmacological studies of BACE1 inhibitors in mouse models of AD have shown potent effects on the production of Aβ. The majority of previously reported BACE1 inhibitors have used peptidomimetic compounds, notably peptidic transition-state isosteres and derivative compounds. The compounds efficiently inhibit BACE, when injected by direct cranial administration [15–17], parenteral dosing [18–21], or orally in combination with p-glycoprotein inhibitors [18–21]. Although these compounds can lower Aβ production, their inability to efficiently cross the blood–brain barrier has been problematic for clinical translation. More recent reports have introduced peripherally administered compounds that can penetrate the blood–brain barrier with greater efficiency. These early preclinical successes have strengthened the support for the eventual use of BACE1 inhibitors in human clinical trials.

The relatively low cost of transgenic mice has led to the widespread adoption of these animals for AD preclinical studies. While the use of these mouse models has proven to be convenient for basic pharmacokinetic studies, and has imparted significant scientific knowledge concerning AD pathology, the differences in biochemistry of rodent models to those of human patients has made it difficult to predict the effectiveness of these therapies when they are extended into human clinical trials [47]. As we will discuss in the next section, although the canine model of aging has not been widely employed for AD preclinical trials, the extensive cognitive repertoire of these animals, exquisite sensitivity to age-related impairments, and a unique biochemistry with age-related degeneration that is surprisingly similar to human patients suggests that the use of dog models is strongly appropriate for advanced preclinical evaluation of BACE1 inhibitors.

7.3 TESTING BACE INHIBITORS IN THE CANINE MODEL OF HUMAN AGING AND AD

Despite successful modeling of numerous aspects of aging and AD, no single animal model has fully replicated *all* aspects of human aging and AD. Thus, it is necessary

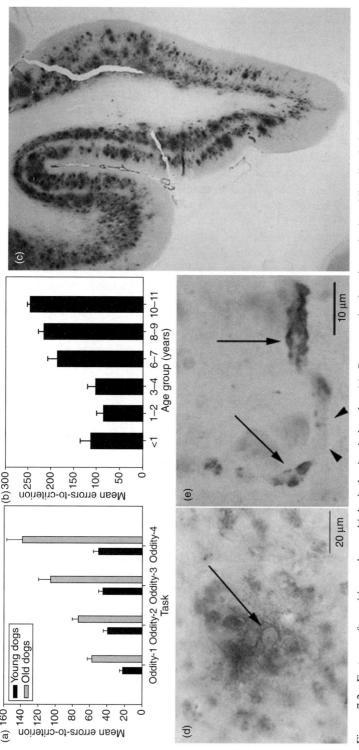

Figure 7.2 Features of cognitive and neurobiological aging in beagles. (a). On a complex learning task, the oddity discrimination problem, aged dogs commit more errors when reaching criterion levels of responding relative to young animals. In addition, progressive increases in error scores for each oddity problem suggest that aged dogs solve each successive problem individually whereas young dogs learn the concept of the task. (b). Acquisition of a spatial memory task is age-dependent in dogs and deficits first appear in middle age (6–7 years). (c). Significant Aβ neuropathology can be observed using antibodies against Aβ$_{1-16}$ and immunohistochemistry in the prefrontal cortex of aged dogs and can accumulate across all cortical layers. (d). A higher magnification photograph showing that intact neurons (arrow) may be surrounded by clouds of diffuse Aβ (brown – Aβ$_{1-16}$ immunostaining) in the aged canine brain (counterstained with cresyl violet). (e). In addition to Aβ in diffuse plaques, subsets of blood vessels also accumulate Aβ (brown – Aβ$_{1-40}$ immunostaining – arrows) whereas other regions of the same vessel may be free of Aβ (arrowheads). Bars in (a) and (b) represent means, and error bars represent standard errors of the mean and reproduced or modified with permission from Elsevier Limited [17, 92].

to continue to develop additional models, to take advantage of unique aspects of each model, and to combine information from convergent studies. Aging research with canines suggests that this model complements existing models but with distinctive characteristics that support unique research opportunities. Indeed, testing BACE inhibitors in the canine model may provide strong support for specific formulations that can be taken to human clinical trials as dogs capture many of the key features of AD, including cognitive decline and neuropathology.

7.3.1   Cognitive Decline in Aging in Canines

Canines are highly trainable animals that are capable of mastering complex learning tasks, making them an excellent model for studying the effects of aging on learning and memory. Age-dependent cognitive deficits in canines can be observed on many different measures of learning and memory. Deficits in complex learning tasks such as size concept learning [48, 49], oddity discrimination learning [50, 51] (Fig. 7.2a), size discrimination learning [52, 53], and spatial learning [54] with age in dogs has been demonstrated. Tasks sensitive to prefrontal cortex function, including reversal learning and visuospatial working memory, also deteriorate with age [52, 53, 55]. Furthermore, egocentric spatial learning and reversal, measuring the ability of animals to select a correct object based on their own body orientation, is age-sensitive [54]. In canines, a measure of spatial attention that was originally developed in nonhuman primates was also vulnerable to aging [56, 57]. Interestingly, on simple learning tasks and procedural learning measures, aged dogs performed equally as well as younger animals [58], suggesting that a subset of cognitive functions remains intact with age as it does in aging humans.

Memory also declines with age in dogs both for information about objects and location in space (spatial) [58–60]. The spatial memory task, in particular, will be useful for preclinical studies of BACE inhibitors as it can be used repeatedly with minimal practice effects in longitudinal studies to determine if memory improvements can occur in response to treatment [61]. Furthermore, studies of the time course of the development of cognitive decline demonstrate that deterioration in spatial ability occurs early in the aging process in canines, between 6 and 7 years of age [55] (Fig. 7.2b), and provides researchers with guidelines for ages at which to start a treatment study. For example, using BACE inhibitors to prevent cognitive decline might be best implemented when animals are younger than 6 years. Studies that are intended to test the hypothesis that BACE inhibitors can be used as treatments for AD might be best administered in animals that are over 8 years of age.

Another key feature of canines that is similar to that observed in humans is that cognitive dysfunction is not an inevitable consequence of aging in humans [62]; recent research has focused on the distinction between those who retain function and those who show decline such as mild cognitive impairment (MCI) [63, 64]. Using a battery of cognitive tests, aged canines are clearly separable into three groups, categorized as (1) successful agers, (2) impaired canines, whose scores fell two standard deviations above the mean of the young animals, and (3) severely impaired canines, who failed to learn [65]. This clustering of aged canines on the basis of cognitive ability is consistent with cognitive aging in rats, nonhuman primates [66–70], and humans [71]. In terms of the pattern and severity of cognitive decline, the canine may parallel normal aging, MCI, and potentially mild AD in humans, which will be very useful for preclinical studies of BACE inhibition.

7.3.2   Aβ and Aging in Canines

Aged canines are an excellent model for testing therapeutics that target Aβ as aging dogs naturally accumulate Aβ without requiring the overexpression of mutant human genes. Extracellular deposits of human-type Aβ [72, 73] develop during the aging process. Both BACE1 and canine β-APP are virtually identical to human APP (~98% homology), as established from the sequence published online for the canine genome (http://www.ensembl.org/Canis_familiaris/). The typical levels of canine Aβ that can be detected in the brain biochemically, are similar to reports in human brain [61]. Most of the Aβ deposits in the canine brain are of the diffuse subtype at the immunohistochemical level (Fig. 7.2c,d), but are fibrillar at the ultrastructural level and at an advanced stage, modeling early plaque formation in humans [74–76]. Similar to human AD, intracellular Aβ is also detectable with immunohistochemistry [77].

Paralleling the aged human brain, specific brain regions show differential vulnerabilities to Aβ [73, 78–85]. When Aβ plaques are characterized in different areas of the brain, each region shows a different age of onset [81]. Initial Aβ deposits occur in a 3- to 4-year time window that starts between the ages of 8 and 9 years in canines, suggesting that longitudinal studies for evaluating interventions to slow or halt Aβ are feasible. Thus, as with information gained from cognitive testing procedures, it is possible to target BACE inhibition either using preventative approaches (i.e., before dogs are 8 years of age) or treatment approaches (dogs over 9 years of age) to test for reductions in Aβ.

Age and cognitive status can predict Aβ pathology in discrete brain structures in canines. For example, canines with prefrontal cortex-dependent reversal learning deficits show significantly higher amounts of Aβ in this brain region [52]. On the other hand, canines deficient on a size discrimination learning task, thought to be sensitive to temporal lobe function, show large amounts of Aβ deposition in the entorhinal cortex [52]. Thus, cognitive decline in aged canines is associated with the accumulation of Aβ, similar to observations in human patients with AD [52, 86–93]. Thus, if BACE inhibition leads to decreases in Aβ deposition, cognitive outcomes might also be expected to improve if these two events are linked.

A common type of amyloidogenic pathology observed in both normal human brain aging and particularly in AD is the accumulation of cerebrovascular amyloid angiopathy (CAA) [94–96]. CAA may compromise the blood–brain barrier, impair vascular function (constriction and dilation) [97], and cause microhemorrhages [98]. Vascular and perivascular abnormalities and cerebrovascular Aβ pathology are frequently found in aged dogs [82, 99–105] (Fig. 7.2e). Vascular Aβ is primarily the shorter 1-40 species, which is identical in dogs and humans [106]. Overall, canines are thought to be a good natural model for examining CAA and treatments for CAA [107]. Thus, if BACE inhibitors are hypothesized to reduce Aβ, then the dog model might be very useful to determine whether the cerebrovasculature might also benefit from reduced pathology.

In summary, aged dogs may be a very useful preclinical testing system in which to determine if BACE inhibitors may be efficacious and safe for use in human clinical trials. Due to similarities between the dog and humans in terms of responsiveness and in drug handling and metabolism, the dog can be considered to be a useful model for chronic BACE treatment in humans. Indeed, dogs are unique in that they were used to establish efficacy and safety in the majority of several drugs commonly used in humans. For example, most statins currently on the market were developed in canines and have been used in chronic studies of over 2 years in length at doses relevant for humans [108, 109]. There is sufficient model development currently such that appropriately aged animals can be selected to measure outcomes on cognitive function and Aβ neuropathology either in prevention or treatment studies. Furthermore, longitudinal studies that can last many years, as is required in human clinical trials, can also be completed successfully in aged dogs as they are a long-lived species, and there are cognitive tasks that can be used repeatedly. Last, there have been several treatment studies completed using the canine model system and illustrate that it is possible to not only measure cognitive improvements [50, 57] but also to detect maintenance of cognitive function [61, 110] as well as reductions of Aβ [61] with the appropriate interventions.

7.4   BACE INHIBITORS AND NONHUMAN PRIMATES

Nonhuman primates are the closest to humans evolutionarily in brain organization and possibly function, and as such are an essential animal model system for the development of interventions to promote successful aging in humans. A variety of monkeys, including chimpanzees and rhesus monkeys, progressively accumulate amyloid and develop senile plaques, similar to that of aging humans [111–113]. However, subsequent studies now show that nonhuman primates accumulate the shorter, less toxic species of $A\beta_{1-40}$, which contrasts with the deposition of the longer, more toxic species $A\beta_{1-42}$ in humans and canines [114]. The latter Aβ type has been implicated in familial and sporadic forms of AD [115]. Furthermore, several newly identified compounds that reduce Aβ selectively reduce $A\beta_{1-42}$ but not $A\beta_{1-40}$, which is important when considering testing potential clinical therapeutics in nonhuman primates [116]. In humans, several studies show a link between the extent of Aβ deposition and dementia severity in AD [117]. Although a similar association has been observed in the canine model [118], there is a lack of evidence for a similar link in nonhuman primates [119].

However, there are significant biochemical and genetic similarities between humans and other primates, and thus there is a rationale for preclinical evaluation of BACE1 inhibitors in these animals, since the results of these studies may predict treatment in human patients. Until recently, the poor pharmacokinetic properties and lack of blood–brain barrier permeablity of BACE1 inhibitors precluded testing in primates. A new class of BACE1 tertiary carbinamine inhibitors, developed from previous isonicotinamide and isophthalate oxadiazole inhibitors, was recently reported as the first class of compounds capable of inhibiting BACE in higher animal species. One compound from this class, called TC-1, was demonstrated to be a selective and potent BACE1 inhibitor, with good membrane permeability and a lack of p-glycoprotein substrate. In rhesus monkey models, oral administration of TC-1, when coupled with ritonavir, an inhibitor of the TC-1 metabolizing enzyme CYP3A4, effectively lowered Aβ production in these animals [120]. Although this study represents the first publication of successful BACE1 inhibition in higher mammals, this area is under active investigation. A variety of new BACE inhibitors is likely to be on the horizon with improvements in metabolic stability and brain penetration.

7.5   FINAL REMARKS

AD is a devastating neurodegenerative disorder that is characterized by the development of extracellular senile plaques and intracellular neurofibrillary tangles in the brain. Generation of the amyloid beta peptide (Aβ), following proteolytic processing of the APP by β-secretase and γ-secretase, is thought to be central to the etiology of AD, and inhibition of these enzymes has become a focus of drug development efforts. In comparison to γ-secretase inhibition, the loss of β-secretase, a rate-limiting enzyme in the production of Aβ, appears to have few reported side effects *in vivo*. Consequently, this protein has become an attractive drug target for the treatment of AD, but the development of potent and selective β-secretase inhibitors with good brain permeability has been a challenge. A critical next step in the development of β-secretase inhibitors is testing in appropriate animal model systems. This chapter reviews several *in vivo* animal models, both genetically manipulated and spontaneous, which are suitable for testing β-secretase inhibitors in preclinical studies.

BACE1, also known as Asp2 and Memapsin2, is highly expressed in the neurons of the brain and is responsible for the production of β-secretase cleavage products sAPPβ, CTFβ, and Aβ; mice, canines, and nonhuman primates express highly conserved orthologs of human BACE1. The development of potent and highly penetrant BACE1 inhibitors has proven to be challenging in preclinical testing with animal models because of the unusually large active site within the enzyme. While a large variety of BACE1 inhibitors have excellent activity *in vitro*, in the past, they have typically displayed poor *in vivo* activity because of limited membrane permeability and inhibition by p-glycoprotein transport. In order to overcome some of these barriers, the administration of BACE1 inhibitors can be coadministered with selective metabolic inhibitors to enhance their availability and uptake [120].

Based upon data in mouse and nonhuman primates, there are several potent and selective families of BACE1 inhibitors that may be able to effectively lower CSF Aβ levels in human patients in clinical trials. The future preclinical development of BACE1 inhibitors in mouse, canines, and nonhuman primate models should focus on maintaining the potency of these compounds while improving overall metabolic stability and increasing properties of brain penetration. Although there are multiple anti-amyloid therapies that have been tested in preclinical trials, including γ-secretase inhibitors and immunization strategies to eliminate accumulation of Aβ protein, there is a strong hope that small molecule BACE1 inhibitors will soon be on the horizon for the treatment of human AD.

ACKNOWLEDGMENT

The authors wish to acknowledge funding support provided by NS058382, NS061933, and NIH/NIA AG12694, and NIH/NINDS R21NS057651.

REFERENCES

1. Scheff, S.W. and Price, D.A. 2006. Alzheimer's disease-related alterations in synaptic density: neocortex and hippocampus. *J Alzheimers Dis* **9**(Suppl 3):101-115.
2. Trojanowski, J.Q., Shin, R.W., Schmidt, M.L., and Lee, V.M. 1995. Relationship between plaques, tangles, and dystrophic processes in Alzheimer's disease. *Neurobiol Aging* **16**(3):335–340; discussion 41–45.
3. Goate A. 2006. Segregation of a missense mutation in the amyloid beta-protein precursor gene with familial Alzheimer's disease. *J Alzheimers Dis* **9**(Suppl 3):341–347.
4. Vassar R. 2005. Beta-secretase, APP and Abeta in Alzheimer's disease. *Subcell Biochem* **38**:79–103.
5. Kojro, E. and Fahrenholz, F. 2005. The non-amyloidogenic pathway: structure and function of alpha-secretases. *Subcell Biochem* **38**:105–127.
6. Hardy, J. and Selkoe, D.J. 2002. The amyloid hypothesis of Alzheimer's disease: progress and problems on the road to therapeutics. *Science* **297**(5580): 353–356.
7. Walsh, D.M. and Selkoe, D.J. 2004. Deciphering the molecular basis of memory failure in Alzheimer's disease. *Neuron* **44**(1):181–193.
8. De Strooper, B. Loss-of-function presenilin mutations in Alzheimer disease. 2007. Talking point on the role of presenilin mutations in Alzheimer disease. *EMBO Rep* **8**(2):141–146.
9. Wolfe, M.S. 2007. When loss is gain: reduced presenilin proteolytic function leads to increased Abeta42/Abeta40. Talking Point on the role of presenilin mutations in Alzheimer disease. *EMBO Rep* **8**(2):136–140.
10. De Strooper, B., Annaert, W., Cupers, P., Saftig, P., Craessaerts, K., Mumm, J.S., Schroeter, E.H., Schrijvers, V., Wolfe, M.S., Ray, W.J., Goate, A., and Kopan, R.A. 1999. Presenilin-1-dependent gamma-secretase-like protease mediates release of Notch intracellular domain. *Nature* **398**(6727):518–522.
11. Doerfler, P., Shearman, M.S., and Perlmutter, R.M. 2001. Presenilin-dependent gamma-secretase activity modulates thymocyte development. *Proc Natl Acad Sci U S A* **98**(16):9312–9317.
12. Hadland, B.K., Manley, N.R., Su, D., Longmore, G.D., Moore, C.L., Wolfe, M.S., Schroeter, E.H., and Kopan, R. 2001. Gamma-secretase inhibitors repress thymocyte development. *Proc Natl Acad Sci U S A* **98**(13):7487–7491.
13. Ghosh, A.K., Bilcer, G., Hong, L., Koelsch, G., and Tang, J. 2007. Memapsin 2 (beta-secretase) inhibitor drug, between fantasy and reality. *Curr Alzheimer Res* **4**(4):418–422.
14. Hong, L., Koelsch, G., Lin, X., Wu, S., Terzyan, S., Ghosh, A.K., Zhang, X.C., and Tang, J. 2000. Structure of the protease domain of memapsin 2 (beta-secretase) complexed with inhibitor. *Science* **290**(5489):150–153.
15. Asai, M., Hattori, C., Iwata, N., Saido, T.C., Sasagawa, N., Szabo, B., Hashimoto, Y., Maruyama, K., Tanuma, S., Kiso, Y., and Ishiura, S. 2006. The novel beta-secretase inhibitor KMI-429 reduces amyloid beta peptide production in amyloid precursor protein transgenic and wild-type mice. *J Neurochem* **96**(2):533–540.
16. Nishitomi, K., Sakaguchi, G., Horikoshi, Y., Gray, A.J., Maeda, M., Hirata-Fukae, C., Becker, A.G., Hosono, M., Sakaguchi, I., Minami, S.S., Nakajima, Y., Li, H.F., Takeyama, C., Kihara, T., Ota, A., Wong, P.C., Aisen, P.S., Kato, A., Kinoshita, N., and Matsuoka, Y. 2006. BACE1 inhibi-

tion reduces endogenous Abeta and alters APP processing in wild-type mice. *J Neurochem* **99**(6): 1555–1563.

17. Sankaranarayanan, S., Price, E.A., Wu, G., Crouthamel, M.C., Shi, X.P., Tugusheva, K., Tyler, K.X., Kahana, J., Ellis, J., Jin, L., Steele, T., Stachel, S., Coburn, C., and Simon, A.J. 2008. In vivo beta-secretase 1 inhibition leads to brain Abeta lowering and increased alpha-secretase processing of amyloid precursor protein without effect on neuregulin-1. *J Pharmacol Exp Ther* **324**(3): 957–969.

18. Chang, W.P., Koelsch, G., Wong, S., Downs, D., Da, H., Weerasena, V., Gordon, B., Devasamudram, T., Bilcer, G., Ghosh, A.K., and Tang. J. 2004. In vivo inhibition of Abeta production by memapsin 2 (beta-secretase) inhibitors. *J Neurochem* **89**(6):1409–1416.

19. Hussain, I., Hawkins, J., Harrison, D., Hille, C., Wayne, G., Cutler, L., Buck, T., Walter, D., Demont, E., Howes, C., Naylor, A., Jeffrey, P., Gonzalez, M.I., Dingwall, C., Michel, A., Redshaw, S., and Davis, J.B. 2007. Oral administration of a potent and selective non-peptidic BACE-1 inhibitor decreases beta-cleavage of amyloid precursor protein and amyloid-beta production in vivo. *J Neurochem* **100**(3):802–809.

20. Stachel, S.J., Coburn, C.A., Sankaranarayanan, S., Price, E.A., Wu, G., Crouthamel, M., Pietrak, B.L., Huang, Q., Lineberger, J., Espeseth, A.S., Jin, L., Ellis, J., Holloway, M.K., Munshi, S., Allison, T., Hazuda, D., Simon, A.J., Graham, S.L., and Vacca, J.P. 2006. Macrocyclic inhibitors of beta-secretase: functional activity in an animal model. *J Med Chem* **49**(21):6147–6150.

21. Stanton, M.G., Stauffer, S.R., Gregro, A.R., Steinbeiser, M., Nantermet, P., Sankaranarayanan, S., Price, E.A., Wu, G., Crouthamel, M.C., Ellis, J., Lai, M.T., Espeseth, A.S., Shi, X.P., Jin, L., Colussi, D., Pietrak, B., Huang, Q., Xu, M., Simon, A.J., Graham, S.L., Vacca, J.P., and Selnick, H. 2007. Discovery of isonicotinamide derived beta-secretase inhibitors: in vivo reduction of beta-amyloid. *J Med Chem* **50**(15):3431–3433.

22. Lindsley, S.R., Moore, K.P., Rajapakse, H.A., Selnick, H.G., Young, M.B., Zhu, H., Munshi, S., Kuo, L., McGaughey, G.B., Colussi, D., Crouthamel, M.C., Lai, M.T., Pietrak, B., Price, E.A., Sankaranarayanan, S., Simon, A.J., Seabrook, G.R., Hazuda, D.J., Pudvah, N.T., Hochman, J.H., Graham, S.L., Vacca, J.P., and Nantermet, P.G. 2007. Design, synthesis, and SAR of macrocyclic tertiary carbinamine BACE-1 inhibitors. *Bioorg Med Chem Lett* **17**(14):4057–4061.

23. Moore, K.P., Zhu, H., Rajapakse, H.A., McGaughey, G.B., Colussi, D., Price, E.A., Sankaranarayanan, S., Simon, A.J., Pudvah, N.T., Hochman, J.H., Allison, T., Munshi, S.K., Graham, S.L., Vacca, J.P., and Nantermet, P.G. 2007. Strategies toward improving the brain penetration of macrocyclic tertiary carbinamine BACE-1 inhibitors. *Bioorg Med Chem Lett* **17**(21):5831–5835.

24. Rajapakse, H.A., Nantermet, P.G., Selnick, H.G., Munshi, S., McGaughey, G.B., Lindsley, S.R., Young, M.B., Lai, M.T., Espeseth, A.S., Shi, X.P., Colussi, D., Pietrak, B., Crouthamel, M.C., Tugusheva, K., Huang, Q., Xu, M., Simon, A.J., Kuo, L., Hazuda, D.J., Graham, S., and Vacca, J.P. 2006. Discovery of oxadiazoyl tertiary carbinamine inhibitors of beta-secretase (BACE-1). *J Med Chem* **49**(25):7270–7273.

25. Stauffer, S.R., Stanton, M.G., Gregro, A.R., Steinbeiser, M.A., Shaffer, J.R., Nantermet, P.G., Barrow, J.C., Rittle, K.E., Collusi, D., Espeseth, A.S., Lai, M.T., Pietrak, B.L., Holloway, M.K., McGaughey, G.B., Munshi, S.K., Hochman, J.H., Simon, A.J., Selnick, H.G., Graham, S.L., and Vacca, J.P. 2007. Discovery and SAR of isonicotinamide BACE-1 inhibitors that bind beta-secretase in a N-terminal 10s-loop down conformation. *Bioorg Med Chem Lett* **17**(6): 1788–1792.

26. Harrison, S.M., Harper, A.J., Hawkins, J., Duddy, G., Grau, E., Pugh, P.L., Winter, P.H., Shilliam, C.S., Hughes, Z.A., Dawson, L.A., Gonzalez, M.I., Upton, N., Pangalos, M.N., and Dingwall, C. 2003. BACE1 (beta-secretase) transgenic and knockout mice: identification of neurochemical deficits and behavioral changes. *Mol Cell Neurosci* **24**(3):646–655.

27. Roberds, S.L., Anderson, J., Basi, G., Bienkowski, M.J., Branstetter, D.G., Chen, K.S., Freedman, S.B., Frigon, N.L., Games, D., Hu, K., Johnson-Wood, K., Kappenman, K.E., Kawabe, T.T., Kola, I., Kuehn, R., Lee, M., Liu, W., Motter, R., Nichols, N.F., Power, M., Robertson, D.W., Schenk, D., Schoor, M., Shopp, G.M., Shuck, M.E., Sinha, S., Svensson, K.A., Tatsuno, G., Tintrup, H., Wijsman, J., Wright, S., and McConlogue, L. 2001. BACE knockout mice are healthy despite lacking the primary beta-secretase activity in brain: implications for Alzheimer's disease therapeutics. *Hum Mol Genet* **10**(12):1317–1324.

28. Cai, H., Wang, Y., McCarthy, D., Wen, H., Borchelt, D.R., Price, D.L., and Wong, P.C. 2001. BACE1 is the major beta-secretase for generation of Abeta peptides by neurons. *Nat Neurosci* **4**(3):233–234.

29. Luo, Y., Bolon, B., Kahn, S., Bennett, B.D., Babu-Khan, S., Denis, P., Fan, W., Kha, H., Zhang, J., Gong, Y., Martin, L., Louis, J.C., Yan, Q., Richards, W.G., Citron, M., and Vassar, R. 2001. Mice deficient in BACE1, the Alzheimer's beta-secretase, have normal phenotype and abolished beta-amyloid generation. *Nat Neurosci* **4**(3):231–232.

30. Ohno, M., Sametsky, E.A., Younkin, L.H., Oakley, H., Younkin, S.G., Citron, M., Vassar, R., and Disterhoft, J.F. 2004. BACE1 deficiency rescues memory deficits and cholinergic dysfunction in a mouse model of Alzheimer's disease. *Neuron* **41**(1):27–33.

31. McGowan, E., Eriksen, J., and Hutton, M. 2006. A decade of modeling Alzheimer's disease in transgenic mice. *Trends Genet* **22**(5):281–289.

32. Games, D., Adams, D., Alessandrini, R., Barbour, R., Berthelette, P., Blackwell, C., Carr, T., Clemens, J., Donaldson, T., Gillespie, F., Guido, T., Hagoplan, S., Johnson-Wood, K., Khan, K., Lee, M., Leibowitz, P., Lieberburg, I., Little, S., Masliah, E., McConlogue, L., Montoya-Zavala, M., Mucke, L., Paganini, L., Penniman, E., Power, M., Schenk, D., Seubert, P., Snyder, B., Sorlano, F., Tan, H., Vitale, J., Wadsworth, S., Wolozin, B., and Zhao, J. 1995. Alzheimer-type neuropathology in transgenic mice overexpressing V717F β-amyloid precursor protein. *Nature* **373**: 523–527.

33. Hsiao, K., Chapman, P., Nilsen, S., Eckman, C., Harigaya, Y., Younkin, S., Yang, F., and Cole, G. 1996. Correlative memory deficits, Abeta elevation, and amyloid plaques in transgenic mice. *Science* **274**(5284):99–102.

34. Borchelt, D.R., Ratovitski, T., van Lare, J., Lee, M.K., Gonzales, V., Jenkins, N.A., Copeland, N.G., Price, D.L., and Sisodia, S.S. 1997. Accelerated amyloid deposition in the brains of transgenic mice coexpressing mutant presenilin 1 and amyloid precursor proteins. *Neuron* **19**(4):939–945.

35. Duff, K., Eckman, C., Zehr, C., Yu, X., Prada, C.M., Perez-tur, J., Hutton, M., Buee, L., Harigaya, Y., Yager, D., Morgan, D., Gordon, M.N., Holcomb, L., Refolo, L., Zenk, B., Hardy, J., and Younkin, S. 1996. Increased amyloid-beta42(43) in brains of mice expressing mutant presenilin 1. *Nature* **383**(6602):710–713.

36. Holcomb, L., Gordon, M.N., McGowan, E., Yu, X., Benkovic, S., Jantzen, P., Wright, K., Saad, I., Mueller, R., Morgan, D., Sanders, S., Zehr, C., O'Campo, K., Hardy, J., Prada, C.M., Eckman, C., Younkin, S., Hsiao, K., and Duff, K. 1998. Accelerated Alzheimer-type phenotype in transgenic mice carrying both mutant amyloid precursor protein and presenilin 1 transgenes. *Nature Medicine* **4**(1):97–100.

37. Irizarry, M.C., McNamara, M., Fedorchak, K., Hsiao, K., and Hyman, B.T. 1997. APPSw transgenic mice develop age-related A beta deposits and neuropil abnormalities, but no neuronal loss in CA1. *J Neuropathol Exp Neurol* **56**(9):965–973.

38. Irizarry, M.C., Soriano, F., McNamara, M., Page, K.J., Schenk, D., Games, D., and Hyman, B.T. 1997. Abeta deposition is associated with neuropil changes, but not with overt neuronal loss in the human amyloid precursor protein V717F (PDAPP) transgenic mouse. *J Neurosci* **17**(18): 7053–7059.

39. Takeuchi, A., Irizarry, M.C., Duff, K., Saido, T.C., Hsiao Ashe, K., Hasegawa, M., Mann, D.M., Hyman, B.T., and Iwatsubo, T. 2000. Age-related amyloid beta deposition in transgenic mice overexpressing both Alzheimer mutant presenilin 1 and amyloid beta precursor protein Swedish mutant is not associated with global neuronal loss. *Am J Pathol* **157**(1):331–339.

40. Laird, F.M., Cai, H., Savonenko, A.V., Farah, M.H., He, K., Melnikova, T., Wen, H., Chiang, H.C., Xu, G., Koliatsos, V.E., Borchelt, D.R., Price, D.L., Lee, H.K., and Wong, P.C. 2005. BACE1, a major determinant of selective vulnerability of the brain to amyloid-beta amyloidogenesis, is essential for cognitive, emotional, and synaptic functions. *J Neurosci* **25**(50):11693–11709.

41. Oakley, H., Cole, S.L., Logan, S., Maus, E., Shao, P., Craft, J., Guillozet-Bongaarts, A., Ohno, M., Disterhoft, J., Van Eldik, L., Berry, R., and Vassar, R. 2006. Intraneuronal beta-amyloid aggregates, neurodegeneration, and neuron loss in transgenic mice with five familial Alzheimer's disease mutations: potential factors in amyloid plaque formation. *J Neurosci* **26**(40):10129–10140.

42. Ohno, M., Chang, L., Tseng, W., Oakley, H., Citron, M., Klein, W.L., Vassar, R., and Disterhoft, J.F. 2006. Temporal memory deficits in Alzheimer's mouse models: rescue by genetic deletion of BACE1. *Eur J Neurosci* **23**(1):251–260.

43. Ohno, M., Cole, S.L., Yasvoina, M., Zhao, J., Citron, M., Berry, R., Disterhoft, J.F., and Vassar, R. 2007. BACE1 gene deletion prevents neuron loss and memory deficits in 5XFAD APP/PS1 transgenic mice. *Neurobiol Dis* **26**(1):134–145.

44. Dominguez, D., Tournoy, J., Hartmann, D., Huth, T., Cryns, K., Deforce, S., Serneels, L., Camacho, I.E., Marjaux, E., Craessaerts, K., Roebroek, A.J., Schwake, M., D'Hooge, R., Bach, P., Kalinke, U., Moechars, D., Alzheimer, C., Reiss, K., Saftig, P., and De Strooper, B. 2005. Phenotypic and biochemical analyses of BACE1- and BACE2-deficient mice. *J Biol Chem* **280**(35):30797–30806.

45. Hu, X., Hicks, C.W., He, W., Wong, P., Macklin, W.B., Trapp, B.D., and Yan, R. 2006. Bace1 modulates myelination in the central and peripheral nervous system. *Nat Neurosci* **9**(12): 1520–1525.

46. Willem, M., Garratt, A.N., Novak, B., Citron, M., Kaufmann, S., Rittger, A., DeStrooper, B., Saftig, P., Birchmeier, C., and Haass, C. 2006. Control of peripheral nerve myelination by the beta-secretase BACE1. *Science* **314**(5799):664–666.

47. Williams, M. 2009. Progress in Alzheimer's disease drug discovery: an update. *Curr Opin Investig Drugs* **10**(1):23–34.

48. Siwak, C.T., Tapp, P.D., Head, E., Zicker, S.C., Murphey, H.L., Muggenburg, B.A., Ikeda-Douglas, C.J., Cotman, C.W., and Milgram, N.W. 2005. Chronic antioxidant and mitochondrial cofactor administration improves discrimination learning in aged but not young dogs. *Prog Neuropsychopharmacol Biol Psychiatry* **29**(3):461–469.

49. Tapp, P.D., Siwak, C., Head, E., Cotman, C.W., Murphey, H., Muggenburg, B.A., Ikeda-Douglas, C., and Milgram, N.W. 2004. Concept abstraction in the aging dog: development of a protocol using successive discrimination and size concept tasks. *Behav Brain Res* **153**:199–210.

50. Cotman, C.W., Head, E., Muggenburg, B.A., Zicker, S., and Milgram, N.W. 2002. Brain aging in the canine: a diet enriched in antioxidants reduces cognitive dysfunction. *Neurobiol Aging* **23**(5):809–818.

51. Milgram, N.W., Zicker, S.C., Head, E., Muggenburg, B.A., Murphey, H., Ikeda-Douglas, C., and Cotman, C.W. 2002. Dietary enrichment counteracts age-associated cognitive dysfunction in canines. *Neurobiol Aging* **23**:737–745.

52. Head, E., Callahan, H., Muggenburg, B.A., Cotman, C.W., and Milgram, N.W. 1998. Visual-discrimination learning ability and beta-amyloid accumulation in the dog. *Neurobiol Aging* **19**(5):415–425.

53. Tapp, P.D., Siwak, C.T., Estrada, J., Muggenburg, B.A., Head, E., Cotman, C.W., and Milgram, N.W. 2003. Size and reversal learning in the beagle dog as a measure of executive function and inhibitory control in aging. *Learn Mem* **10**(1):64–73.

54. Christie, L.A., Studzinski, C.M., Araujo, J.A., Leung, C.S., Ikeda-Douglas, C.J., Head, E., Cotman, C.W., and Milgram, N.W. 2005. A comparison of egocentric and allocentric age-dependent spatial learning in the beagle dog. *Prog Neuropsychopharmacol Biol Psychiatry* **29**(3):361–369.

55. Studzinski, C.M., Christie, L.A., Araujo, J.A., Burnham, W.M., Head, E., Cotman, C.W., and Milgram, N.W. 2006. Visuospatial function in the beagle dog: an early marker of cognitive decline in a model of human aging and dementia. *Neurobiol Learn Mem* **86**(2):197–204.

56. Milgram, N.W., Adams, B., Callahan, H., Head, E., Mackay, W., Thirlwell, C., and Cotman, C.W. 1999. Landmark discrimination learning in the dog. *Learn Memory* **6**(1):54–61.

57. Milgram, N.W., Head, E., Muggenburg, B.A., Holowachuk, D., Murphey, H., Estrada, J., Ikeda-Douglas, C.J., Zicker, S.C., and Cotman, C.W. 2002. Landmark discrimination learning in the dog: effects of age, an antioxidant fortified diet, and cognitive strategy. *Neurosci Biobehav Rev* **26**(6):679–695.

58. Milgram, N.W., Head, E., Weiner, E., and Thomas, E. 1994. Cognitive functions and aging in the dog: acquisition of nonspatial visual tasks. *Behav Neurosci* **108**:57–68.

59. Chan, A.D., Nippak, P.M., Murphey, H., Ikeda-Douglas, C.J., Muggenburg, B., Head, E., Cotman, C.W., and Milgram, N.W. 2002. Visuospatial impairments in aged canines (*Canis familiaris*): the role of cognitive-behavioral flexibility. *Behav Neurosci* **116**(3):443–454.

60. Head, E., Mehta, R., Hartley, J., Kameka, A.M., Cummings, B.J., Cotman, C.W., Ruehl, W.W., and Milgram, N.W. 1995. Spatial learning and memory as a function of age in the dog. *Behav Neurosci* **109**:851–858.

61. Head, E., Pop, V., Vasilevko, V., Hill, M., Saing, T., Sarsoza, F., Nistor, M., Christie, L.A., Milton, S., Glabe, C., Barrett, E., and Cribbs, D. 2008. A two-year study with fibrillar beta-amyloid (Abeta) immunization in aged canines: effects on cognitive function and brain Abeta. *J Neurosci* **28**(14):3555–3566.

62. Albert, M.S. and Funkenstein, H.H. 1992. The effects of age: normal variation and its relation to disease. In: *Disorders of the Nervous System: Clinical Neurology*, 2nd ed. (A.K. Asburg, G.M. McKhanney, and W.I. McDonald, eds.). Philadelphia, PA: Saunders, pp. 598–611.

63. Petersen, R.C., Smith, G.E., Waring, S.C., Ivnik, R.J., Kokmen, E., and Tangelos, E.G. 1997. Aging, memory, and mild cognitive impairment. *Int Psychogeriatr* **9**(Suppl 1):65–69.

64. Petersen, R.C., Smith, G.E., Waring, S.C., Ivnik, R.J., Tangalos, E.G., and Kokmen, E. 1999. Mild cognitive impairment: clinical characterization and outcome. *Arch Neurol* **56**(3):303–308.

65. Head, E., Milgram, N.W. and Cotman, C.W. 2001. Neurobiological models of aging in the dog and other vertebrate species. In *Functional Neurobiology of Aging* (P. Hof and C. Mobbs, eds.). San Diego, CA: Academic Press, pp. 457–468.

66. Baxter, M.G. and Gallagher, M. 1996. Neurobiological substrates of behavioral decline: models and data analytic strategies for individual differences in aging. *Neurobiol Aging* **17**:491–495.

67. Markowska, A.L., Stone, W.S., Ingram, D.K., Reynolds, J., Gold, P.E., Conti, L.H., Pontecorvo, M.J., Wenk, G.L., and Olton, D.S. 1989. Individual differences in aging: behavioral and neurobiological correlates. *Neurobiol Aging* **10**:31–43.

68. Rapp, P.R. 1993. Neuropsychological analysis of learning and memory in aged nonhuman primates. *Neurobiol Aging* **14**:627–629.

69. Rapp, P.R. and Amaral, D.G. 1991. Recognition memory deficits in a subpopulation of aged monkeys resemble the effects of medial temporal lobe damage. *Neurobiol Aging* **12**:481–486.

70. Rapp, P.R., Kansky, M.T., Roberts, J.A., and Eichenbaum, H. 1994. New directions for studying cognitive decline in old monkeys. *Seminars in the Neurosciences* **6**:369–377.

71. Rowe, J.W. and Kahn, R.L. 1987. Human aging: usual and successful. *Science* **237**(4811): 143–149.

72. Johnstone, E.M., Chaney, M.O., Norris, F.H., Pascual, R., and Little, S.P. 1991. Conservation of the sequence of the Alzheimer's disease amyloid peptide in dog, polar bear and five other mammals by cross-species polymerase chain reaction analysis. *Brain Res Mol Brain Res* **10**(4):299–305.

73. Selkoe, D.J., Bell, D.S., Podlisny, M.B., Price, D.L., and Cork, L.C. 1987. Conservation of brain amyloid proteins in aged mammals and humans with Alzheimer's disease. *Science* **235**:873–877.

74. Torp, R., Head, E., and Cotman, C.W. 2000. Ultrastructural analyses of beta-amyloid in the aged dog brain: neuronal beta-amyloid is localized to the plasma membrane. *Prog Neuropsychopharmacol Biol Psychiatry* **24**:801–810.

75. Torp, R., Head, E., Milgram, N.W., Hahn, F., Ottersen, O.P., and Cotman, C.W. 2000. Ultrastructural evidence of fibrillar b-amyloid associated with neuronal membranes in behaviorally characterized aged dog brains. *Neuroscience* **93**(3):495–506.

76. Torp, R., Ottersen, O.P., Cotman, C.W., and Head E. 2003. Identification of neuronal plasma membrane microdomains that colocalize beta-amyloid and presenilin: implications for beta-amyloid precursor protein processing. *Neuroscience* **120**(2):291–300.

77. Cummings, B.J., Head, E., Ruehl, W., Milgram, N.W., and Cotman, C.W. 1996. The canine as an animal model of human aging and dementia. *Neurobiol Aging* **17**(2):259–268.

78. Braak, H. and Braak, E. 1991. Neuropathological stageing of Alzheimer-related changes. *Acta Neuropathol* **82**(4):239–259.

79. Braak, H., Braak, E., and Bohl, J. 1993. Staging of Alzheimer-related cortical destruction. *Review in Clin Neurosci* **33**:403–408.

80. Giaccone, G., Verga, L., Finazzi, M., Pollo, B., Tagliavini, F., Frangione, B., and Bugiani, O. 1990. Cerebral preamyloid deposits and congophilic angiopathy in aged dogs. *Neurosci Lett* **114**:178–183.

81. Head, E., McCleary, R., Hahn, F.F., Milgram, N.W., and Cotman, C.W. 2000. Region-specific age at onset of beta-amyloid in dogs. *Neurobiol Aging* **21**(1):89–96.

82. Ishihara, T., Gondo, T., Takahashi, M., Uchino, F., Ikeda, S., Allsop, D., and Imai, K. 1991. Immunohistochemical and immunoelectron microscopial characterization of cerebrovascular and senile plaque amyloid in aged dogs' brains. *Brain Res* **548**:196–205.

83. Thal, D.R., Rub, U., Orantes, M., and Braak, H. 2002. Phases of A beta-deposition in the human brain and its relevance for the development of AD. *Neurology* **58**(12):1791–1800.

84. Wisniewski, H.M., Johnson, A.B., Raine, C.S., Kay, W.J., and Terry, R.D. 1970. Senile plaques and cerebral amyloidosis in aged dogs. *Lab Invest* **23**:287–296.

85. Wisniewski, H.M., Wegiel, J., Morys, J., Bancher, C., Soltysiak, Z., and Kim, K.S. 1990. Aged dogs: an animal model to study beta-protein amyloidogenesis. In *Alzheimer's disease Epidemiology, Neuropathology, Neurochemistry and Clinics* (K. Maurer, P. Riederer, and H. Beckman, eds.). New York: Springer-Verlag, pp. 151–167.

86. Alafuzoff, L., Iqbal, K., Friden, H., Adolfsson, R., and Winblad, B. 1987. Histopathological criteria for progressive dementia disorders: clinical-pathological correlation and classification by multivariate analysis. *Acta Neuropatholog (Berlin)* **74**:209–225.

87. Cummings, B.J. and Cotman, C.W. 1995. Image analysis of beta-amyloid "load" in Alzheimer's disease and relation to dementia severity. *Lancet* **346**:1524–1528.

88. Dayan, A.D. 1970. Quantitative histological studies on the aged human brain. I. Senile plaques and neurofibrillary tangles in "normal" patients. *Acta Neuropathol (Berlin)* **16**:85–94.

89. Delaere, P., Duyckaerts, C., Masters, C., Beyreuther, K., Piette, F., and Hauw, J-J. 1990. Large amounts of neocortical beta A4 deposits without neuritic plaques nor tangles in a psychometrically assessed, non-demented person. *Neurosci Lett* **116**:87–93.

90. Dickson, D.W., Crystal, H.A., Bevona, C., Honer, W., Vincent, I., and Davies, P. 1995. Correlations of synaptic and pathological markers with cognition of the elderly. *Neurobiol Aging* **16**(3):285–304.

91. Langui, D., Probst, A., and Ulrich, J. 1995. Alzheimer's changes in non-demented and demented patients: a statistical approach to their relationships. *Acta Neuropathol* **89**:57–62.

92. Tomlinson, B.E., Blessed, G., and Roth, M. 1968. Observations on the brains of non-demented old people. *J Neurol Sci* **7**:331–356.

93. Wisniewski, H.M. 1979. The aging brain. In *Spontaneous Animal Models of Human Disease* (E.J. Andrews, B.C. Ward, and N.H. Altman, eds.). New York: Academic Press, pp. 148–152.

94. Attems, J. 2005. Sporadic cerebral amyloid angiopathy: pathology, clinical implications, and possible pathomechanisms. *Acta Neuropathol* **110**(4):345–359.

95. Attems, J., Jellinger, K.A., and Lintner, F. 2005. Alzheimer's disease pathology influences severity and topographical distribution of cerebral amyloid angiopathy. *Acta Neuropathol* **110**(3):222–231.

96. Herzig, M.C., Van Nostrand, W.E., and Jucker, M. 2006. Mechanism of cerebral beta-amyloid angiopathy: murine and cellular models. *Brain Pathol* **16**(1):40–54.

97. Prior, R., D'Urso, D., Frank, R., Prikulis, I., and Pavlakovic, G. 1996. Loss of vessel wall viability in cerebral amyloid angiopathy. *NeuroReport* **7**:562.

98. Deane, R. and Zlokovic, B.V. 2007. Role of the blood–brain barrier in the pathogenesis of Alzheimer's disease. *Curr Alzheimer Res* **4**(2):191–197.

99. Shimada, A., Kuwamura, M., Akawkura, T., Umemura, T. , Takada, K., Ohama, E., and Itakura, C. 1992. Topographic relationship between senile plaques and cerebrovascular amyloidosis in the brain of aged dogs. *J Vet Med Sci* **54**(1):137–144.

100. Uchida, K., Kuroki, K., Yoshino, T., Yamaguchi, R., and Tateyama, S. 1997. Immunohistochemical study of constituents other than beta-protein in canine senile plaques and cerebral amyloid angiopathy. *Acta Neuropathol* **93**(3):277–284.

101. Uchida, K., Miyauchi, Y., Nakayama, H., and Goto, N. 1990. Amyloid angiopathy with cerebral hemorrhage and senile plaque in aged dogs. *Nippon Juigaku Zasshi* **52**(3):605–611.

102. Uchida, K., Nakayama, H., and Goto, N. 1991. Pathological studies on cerebral amyloid angiopathy, senile plaques and amyloid deposition in visceral organs in aged dogs. *J Vet Med Sci* **53**(6):1037–1042.

103. Uchida, K., Okuda, R., Yamaguchi, R., Tateyama, S., Nakayama, H., and Goto, N. 1993. Double-labeling immunohistochemical studies on canine senile plaques and cerebral amyloid angiopathy. *J Vet Med Sci* **55**(4):637–642.

104. Uchida, K., Tani, Y., Uetsuka, K., Nakayama, H., and Goto, N. 1992. Immunohistochemical studies on canine cerebral amyloid angiopathy and senile plaques. *J Vet Med Sci* **54**(4):659–667.

105. Yoshino, T., Uchida, K., Tateyama, S., Yamaguchi, R., Nakayama, H., and Goto, N. 1996. A retrospective study of canine senile plaques and cerebral amyloid angiopathy. *Vet Pathol* **33**:230–234.

106. Wisniewski, T., Lalowski, M., Bobik, M., Russell, M., Strosznajder, J., and Frangione, B. 1996. Amyloid Beta 1-42 deposits do not lead to Alzheimer's neuritic plaques in aged dogs. *Biochem J* **313**:575–580.

107. Walker, L.C. 1997. Animal models of cerebral beta-amyloid angiopathy. *Brain Res Rev* **25**:70–84.

108. Alberts, A.W. 1990. Lovastatin and simvastatin – inhibitors of HMG CoA reductase and cholesterol biosynthesis. *Cardiology* **77**(4):14–21.

109. Gerson, R.J., MacDonald, J.S., Alberts, A.W., Kornbrust, D.J., Majka, J.A., Stubbs, R.J., and Bokelman, D.L. 1989. Animal safety and toxicology of simvastatin and related hydroxy-methylglutaryl-coenzyme A reductase inhibitors. *Am J Med* **87**(4A):28S–38S.

110. Milgram, N.W., Head, E., Zicker, S.C., Ikeda-Douglas, C.J., Murphey, H., Muggenburg, B., Siwak, C., Tapp, D., and Cotman, C.W. 2005. Learning ability in aged beagle dogs is preserved by behavioral enrichment and dietary fortification: a two-year longitudinal study. *Neurobiol Aging* **26**(1):77–90.

111. Cork, L.C., Kitt, C.A., Struble, R.G., Griffin, J.W., and Price, D.L. 1987. Animal models of degenerative neurological disease. *Prog Clin Biol Res* **229**:241–269.

112. Fainman, J., Eid, M.D., Ervin, F.R., and Palmour, R.M. 2007. A primate model for Alzheimer's disease: investigation of the apolipoprotein E profile of the vervet monkey of St. Kitts. *Am J Med Genet B Neuropsychiatr Genet* **144B**(6):818–819.

113. Walker, L.C. 1997. Animal models of cerebral beta-amyloid angiopathy. *Brain Res Brain Res Rev* **25**(1):70–84.

114. Gearing, M., Tigges, J., Mori, H., and Mirra, S.S. 1996. Ab40 is a major form of b-amyloid in nonhuman primates. *Neurobiol Aging* **17**:903–908.

115. Selkoe, D.J. and Schenk, D. 2003. Alzheimer's disease: molecular understanding predicts amyloid-based therapeutics. *Annu Rev Pharmacol Toxicol* **43**:545–584.

116. Weggen, S., Eriksen, J.L., Das, P., Sagi, S.A., Wang, R., Pietrzik, C.U., Findlay, K.A., Smith, T.E., Murphy, M.P., Bulter, T., Kang, D.E., Marquez-Sterling, N., Golde, T.E., and Koo, E.H. 2001. A subset of NSAIDs lower amyloidogenic Abeta42 independently of cyclooxygenase activity. *Nature* **414**(6860):212–216.

117. Cummings, B.J. 1997. Plaques and tangles: searching for primary events in a forest of data. *Neurobiol Aging* **18**(4):358–362.

118. Cummings, B.J., Head, E., Afagh, A.J., Milgram, N.W., and Cotman, C.W. 1996. Beta-amyloid accumulation correlates with cognitive dysfunction in the aged canine. *Neurobiol Learn Mem* **66**(1):11–23.

119. Cork, L.C. 1993. Plaques in prefrontal cortex of aged, behaviorally-tested Rhesus monkeys: incidence, distribution and relationship to task performance. *Neurobiol Aging* **1993**:675–676.

120. Sankaranarayanan, S., Holahan, M.A., Colussi, D., Crouthamel, M.C., Devanarayan, V., Ellis, J., Espeseth, A., Gates, A.T., Graham, S.L., Gregro, A.R., Hazuda, D., Hochman, J.H., Holloway, K., Jin, L., Kahana, J., Lai, M.T., Lineberger, J., McGaughey, G., Moore, K.P., Nantermet, P., Pietrak, B., Price, E.A., Rajapakse, H., Stauffer, S., Steinbeiser, M.A., Seabrook, G., Selnick, H.G., Shi, X.P., Stanton, M.G., Swestock, J., Tugusheva, K., Tyler, K.X., Vacca, J.P., Wong, J., Wu, G., Xu, M., Cook, J.J., and Simon, A.J. 2009. First demonstration of cerebrospinal fluid and plasma A beta lowering with oral administration of a beta-site amyloid precursor protein-cleaving enzyme 1 inhibitor in nonhuman primates. *J Pharmacol Exp Ther* **328**(1):131–140.

ADSORPTION, DISTRIBUTION, METABOLISM, EXCRETION (ADME), EFFICACY, AND TOXICOLOGY FOR BACE INHIBITORS

Ishrut Hussain[1] *and Emmanuel Demont*[2]
[1]GlaxoSmithKline R&D, Harlow, United Kingdom and [2]GlaxoSmithKline R&D, Hertfordshire, United Kingdom

8.1 INTRODUCTION

Alzheimer's disease (AD) is a devastating neurodegenerative disorder characterized pathologically by the presence of extracellular senile plaques and intracellular neurofibrillary tangles [1, 2]. Although currently marketed drugs for the treatment of AD provide some symptomatic relief from the neurotransmission deficits observed in these patients, they fail to halt disease progression. Consequently, there is a large unmet clinical need for disease-modifying therapies.

The identification of BACE (β-site APP cleaving enzyme) as the elusive β-secretase, a key enzyme in the production of Aβ peptides, was a major advance in the field of AD [3–6]. Due to the potential for disease modification, many pharmaceutical companies and academic institutions have been actively developing BACE inhibitors for the treatment of AD. An ideal BACE inhibitor would exhibit selectivity against other aspartic proteases, potently and effectively lower Aβ in preclinical models, cross the blood–brain barrier, and exhibit a good pharmacokinetic (PK) profile. The PK characteristics of a drug encompass its absorption, distribution, metabolism, excretion (ADME) and its toxicological properties which are all critical as they influence the drug levels achieved in target tissues and thereby influence the pharmacological activity of compounds. Despite intense efforts, nearly a decade since the discovery of BACE, only one BACE inhibitor has reportedly entered clini-

BACE: Lead Target for Orchestrated Therapy of Alzheimer's Disease, Edited by Varghese John
Copyright © 2010 John Wiley & Sons, Inc.

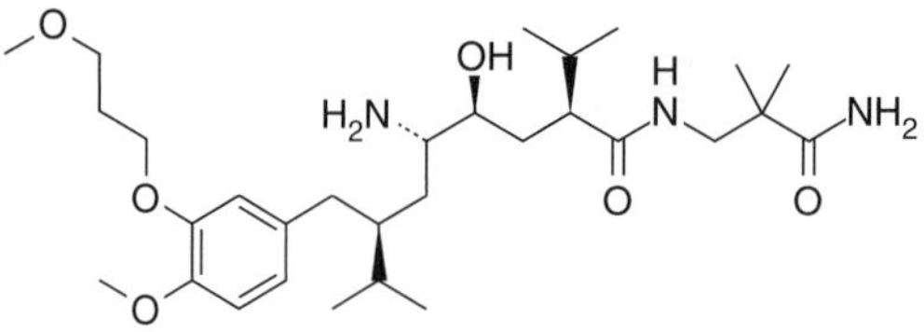

Figure 8.1   Structure of Aliskiren.

cal trials. This exemplifies the challenges in the development of drug-like brain-penetrant BACE inhibitors.

BACE is a transmembrane aspartic protease with a large open active site containing numerous charged residues [7]. Prior to its discovery, only two other aspartic proteases had been the focus of medicinal chemistry programs [8]: renin, for the treatment of hypertension, and HIV protease, as part of the treatment of AIDS. Only one renin inhibitor, Aliskiren (Novartis) [9] (Fig. 8.1), has been launched so far, in 2008, despite over 900 patents published in this area. In the case of HIV protease inhibitors, due to the life-threatening condition of the disease, nine inhibitors have reached the market [10], but none of these are devoid of side effects and ADME liabilities.

The ADME profile of marketed HIV protease inhibitors highlights the difficulty of aspartic proteases as a target class and also clearly illustrates the challenges researchers have faced in the development of drug-like BACE inhibitors. In general, HIV protease inhibitors are lipophilic molecules of high molecular weight (Fig. 8.2; Table 8.1). All of them, with the notable exception of Lopinavir (Abbott Laboratories), are based on a transition-state mimetic scaffold and bear many functionalities, leading to a high polar surface area (PSA) (Table 8.1). Poor aqueous solubility, low membrane permeability, and rapid metabolism by liver cytochrome P450 (CYP) enzymes (in most cases CYP3A4) all contribute to the low oral bioavailability of these compounds. Most HIV protease inhibitors have also been shown to be substrates for the drug transporter, P-glycoprotein (P-gp), which significantly impacts their distribution *in vivo* [11].

Akin to the HIV protease inhibitor field, the majority of BACE inhibitors are also based on a transition-state mimetic approach. Consequently, it is not totally unexpected that the development of drug-like BACE inhibitors has been plagued by similar ADME problems as those faced by HIV protease inhibitors. Coadministration of a subtherapeutic dose of Ritonavir (Abbott Laboratories) has been adopted to circumvent some of the ADME issues faced by HIV protease inhibitors. Ritonavir improves the oral bioavailability and prolongs the half-life of HIV protease inhibitors, primarily via inhibition of CYP3A4 [12]. This drug–drug interaction is beneficial as it reduces both the dose and frequency of administration required to achieve clinical efficacy. Such an approach to boost the ADME properties of BACE inhibitors would be less attractive for the target AD population who is elderly and most likely on polypharmacy. Since BACE is the first aspartic protease identified as a central nervous system target for drug discovery and given the fact that Aβ production and deposition in AD occurs in the brain, BACE inhibitors need to effectively

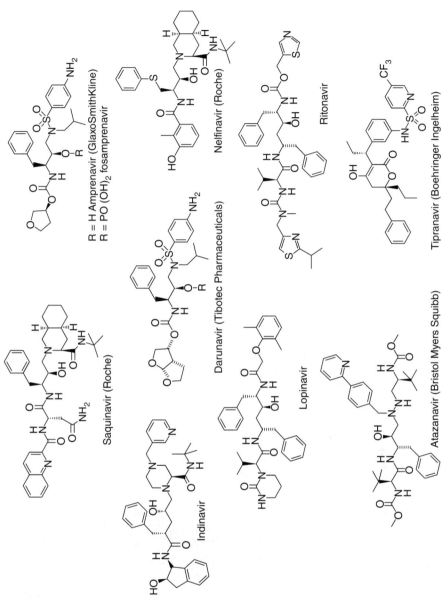

Figure 8.2 Structures of marketed HIV protease inhibitors.

179

TABLE 8.1   Calculated Physiochemical Properties of HIV Protease Inhibitors

Drug	MW	HBA	HBD	PSA	CMR	ACD LogP
Ritonavir	721.03	6	4	145.78	20.118	2.3
Atazanavir	690.98	7	5	154.15	19.65	4.4
Saquinavir	670.94	6	5	166.75	19.046	5.1
Lopinavir	628.89	4	4	120	18.234	5.4
Indinavir	613.88	5	4	118.03	17.81	3.4
Tipranavir	602.73	5	1	105.6	15.496	6.9
Nelfinavir	567.86	4	4	101.9	16.328	7.3
Darunavir	547.73	6	3	140.42	14.346	3.2
Amprenavir	505.69	5	3	131.19	13.525	2.7

MW, molecular weight; HBA, hydrogen bond acceptors; HBD, hydrogen bond donors; PSA, polar surface area; CMR, calculated molar refractivity; ACD LogP, lipophilicity

cross the blood–brain barrier if they are to demonstrate efficacy. This represents another major challenge for BACE inhibitor development as the majority of aspartic protease inhibitors exhibit P-gp liabilities that render them non-brain penetrant.

In this chapter we will review published ADME characteristics of BACE inhibitors, and we will highlight how these compounds bear the same ADME issues as those observed in the development of HIV protease inhibitors. In addition, we will discuss bioavailability and brain uptake of known BACE inhibitors in relation to their reported efficacy in preclinical models. We will focus primarily on compounds that have demonstrated central Aβ lowering as these are the most clinically relevant.

8.2   DEVELOPMENT OF BACE INHIBITORS WITH OPTIMIZED ADME PROPERTIES

In general, high-throughput screens failed to identify tractable hits for BACE inhibitor development. Consequently, the first generation of BACE inhibitors were developed using a "rational drug design" approach. These compounds were based upon the amyloid precursor protein (APP) substrate sequence in which residues at the cleavage site were replaced with a non-hydrolyzable group such as a hydroxyethylene (HE), hydroxyethylamine (HEA) or a statine group [13, 14]. The resulting peptidomimetic BACE inhibitors such as OM99-2 [7] potently inhibited BACE activity *in vitro*. However, these compounds were large in size with molecular weights ranging from 700 to >1000 Da and they lacked activity in cells. To overcome some of these issues, structure–activity relationship (SAR) focused on the generation of BACE inhibitors with lower molecular weight, reduced PSA, and more optimal physiochemical properties. This approach did result in the generation of compounds that were weakly active in cells [15, 16]. However, the resulting compounds were still peptidomimetic and lacked the required drug-like properties.

Significant efforts focused on the identification and generation of potent small molecule non-peptidic BACE inhibitors with more desirable ADME characteristics. To illustrate progress in this area and highlight the common challenges faced by all groups who were actively trying to develop drug-like BACE inhibitors, we have chosen to focus our review on the ADME properties of BACE inhibitors developed by researchers at Merck and GlaxoSmithKline.

8.2.1 Progress at Merck

Rather than using a substrate-based polypeptide bearing a non-cleavable transition-state isosteres as an entry point, researchers at Merck managed to identify compound **1** (Fig. 8.3), as a reversible "low" molecular weight (MW = 506) BACE-1 inhibitor (IC$_{50}$ = 25 μM) from their high-throughput screening campaign [17]. The potency of this hit was further increased to generate compound **2**. Subsequent modifications, including the incorporation of a HEA transition-state mimetic led to compound **3** with nanomolar potency in an enzyme and cell-based assay [18]. Unfortunately, this compound exhibited significant PK liabilities. Its membrane permeability (apparent permeability coefficient; Papp) was poor (Papp = 0.6 × 10^{-6} cm/s). In addition, it was found to be a strong substrate of P-gp transport, which would preclude any chance of significant brain penetration [19]. These properties were most likely associated with the high number of hydrogen bond acceptors/donors in compound **3** and so efforts were directed toward removal of the α-methyl benzamide functionality. This led to the synthesis of compound **4**, with significantly improved membrane permeability (Papp = 14 × 10^{-6} cm/s). However, this compound was still a moderate P-gp substrate (B/A – A/B mdr1a = 8), probably due to the presence of the remaining HEA moiety, amide bond, and sulfonamide [19].

Attempts to improve the physiochemical properties of compounds were further exemplified with the use of reduced amide isosteres in a series analogous to compound **3** [20]. In this series, analogues with polar warheads were as potent against BACE enzyme as their more lipophylic analogues. However, they failed to show significant cell activity, probably due to their poor membrane permeability. In contrast, removal of an amide functionality lead to increased membrane permeability (Papp = 24 × 10^{-6} cm/s). Unfortunately, all of these compounds remained P-gp substrates.

As blood–brain barrier permeability was one of the key properties required for a candidate BACE inhibitor, interactions with P-gp needed to be minimized. This was achieved to some extent by the formation of macrocycles [21]. This effort resulted in the generation of a potent BACE inhibitor (Fig. 8.4) with reasonable cell potency (IC$_{50}$ = 76 nM) and reduced P-gp susceptibility (B/A – A/B = 5.5 mdr1a).

This series of modifications, however, were not sufficient to deliver an orally efficacious BACE inhibitor and further modifications were conducted in order to improve both permeability and *in vivo* stability, as well as lowering affinity for P-gp. It was first possible to modify very significantly the nature of the functionality binding not only to the active site but to the loop as well [22]. Inhibitor **6** proved more potent against BACE than inhibitor **5** (Fig. 8.5) and showed good activity in

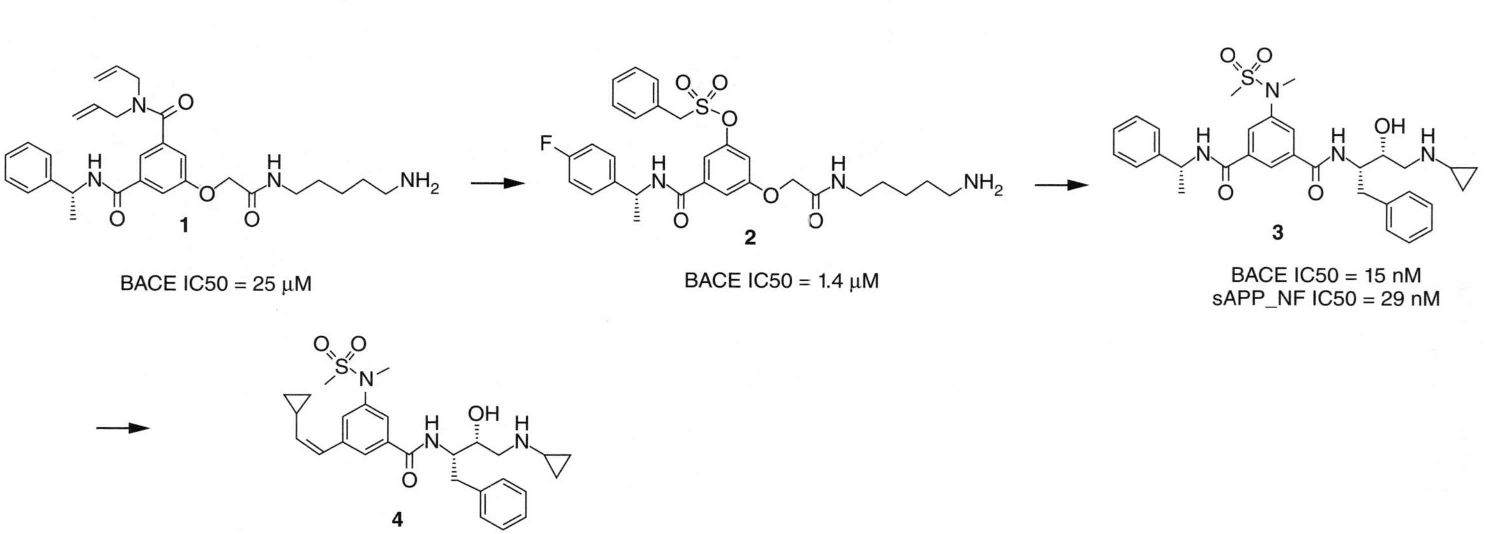

Figure 8.3 Identification of cell permeable BACE inhibitors.

BACE IC50 = 25 μM

BACE IC50 = 1.4 μM

BACE IC50 = 15 nM
sAPP_NF IC50 = 29 nM

1

2

3

4

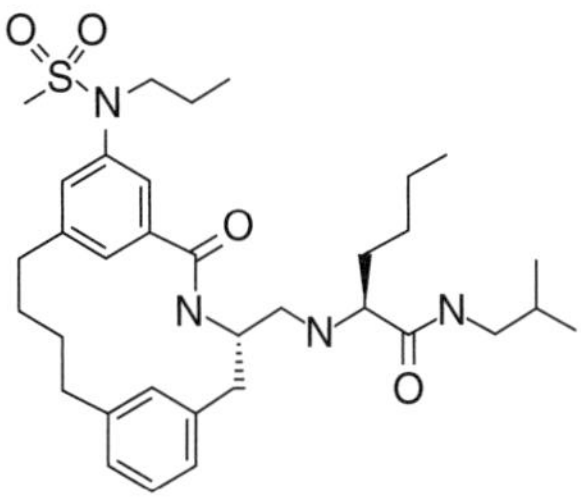

Figure 8.4   Macrocyclic BACE inhibitor.

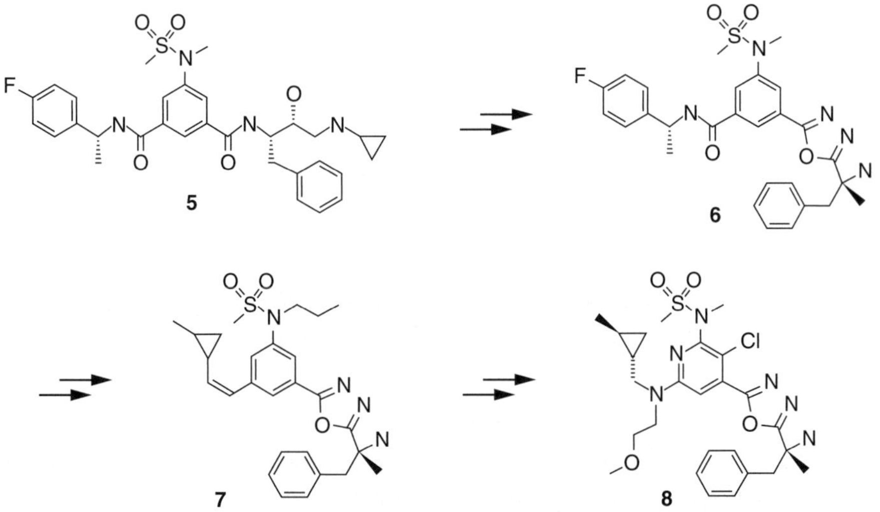

Figure 8.5   Discovery of isonicotinamide and tertiary carbamine BACE inhibitors.

a cell-based assay (IC_{50} = 65 nM). As it was still a P-gp substrate, replacement of the left-hand side benzamide was undertaken to yield compound **7** [23]. Subsequent replacement of the disubstituted styrene present in **7** with an isonicotinamide moiety [24] led to compound **8** (TC-1) [25]. This tertiary carbinamine derivative showed good enzyme and cell potencies (IC_{50}s = 0.4 and 40 nM, respectively) as well good permeability (Papp = 22×10^{-6} cm/s). Importantly, it also exhibited minimal interactions with P-gp in various species (B-A/A-B ratio = 2.3 [mouse], 1.9 [human], 2.5 [monkey]), which would favor good brain penetration. Unfortunately, this compound exhibited very poor oral bioavailability [25].

SAR in the isonicotinamide series also led to BACE inhibitors with improved potency in cells, increased permeability and a decreased affinity for P-gp efflux [26]. However, PK studies in the rat demonstrated these compounds displayed high clearance, high volumes of distribution, moderate half-lives and, with the notable exception of one compound **9a**, poor oral bioavailability (Table 8.2). Unfortunately, the cell potency of this compound was not good enough to justify further progression to an animal model.

TABLE 8.2 *In Vivo* Pharamacokinetic Properties of Isonicotinamide BACE Inhibitors

9a-c

Cmpd	R^1	R^2	R^3	Cl^a (mg/ min/kg)	Vd^a (L/kg)	$t\frac{1}{2}^b$ (h)	$Cmax^b$ (μM)	%F
9a	CH_3	CH_3	CH_2OCH_3	42.6	5.3	2.7	2.7	69
9b	$CH(CH_3)_2$	CH_3	CH_2F	59.1	4.2	1.6	0.2	8
9c	$CH(CH_3)_2$	H	CH_2F	45.8	3.9	1.6	0.3	13

^{a} 2 mg/kg iv dose (solution in 25%DMSO/75%H_2O). ^{b} 10 mg/kg oral dose (solution in 1% methyl cellulose).

Overall, the studies published by Merck clearly demonstrated the challenges in generating BACE inhibitors with optimal ADME properties.

8.2.2 Progress at GlaxoSmithKline

Researchers at GlaxoSmithKline faced similar challenges in the development of drug-like BACE inhibitors. The micromolar hit **10** (Fig. 8.6) was obtained from a focused library [27] based on a transition-state HEA mimetic and was further optimized to deliver compounds of nanomolar potency in enzyme assays [28]. These inhibitors were active in cell-based assays but exhibited cytochrome P450 liabilities, mainly at CYP3A4, high *in vitro* clearance, and high PSA (Table 8.3). It proved possible to overcome the CYP and *in vitro* clearance liability by decreasing lipophilicity (LogD) as exemplified by compound **14**. However, the high PSA and low membrane permeability of this compound resulted in poor oral bioavailability (Fpo). Typically, compound **14** exhibited Fpo of 0.2% at 100 mg/kg po in rat despite moderate blood clearance (64 mL/min/kg).

In general, most of these BACE inhibitors demonstrated rapid clearance *in vivo*, with a few exceptions such as compound **13** (Table 8.4). Following intravenous administration via the hepatic portal vein, compound **13** was moderately cleared and well distributed but with suboptimal bioavailability, implying some first-pass elimination. The oral bioavailability of compound **13** at 3 mg/kg dose was identical to what was observed with intravenous administration suggesting complete absorption (probably related to a "low" PSA and appropriate formulation). Oral bioavailability was much higher at the 10 mg/kg dose and the nonlinear kinetics was most likely due to saturation of liver clearance at this dose. Like many other BACE inhibitors in this series, the brain penetration of this compound was low (Bl: Br ≈ 0.1:1) due

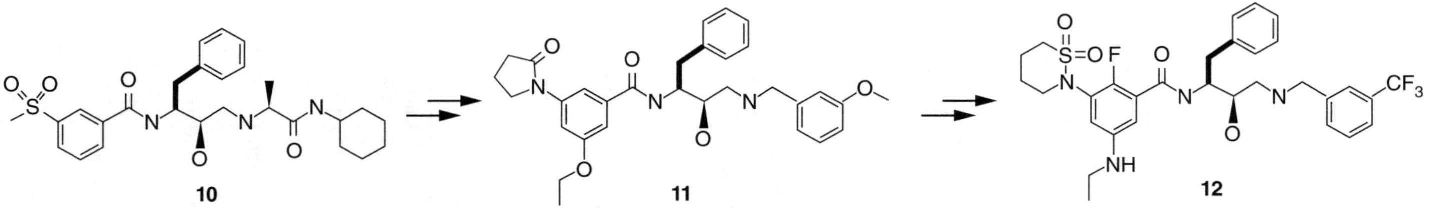

Figure 8.6 Discovery of GSK188909.

TABLE 8.3 *In Vitro* **Profile of Representative BACE Inhibitors**

Cmpd	BACE IC$_{50}$ (μM)	Aβ40 IC$_{50}$ (μM)	CYP IC$_{50}$ (μM)[a]	Cli (m, r, h)[b]	CHI LogD	PSA
11	9	35	14, 70, 61, 17, 3.0, 9.4	nd	1.93	100
12	2	5	>100, 9, 10, 6.2, 0.4, 1.6	46, 17, 18	2.82	111
13	9	35	75, 60, 15, 11, 75, 6.3	37, 8.7, 15	2.39	94
14	10	75	All > 89 (3A4 DEF)	5.4, 1.7, 4.2	1.36	129

[a] 1A2, 2C9, 2C19, 2D6, 3A4 (DEF, PPR); [b] ml/min/g liver. nd, not determined.

TABLE 8.4 *In Vivo* **PK Parameters of BACE Inhibitors**

Dose Route	Parameter	13	12
Intravenous[a] (n = 3/4)	CLb (mL/min/kg)	51 ± 9	83 ± 5
	Vss (L/kg)	4.5 ± 0.7	5.5 ± 0.6
	t½ (iv) (h)	1.9 ± 0.3	1.5 ± 0.3
	Fipv (%)	38 ± 11	nd
Oral[b] @ 3 mg/kg (n = 4)	Fpo (%)	35 ± 15	nd
	t½ (po) (h)	2.1, nd, 1.8, nd	nd
	AUC/Dose (min.kg/L)	6.9 ± 2.9	nd
Oral[b] @ 10 mg/kg (n = 3/4)	Fpo (%)	67 ± 45	7 ± 2
	t½ (po) (h)	1.8, 3.1, nd, nd	nd
	AUC/Dose (min.kg/L)	17.3 ± 14.8	0.86 ± 0.24

[a] For 13: 1 mg/kg/h infusion in hepatic portal vein for 1 h then in femoral vein for 1 h (solution in 2% DMSO, 0.9% (w/v) saline containing 10% (w/v) Kleptose. For 12: 1 mg/kg/h infusion in femoral vein for 1 h (solution 0.9% (w/v) saline containing 10% (w/v) Kleptose). [b] For 13: solution in 5% (v/v) Ethanol, Capmul MCM C8 and solutol HS 15 (20:80); For 12: solution 1% (v/v) Tween 80 and 1% (v/v) methylcellulose aq. nd, not determined.

to efficient efflux by the P-gp transporter. A related BACE inhibitor, compound **12** (GSK188909) [29] exhibited lower oral bioavailability than compound **13** and was also a strong P-gp substrate. However, its increased cell potency favored its selection for proof of mechanism studies *in vivo*.

In an attempt to increase the metabolic stability of this series, qualitative studies performed on GSK188909 (compound **12**) revealed that the main route of metabolism was de-alkylation of the left-hand side aniline and oxidation of the benzylic position [30]. Initial attempts to block these positions failed to improve metabolic stability. Moreover, a predictive model of absorption based on calculated molar refractivity (CMR) and lipophilicity (Fig. 8.7) suggested that most of the

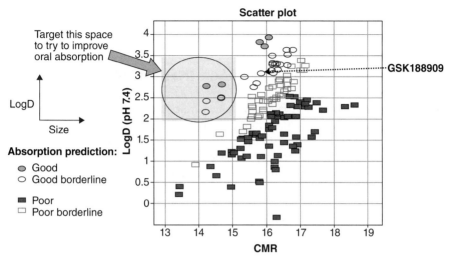

Figure 8.7   Scatter plot of predicted permeability of BACE inhibitors.

TABLE 8.5   *In Vivo* Pharmacokinetics of Compound 15

Species	$Cl_{blood}{}^a$ (mL/min/kg)	Vd^a (L/kg)	$t\frac{1}{2}{}^a$ (h)	$Cmax^b$ (µM)	%F
Rat (*n* = 2/3)	72, 62	11, 8	3, 2.8	0.184 ± 0.082	17, 22
Dog (*n* = 3)	23 ± 5	4.9 ± 0.9	4.2 ± 0.2	2.969 ± 0.787	79 ± 50
Monkey (*n* = 3)	29 ± 7	3.8 ± 0.9	2.0 ± 0.12	2.127 ± 0.095	73 ± 20

^{a} 1 mg/kg/h iv dose (solution of mesylate salt in 0.9 w/v saline containing 10% w/v Kleptose); ^{b} 10 mg/kg dose (solubtion of mesylate salt in 1% v/v Tween-80 and 1% w/v methylcellulose aqueous).

inhibitors in this series were predicted to be poorly absorbed. A novel series was needed and further SAR led to the discovery of a novel tricyclic non-prime side [30]. In particular, compound **15** was identified and shown to display good cellular activity and good PK properties in multiple species (Table 8.5). Encouragingly, this compound also exhibited increased brain penetration compared with the first generation of HEA inhibitors (Br:Bl ratio: ~0.37:1).

Overall, the work published by researchers at Merck, GlaxoSmithKline, and other groups [31] demonstrated that as in the case of HIV protease inhibitors, surmounting the combination of PK issues displayed by BACE inhibitors was extremely difficult. However, these efforts did lead to the identification of tool compounds that were shown to be efficacious in animal models.

8.3   *IN VIVO* EFFICACY OF BACE INHIBITORS

It is imperative that a BACE inhibitor demonstrates significant Aβ lowering in the brain of a preclinical disease-relevant model prior to its selection as a candidate compound. In addition, as oral administration is the preferred route for delivery of BACE inhibitors to AD patients, a pharmacological effect on Aβ needs to be established following oral administration of compound. In general, transgenic mice over-expressing an APP transgene, which results in the overproduction of Aβ peptides in the brain and their subsequent accumulation and deposition as plaques, are utilized for these pharmacodynamic studies [32]. More recently, *in vivo* models of endogenous Aβ production and clearance such as the mouse and rat have been developed and used for efficacy studies [33, 34]. Ideally, potential clinical candidates would also be evaluated in higher species such as a primate model to investigate the dynamics of Aβ lowering before progressing to clinical studies.

The first demonstration that a BACE inhibitor could lower brain Aβ *in vivo* was reported for a potent transition-state HE isostere inhibitor, OM00-3 [35]. This tool compound exhibited no drug-like properties and due to its large size (MW = 936) was not predicted to cross the blood–brain barrier. Consequently, it was conjugated to a poly D-arginine carrier peptide to increase its membrane permeability and facilitate brain penetration. Intraperitoneal administration of conjugated OM00-3 led to a reduction in plasma and brain Aβ40, thereby providing proof of mechanism for a BACE inhibitor. In subsequent reports, Aβ lowering was reported for a number of other tool BACE inhibitors that also exhibited inadequate PK properties. In these studies, compounds with poor oral bioavailability were administered via nonoptimal peripheral dose routes such as intravenous injection [21, 26] whereas direct delivery into the brain was required for compounds that were non-brain penetrant [33, 34, 36]. The requirement for brain penetration was clearly illustrated with Merck-3, a HEA isostere. If delivered peripherally via intravenous injection, this compound failed to lower brain Aβ due to its poor membrane permeability and its interactions with the P-gp transporter [36]. However, direct delivery into the brain by intracerebroventricular administration circumvented this problem, allowing adequate compound exposure at the target site to lower brain Aβ. Other groups used plasma Aβ as a readout to the assess efficacy of BACE inhibitors with limited brain penetration [31, 37, 38]. Although a decrease in plasma Aβ was consistent with inhibition of BACE in the periphery, it gave no indication of the central efficacy of these compounds.

The first orally bioavailable BACE inhibitor shown to reduce brain Aβ was GSK188909 (compound **12**) [39]. Oral administration of GSK188909 (250 mg/kg twice daily for 5 days) significantly decreased brain Aβ40 (18%) and Aβ42 (23%) in mutant APP, PS-1 transgenic (TASTPM) mice with a brain exposure of $0.17 \pm 0.09 \mu M$ (Fig. 8.8). Although this compound had a PK profile providing good oral exposure at high oral doses, it was found to exhibit low brain penetration

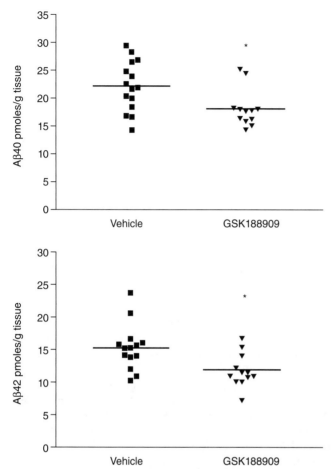

Figure 8.8 Subchronic dosing of GSK188909 lowers brain Aβ in TASTPM mice. Brain Aβ levels in TASTPM mice dosed with GSK188909 (250 mg/kg po bid) for 5 days. A significant decrease in Aβ40 and Aβ42 was observed in mice treated with GSK188909 (*$p < 0.01$ vs. vehicle). Reproduced from Hussain et al. 2007 [39] with permission of the International Society for Neurochemistry.

(blood : brain ratio ≤1:0.06) due to a strong interaction with the P-gp transporter. Increasing the brain exposure of GSK188909 by employing a P-gp inhibitor, GF120918 significantly enhanced brain Aβ lowering. Oral administration of GSK188909 (250 mg/kg) following a pre-dose of GF120918 (250 mg/kg) resulted in an approximate nine-fold increase in brain concentration of GSK188909 (blood : brain ratio 1:0.44; brain exposure 5.43 ± 3.5 μM), and this led to a greater reduction in brain Aβ40 (68%) and Aβ42 (55%) (Fig. 8.9). Unfortunately, the low brain penetration of GSK188909, its predicted high plasma protein binding, and the high dose required for efficacy significantly limited the development of this compound. A significant interaction with the P-gp transporter was subsequently reported to reduce the *in vivo* efficacy of other BACE inhibitors [40].

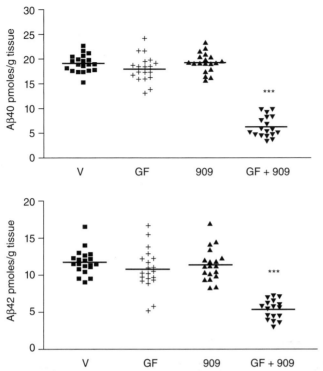

Figure 8.9   P-gp inhibitor enhances brain Aβ lowering activity of GSK188909 in TASTPM mice. Brain Aβ levels in TASTPM mice 9 h after acute oral dosing with vehicle (V) or 250 mg/kg GSK188909 (909) in the absence or presence of an oral pre-dose of 250 mg/kg GF120918 (GF). A significant decrease in Aβ40 and Aβ42 was observed in mice treated with GF120918 and GSK188909 (***$p < 0.000001$ vs. vehicle). Reproduced from Hussain et al. 2007 [39] with permission of the International Society for Neurochemistry.

The Aβ lowering activity of a potent and selective tertiary carbinamine BACE inhibitor TC-1 (compound **8**, Fig. 8.5) in APP transgenic mice and the rhesus monkey was recently published [25]. With regard to its ADME properties, this compound had an MW of 563, exhibited good passive membrane permeability, and was shown to be less susceptible to P-gp transport, suggesting good brain penetration should be achieved. However, when assessed in an acute brain penetration model, this compound was found to be only marginally brain penetrant with a brain : plasma ratio of 9% in rats [41]. In addition, TC-1 demonstrated high protein binding (>98%) in mouse, human, and rhesus monkey plasma, and was found to be rapidly metabolized by the liver cytochrome P450 enzymes CYP3A4, both resulting in poor oral bioavailability and low free drug concentrations. Consequently, intraperitoneal administration at a relatively high dose or intravenous infusion was required to demonstrate efficacy in APP transgenic mice or in rhesus monkeys, respectively.

TABLE 8.6 Effect of Ritonavir on the *In Vivo* PK Profile of TC-1

Cmpd	Cl[a] (mg/min/kg)	t½[a] (h)	AUC[b] (μM/h)	%F[b]
TC-1	24	≈1	0.1	<1
TC-1 + Ritonavir[c]	7	≈3	39	≈83

[a] 1 mg/kg TC-1 iv bolus; [b] 10 mg/kg TC-1 po; [c] 10 mg/kg.

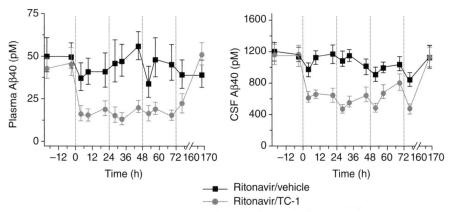

Figure 8.10   Ritonavir enhances the the Aβ lowering activity of TC-1 in primates. Time course of plasma and CSF Aβ40 levels over 3.5 days in primates co-dosed with ritonavir/vehicle (black filled squares) and ritonavir/TC-1 (red filled circles). Significant plasma ($p < 0.001$) and CSF ($p < 0.001$) Aβ40 lowering was observed relative to ritonavir/vehicle group. Reproduced from Sankaranarayanan et al. 2008 [25] with permission of the American Society for Pharmacology and Experimental Therapeutics.

To circumvent the PK issues with this compound and allow oral dosing studies in rhesus monkeys, the effect of Ritonavir, an HIV protease inhibitor that inhibits CYP3A4 metabolism, was investigated. Co-dosing with Ritonavir increased the oral bioavailability of TC-1 from <1% to 80%, decreased plasma clearance of compound more than three-fold, and increased both the plasma half-life of compound and plasma exposures (Table 8.6). In a subsequent efficacy study, oral administration of Ritonavir (10 mg/kg) followed by TC-1 (15 mg/kg) twice daily for 3.5 days resulted in a sustained reduction in plasma Aβ40 (61%) and encouragingly, CSF Aβ40 (42%) and Aβ42 (43%) were also reduced (Fig. 8.10). These Aβ reductions were associated with average plasma and CSF concentrations of TC-1 of $2.7 \pm 0.6 \, \mu M$ and $25 \pm 4 \, nM$, respectively, with a calculated free plasma concentration of approximately 27 nM.

Studies with Ritonavir and GF120918 demonstrated the utility of these drugs in augmenting the ADME properties of BACE inhibitors, thereby allowing the *in vivo* efficacy of BACE inhibitors to be explored in preclinical models. However,

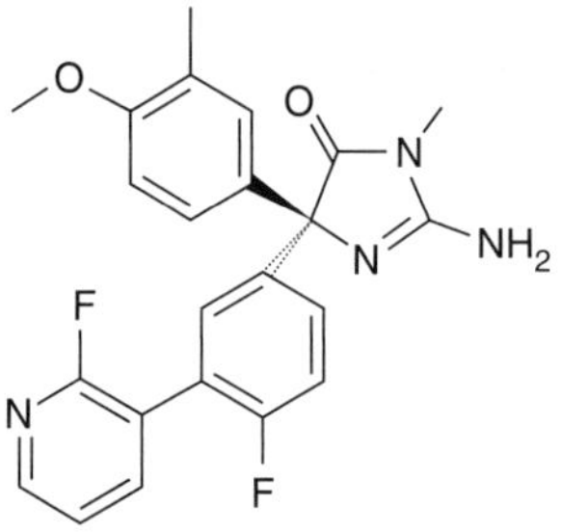

Figure 8.11   Structure of WAY-258131.

this coadministration approach may not be a viable option for the treatment of AD patients due to the potential for adverse events associated with drug–drug interactions, particularly while treating an elderly patient population on polypharmacy.

CTS-21166, a small molecule transition-state BACE inhibitor from Co-Mentis, recently entered clinical trials [42]. Intraperitoneal administration of CTS-21166 (4 mg/kg) for 6 weeks in APP transgenic mice resulted in a decrease in brain Aβ40 (38%) and Aβ42 (35%) and reduced plaque load in the hippocampus and cortex. PK measurements in rats and mice indicated that CTS-21166 displayed good brain penetration (blood : brain ratio 1:0.44) and did not exhibit high plasma protein binding [42]. Based on this positive preclinical efficacy data, Co-Mentis progressed to a Phase I clinical trial in healthy volunteers. The compound was well tolerated and was shown to decrease plasma Aβ levels following a single intravenous injection [42]. Although these are encouraging preliminary findings, evidence of central Aβ lowering following oral administration of CTS-21166 remains to be demonstrated.

The identification of non-transition-state mimetic BACE inhibitors suitable for evaluation in preclinical models has proven to be more challenging. WAY-258131 (Fig. 8.11), a small molecule BACE inhibitor developed by researchers at Wyeth, reportedly lowered brain Aβ in a dose-dependant manner in Tg2576 mice [43]. Details of these studies along with the PK profile of this compound have yet to be published.

The numerous *in vivo* studies clearly illustrate how the inadequate PK properties of BACE inhibitors have significantly limited their efficacy in animal models.

8.4   TOXICOLOGY OF BACE INHIBITORS

Following selection of a BACE inhibitor candidate and prior to its testing in clinical trials, the toxicological properties of a compound are investigated in one or more preclinical species (rat, dog) at high doses to establish the maximum tolerated dose and identify any adverse effects. One BACE inhibitor, CTS-21166, has entered Phase I clinical trials, and although its toxicological profile is not publically available, it must be acceptable to allow dosing in humans up to a dose of 225 mg.

8.5   FINAL REMARKS

In this chapter we have reviewed the ADME properties of BACE inhibitors and highlighted the major hurdles scientists have faced in the development of compounds suitable for clinical evaluation. The generation of potent and selective BACE inhibitors was relatively straightforward. However, like the HIV protease inhibitor field, incorporating drug-like properties into these compounds has been more challenging and resource-intensive. Despite tremendous efforts and several alterations to BACE inhibitor chemotypes, the generation of a brain-penetrant molecule devoid of CYP interactions and with an optimal *in vivo* ADME profile has proven a near impossible hurdle to overcome. Encouragingly, one BACE inhibitor has overcome some of these challenges and entered clinical trials, thereby, giving hope for the future development of BACE therapeutics.

REFERENCES

 1. Glenner, G.G. and Wong, C.W. 1984. Alzheimer's disease: initial report of the purification and characterization of a novel cerebrovascular amyloid protein. *Biochem Biophys Res Comm* **120**:885–890.
 2. Goedert, M., Wischik, C.M., Crowther, R.A., Walker, J.E., and Klug, A. 1988. Cloning and sequencing of the cDNA encoding a core protein of the paired helical filament of Alzheimer disease: identification as the microtubule-associated protein tau. *Proc Natl Acad Sci U S A* **85**:4051–4055.
 3. Hussain, I., Powell, D., Howlett, D.R., Tew, D.G., Meek, T.D., Chapman, C., Gloger, I.S., Murphy, K.E., Southan, C.D., Ryan, D.M., Smith, T.S., Simmons, D.L., Walsh, F.S., Dingwall, C., and Christie, G. 1999. Identification of a novel aspartic protease (Asp2) as β-secretase. *Mol Cell Neurosci* **14**:419–427.
 4. Vassar, R., Bennett, B.D., Babu-Khan, S., Kahn, S., Mendiaz, E.A., Denis, P., Teplow, D.B., Ross, S., Amarante, P., Loeloff, R., Luo, Y., Fisher, S., Fuller, J., Edenson, S., Lile, J., Jarosinski, M.A., Biere, A.L., Curran, E., Burgess, T., Louis, J.C., Collins, F., Treanor, J., Rogers, G., and Citron, M. 1999. β-secretase cleavage of Alzheimer's amyloid precursor protein by the transmembrane aspartic protease BACE. *Science* **286**:735–741.
 5. Yan, R., Bienkowski, M.J., Shuck, M.E., Miao, H., Tory, M.C., Pauley, A.M., Brashier, J.R., Stratman, N.C., Mathews, W.R., Buhl, A.E., Carter, D.B., Tomasselli, A.G., Parodi, L.A., Heinrikson, R.L., and Gurney, M.E. 1999. Membrane-anchored aspartyl protease with Alzheimer's disease β-secretase activity. *Nature* **402**:533–537.
 6. Sinha, S., Anderson, J.P., Barbour, R., Basi, G.S., Caccavello, R., Davis, D., Doan, M., Dovey, H.F., Frigon, N., Hong, J., Jacobson-Croak, K., Jewett, N., Keim, P., Knops, J., Lieburg, I., Power, M., Tan, H., Tatsuno, G., Tung, J., Schenk, D., Seubert, P., Suomensaari, S.M., Wang, S., Walker, D., Zhao, J., McConlogue, L., and John, V. 1999. Purification and cloning of amyloid precursor protein β-secretase from human brain. *Nature* **402**:537–540.
 7. Hong, L., Koelsch, G., Lin, X., Wu, S., Terzyan, S., Ghosh, A.K., Zhang, X.C., and Tang, J. 2000. Structure of the protease domain of memapsin 2 (beta-secretase) complexed with inhibitor. *Science* **290**:150–153.
 8. Eder, J., Hommel, U., Cumin, F., Martoglio, B., and Gerhartz, B. 2007. Aspartic proteases in drug discovery. *Cur Pharm Des* **12**:271–285.
 9. Muller, D.N. and Luft, F.C. 2006. Direct renin inhibition with Aliskiren in hypertension and target organ damage. *Clin J Am Soc Nephrol* **1**:221–228.
10. Abbenante, G. and Fairlie, D.P. 2005. Protease inhibitors in the clinic. *Med Chem* **1**:71–104.
11. Savolainen, J., Edwards, J.E., Morgan, M.E., McNamara, P.J., and Anderson, B.D. 2002. Effects of a P-glycoprotein inhibitor on brain and plasma concentrations of anti-human immunodeficiency virus drugs administered in combination in rats. *Drug Metab Dispos* **30**:479–482.

12. Cooper, C.L., Van Heeswijk, R.P.G., Gallicano, K., and Cameron, D.W. 2003. A review of low-dose ritonavir in protease inhibitor combination therapy. *HIV/AIDS* **36**:1585–1592.

13. Ghosh, A.K., Bilcer, G., Harwood, C., Kawahama, R., Shin, D., Hussain, K.A., Hong, L., Loy, J.A., Nguyen, C., Koelsch, G., Ermolieff, J., and Tang, J. 2001. Structure-based design: potent inhibitors of human brain memapsin 2 (β-secretase). *J Med Chem* **44**:2865–2868.

14. Tung, J.S., Davis, D.L., Anderson, J.P., Walker, D.E., Mamo, S., Jewett, N., Hom, R.K., Sinha, S., Thorsett, E.D., and John, V. 2002. Design of substrate-based inhibitors of human β-secretase. *J Med Chem* **45**:259–262.

15. Hom, R.K., Fang, L.Y., Mamo, S., Tung, J.S., Guinn, A.C., Walker, D.E., Davis, D.L., Gailunas, A.F., Thorsett, E.D., Sinha, S., Knops, J.E., Jewett, N.E., Anderson, J.P., and John, V. 2003. Design and synthesis of statine-based cell-permeable peptidomimetic inhibitors of human β-secretase. *J Med Chem* **46**:1799–1802.

16. Hom, R.K., Gailunas, A.F., Mamo, S., Fang, L.Y., Tung, J.S., Walker, D.E., Davis, D., Thorsett, E.D., Jewett, N.E., Moon, J.B., and John, V. 2004. Design and synthesis of hydroxyethylene-based peptidomimetic inhibitors of human β-secretase. *J Med Chem* **47**:158–164.

17. Coburn, C.A., Stachel, S.J., Li, Y.-M., Rush, D.M., Steele, T.G., Chen-Dodson, E., Holloway, M.K., Xu, M., Huang, Q., Lai, M.-T., Shi, X.-P., Sardana, V., Chen, Z., Munshi, S., Kuo, L., Makara, G.M., Annis, D.A., Tadikonda, P.K., Nash, H.M., Vacca, J.P., and Wang, T. 2004. Identification of a small molecule nonpeptide active site β-secretase inhibitor that displays a non-traditional binding mode for aspartyl proteases. *J Med Chem* **47**:6117–6119.

18. Stachel, S.J., Coburn, C.A., Steele, T.G., Jones, K.G., Loutzenhiser, E.F., Gregro, A.R., Rajapakse, H.A., Lai, M.-T., Crouthamel, M.-C., Xu, M., Tugusheva, K., Lineberger, J.E., Pietrak, B.L., Espeseth, A.S., Shi, X.-P., Chen-Dodson, E., Holloway, M.K., Munshi, S., Simon, A.J., Kuo, L., and Vacca, J.P. 2004. Structure-based design of potent and selective cell-permeable inhibitors of human β-secretase (BACE-1). *J Med Chem* **47**:6447–6450.

19. Stachel, S.J., Coburn, C.A., Steele, T.G., Crouthamel, M.-C., Pietrak, B.L., Lai, M.-T., Holloway, M.K., Munshi, S.K., Graham, S.L., and Vacca, J.P. 2006. Conformationally biased P3 amide replacements of β-secretase inhibitors. *Bioorg Med Chem Lett* **16**:641–644.

20. Coburn, C.A., Stachel, S.J., Jones, K.G., Steele, T.G., Rush, D.M., DiMuzio, J., Pietrak, B.L., Lai, M.-T., Huang, Q., Lineberger, J., Jin, L., Munshi, S., Holloway, M.K., Espeseth, A., Simon, A., Hazuda, D., Graham, S.L., and Vacca, J.P. 2006. BACE-1 inhibition by a series of ψ[CH2NH] reduced amide isosteres. *Bioorg Med Chem Lett* **16**:3635–3638.

21. Stachel, S.J., Coburn, C.A., Sankaranarayanan, S., Price, E.A., Pietrak, B.L., Huang, Q., Lineberger, J., Espeseth, A.S., Jin, L., Ellis, J., Holloway, M.K., Munshi, S., Allison, T., Hazuda, D., Simon, A.J., Graham, S.L., and Vacca, J.P. 2006. Macrocyclic inhibitors of β-secretase: functional activity in an animal model. *J Med Chem* **49**:6147–6150.

22. Rajapakse, H.A., Nantermet, P.G., Selnick, H.G., Munshi, S., McGaughey, G.B., Lindsley, S.R., Young, M.B., Lai, M.-T., Espeseth, A.S., Shi, X.-P., Colussi, D., Pietrak, B., Crouthamel, M.-C., Tugusheva, K., Huang, Q., Xu, M., Simon, A.J., Kuo, L., Hazuda, D.J., Graham, S., and Vacca, J.P. 2006. Discovery of oxadiazoyl tertiary carbinamine inhibitors of β-secreatse (BACE-1). *J Med Chem* **49**:7270–7273.

23. McGauchey, G.B., Colussi, D., Graham, S.L., Lai, M.-T., Munshi, S.K., Nantermet, P.G., Pietrak, B., Rajapakse, H.A., Selnick, H.G., Stauffer, S.R., and Holloway, M.K. 2007. β-secretase (BACE-1) inhibitors: accounting for 10s loop flexibility using rigid active sites. *Bioorg Med Chem Lett* **17**:1117–1121.

24. Stauffer, S.R., Stanton, M.G., Gregro, A.R., Steinbeiser, M.A., Shaffer, J.R., Nantermet, P.G., Barrow, J.C., Rittle, K.E., Colussi, D., Espeseth, A.S., Lai, M.-T., Pietrak, B.L., Holloway, M.K., McGaughey, G.B., Munshi, S.K., Hochman, J.H., Simon, A.J., Selnick, H.G., Graham, S.L., and Vacca, J.P. 2007. Discovery and SAR of isonicotinamide BACE-1 inhibitors that bind β-secretase in an N-terminal 10s-loop down conformation. *Bioorg Med Chem Lett* **17**:1788–1792.

25. Sankaranarayanan, S., Holahan, M.A., Colussi, D., Crouthamel, M.C., Devanarayan, V., Ellis, J., Espeseth, A., Gates, A.T., Graham, S.L., Gregro, A.R., Hazuda, D., Hochman, J.H., Holloway, K., Jin, L., Kahana, J., Lai, M.T., Lineberger, J., McGaughey, G., Moore, K.P., Nantermet, P., Pietrak, B., Price, E.A., Rajapakse, H., Stauffer, S., Steinbeiser, M.A., Seabrook, G., Selnick, H.G., Shi, X.P., Stanton, M.G., Swestock, J., Tugusheva, K., Tyler, K.X., Vacca, J.P., Wong, J., Wu, G., Xu, M.,

Cook, J.J., and Simon, A.J. 2009. First demonstration of CSF and plasma Aβ lowering with oral administration of a BACE1 inhibitor in nonhuman primates. *J Pharmacol Exp Ther* **328**:131–140.

26. Stanton, M.G., Stauffer, S.R., Gregro, A.R., Steinbeiser, M., Nantermet, P., Sankaranarayanan, S., Price, E.A., Wu, G., Crouthamel, M.-C., Ellis, J., Lai, M.-T., Espeseth, A.S., Shi, X.-P., Jin, L., Colussi, D., Pietrak, B., Huang, Q., Xu, M., Simon, A.J., Graham, S.L., Vacca, J.P., and Selnick, H. 2007. Discovery of isonicotinamide derived β-secretase inhibitors: in vivo reduction of γ-amyloid. *J Med Chem* **50**:3431–3433.

27. Clarke, B., Demont, E., Dingwall, C., Dunsdon, R., Faller, A., Hawkins, J., Hussain, I., MacPherson, D., Maile, G., Matico, R., Milner, P., Mosley, J., Naylor, A., O'Brien, A., Redshaw, S., Riddell, D., Rowland, P., Soleil, V., Smith, K.J., Stanway, S., Stemp, G., Sweitzer, S., Theobald, P., Vesey, D., Walter, D.S., Ward, J., and Wayne, G. 2008. BACE-1 inhibitors part 1: identification of novel hydroxy ethylamines (HEAs). *Bioorg Med Chem Lett* **18**:1011–1016.

28. Clarke, B., Demont, E., Dingwall, C., Dunsdon, R., Faller, A., Hawkins, J., Hussain, I., MacPherson, D., Maile, G., Matico, R., Milner, P., Mosley, J., Naylor, A., O'Brien, A., Redshaw, S., Riddell, D., Rowland, P., Soleil, V., Smith, K.J., Stanway, S., Stemp, G., Sweitzer, S., Theobald, P., Vesey, D., Walter, D.S., Ward, J., and Wayne, G. 2008. BACE-1 inhibitors part 2: identification of hydroxy ethylamines (HEAs) with reduced peptidic character. *Bioorg Med Chem Lett* **18**:1017–1021.

29. Beswick, P., Charrier, N., Clarke, B., Demont, E., Dingwall, C., Dunsdon, R., Faller, A., Gleave, R., Hawkins, J., Hussain, I., Johnson, C.N., MacPherson, D., Maile, G., Matico, R., Milner, P., Mosley, J., Naylor, A., O'Brien, A., Redshaw, S., Riddell, D., Rowland, P., Soleil, V., Skidmore, J., Smith, K.J., Stanway, S., Stemp, G., Stuart, A., Sweitzer, S., Theobald, P., Vesey, D., Walter, D.S., Ward, J., and Wayne, G. 2008. BACE-1 inhibitors part 3: identification of hydroxy ethylamines (HEAs) with nanomolar potency in cells. *Bioorg Med Chem Lett* **18**:1022–1026.

30. Charrier, N., Clarke, B., Cutler, L., Demont, E., Dingwall, C., Dunsdon, R., East, P., Hawkins, J., Howes, C., Hussain, I., Jeffrey, P., Maile, G., Matico, R., Mosley, J., Naylor, A., O'Brien, A., Redshaw, S., Rowland, P., Soleil, V., Smith, K.J., Sweitzer, S., Theobald, P., Vesey, D., Walter, D.S., and Wayne, G. 2008. Second generation of hydroxyethylamine BACE-1 inhibitors: optimizing potency and oral bioavailability. *J Med Chem* **51**:3313–3317.

31. Iserloh, U., Pan, J., Stamford, A.W., Kennedy, M.E., Zhang, Q., Zhang, L., Parker, E.M., McHugh, N.A., Favreau, L., Strickland, C., and Voigt, J. 2008. Disocvery of an orally efficacious 4-phenoxy-pyrrolidine-based BACE-1 inhibitor. *Bioorg Med Chem Lett* **18**:418–422.

32. McGowan, E., Eriksen, J., and Hutton, M. 2006. A decade of modeling Alzheimer's disease in transgenic mice. *Trends Genet* **22**:281–289.

33. Asai, M., Hattori, C., Iwata, N., Saido, T.C., Sasagawa, N., Szabó, B., Hashimoto, Y., Maruyama, K., Tanuma, S., Kiso, Y., and Ishiura, S. 2006. The novel beta-secretase inhibitor KMI-429 reduces amyloid beta peptide production in amyloid precursor protein transgenic and wild-type mice. *J Neurochem* **96**:533–540.

34. Nishitomi, K., Sakaguchi, G., Horikoshi, Y., Gray, A.J., Maeda, M., Hirata-Fukae, C., Becker, A.G., Hosono, M., Sakaguchi, I., Minami, S.S., Nakajima, Y., Li, H.F., Takeyama, C., Kihara, T., Ota, A., Wong, P.C., Aisen, P.S., Kato, A., Kinoshita, N., and Matsuoka, Y. 2006. BACE1 inhibition reduces endogenous Abeta and alters APP processing in wild-type mice. *J Neurochem* **99**:1555–1563.

35. Chang, W.P., Koelsch, G., Wong, S., Downs, D., Da, H., Weerasena, V., Gordon, B., Devasamudram, T., Bilcer, G., Ghosh, A.K., and Tang, J. 2004. In vivo inhibition of Abeta production by memapsin 2 (beta-secretase) inhibitors. *J Neurochem* **89**:1409–1416.

36. Sankaranarayanan, S., Price, E.A., Wu, G., Crouthamel, M.C., Shi, X.P., Tugusheva, K., Tyler, K.X., Kahana, J., Ellis, J., Jin, L., Steele, T., Stachel, S., Coburn, C., and Simon, A.J. 2008. In vivo beta-secretase 1 inhibition leads to brain Abeta lowering and increased alpha-secretase processing of amyloid precursor protein without effect on neuregulin-1. *J Pharmacol Exp Ther* **324**:957–969.

37. Baxter, E.W., Conway, K.A., Kennis, L., Bischoff, F., Mercken, M.H., Winter, H.L., Reynolds, C.H., Tounge, B.A., Luo, C., Scott, M.K., Huang, Y., Braeken, M., Pieters, S.M., Berthelot, D.J., Masure, S., Bruinzeel, W.D., Jordan, A.D., Parker, M.H., Boyd, R.E., Qu, J., Alexander, R.S., Brenneman, D.E., and Reitz, A.B. 2007. 2-Amino-3,4-dihydroquinazolines as inhibitors of BACE-1 (beta-site APP cleaving enzyme): use of structure based design to convert a micromolar hit into a nanomolar lead. *J Med Chem* **50**:4261–4264.

38. Cumming, J.N., Le, T.X., Babu, S., Carroll, C., Chen, X., Favreau, L., Gaspari, P., Guo, T., Hobbs, D.W., Huang, Y., Iserloh, U., Kennedy, M.E., Kuvelkar, R., Li, G., Lowrie, J., McHugh, N.A., Ozgur, L., Pan, J., Parker, E.M., Saionz, K., Stamford, A.W., Strickland, C., Tadesse, D., Voigt, J., Wang, L., Wu, Y., Zhang, L., and Zhang, Q. 2008. Rational design of novel, potent piperazinone and imid-azolidinone BACE1 inhibitors. *Bioorg Med Chem Lett* **18**:3236–3241.
39. Hussain, I., Hawkins, J., Harrison, D., Hille, C., Wayne, G., Cutler, L., Buck, T., Walter, D., Demont, E., Howes, C., Naylor, A., Jeffrey, P., Gonzalez, M.I., Dingwall, C., Michel, A., Redshaw, S., and Davis, J.B. 2007. Oral administration of a potent and selective non-peptidic BACE-1 inhibitor decreases beta-cleavage of amyloid precursor protein and amyloid-beta production in vivo. *J Neurochem* **100**:802–809.
40. Meredith, J.E. Jr., Thompson, L.A., Toyn, J.H., Marcin, L., Barten, D.M., Marcinkeviciene, J., Kopcho, L., Kim, Y., Lin, A., Guss, V., Burton, C., Iben, L., Polson, C., Cantone, J., Ford, M., Drexler, D., Fiedler, T., Lentz, K.A., Grace, J.E. Jr., Kolb, J., Corsa, J., Pierdomenico, M., Jones, K., Olson, R.E., Macor, J.E., and Albright, C.F. 2008. P-glycoprotein efflux and other factors limit brain amyloid beta reduction by beta-site amyloid precursor protein-cleaving enzyme 1 inhibitors in mice. *J Pharmacol Exp Ther* **326**:502–513.
41. Nantermet, P.G., Rajapakse, H.A., Stanton, M.G., Stauffer, S.R., Barrow, J.C., Gregro, A.R., Moore, K.P., Steinbeiser, M.A., Swestock, J., Selnick, H.G., Graham, S.L., McGaughey, G.B., Colussi, D., Lai, M.T., Sankaranarayanan, S., Simon, A.J., Munshi, S., Cook, J.J., Holahan, M.A., Michener, M.S., and Vacca, J.P. 2008. Evolution of tertiary carbinamine BACE-1 inhibitors: Abeta reduction in rhesus CSF upon oral dosing. *ChemMedChem* **4**:37–40.
42. Strobel, G. 2008. Keystone Drug News: CoMentis BACE Inhibitor Debuts. Alzheimer Research Forum. Available at http://www.alzforum.org/new/detail.asp?id=1790 (accessed April 5, 2008).
43. Malamas, M., Erdei, J., Gunawan, I., Robichaud, A., Turner, J., Hu, Y., Wagner, E., Aschmies, S., Comery, T., Fan, K., Chopra, R., Magold, R., Pangalos, M., Reinhart, P., Riddell, D., Jacobsen, S., Abou-Gharbia, M., and Bard, J. 2008. Small molecule BACE-1 inhibitors are potent, selective and orally active. *Alzheimer's and Dementia* **4**:T515.

CHAPTER 9

CLINICAL TRIALS FOR DISEASE-MODIFYING DRUGS SUCH AS BACE INHIBITORS

Henry H. Hsu

CoMentis, Inc., South San Francisco, CA

9.1 INTRODUCTION

More than 5 million Americans are estimated to have Alzheimer's disease (AD), and it is the fifth leading cause of death in those older than 65 years [1]. By 2050, the incidence of AD is expected to approach a million people per year, with a prevalence of 11–15 million persons. Fourteen percent of all people aged 71 and older have dementia, with the majority having AD. These statistics point to the huge unmet need for more effective therapies to treat this increasingly common disease.

The development of new drugs to treat AD has evolved substantially as our understanding of the pathogenesis of AD has shifted from approaches targeting the "cholinergic hypothesis" to the "amyloid hypothesis" [2]. Currently approved treatments have targeted modulation of neurotransmitters, particularly acetylcholine, via inhibition of the activity of cholinesterases, as well as the glutamatergic system by blocking N-methyl-D-aspartic acid (NMDA) glutamate receptors [3]. As such, the clinical development of these drugs has focused on demonstration of cognitive benefit over a relatively short time period (from 3 to 6 months), and these drugs have not been demonstrated to alter the underlying course of AD [4]. These therapies, which include donepazil, galantamine, rivastigmine, and memantine, were all approved based upon demonstration of meaningful clinical benefit compared with placebo in AD patients as assessed by a combination of patient-administered cognitive tests, such as the Alzheimer's Disease Assessment Scale (ADAS)-cog, and a clinician-based assessment of change, such as the Clinician's Interview Based Impression of Change (CIBIC)-plus. These tests were administered during randomized placebo-controlled clinical trials over the course of up to 6 months and showed an early improvement in cognition among active treatment recipients followed by a gradual decline that generally paralleled the decline in placebo recipients. Hence, these agents have been categorized as providing "symptomatic" benefits. While

BACE: Lead Target for Orchestrated Therapy of Alzheimer's Disease, Edited by Varghese John
Copyright © 2010 John Wiley & Sons, Inc.

clinically relevant benefits were demonstrated, most clinicians have considered the degree of symptomatic improvement to be modest.

The amyloid hypothesis has greatly expanded our understanding of the pathogenesis of AD and a wide range of new drug targets have emerged as our understanding of the cascade of underlying events associated with AD have been enlarged. The drugs generating the most excitement are those that seek to alter the course of AD by rationally targeting key aspects of this cascade considered critical for progression of the disease [5]. The clinical development of these new drugs requires modified approaches from that of symptomatic therapies as they may or may not show early short-term beneficial effects but would be expected to alter the underlying trajectory of the disease over longer-term treatment. As a result, the concept of "disease modification" has emerged as a goal in the clinical development of new therapeutics for AD [6]. While this concept is a very rational extension of our understanding of the basic science of AD, the practical implementation and demonstration of disease modification poses significant challenges at the operational and regulatory levels, which will be described in this chapter. In addition, these next-generation therapies are associated with substantial drug development challenges during early-phase human clinical testing, particularly in Phase 2 testing, where it is desirable to demonstrate sufficient "proof-of-concept" to justify the large time and financial investment required for conducting pivotal clinical studies.

9.2 UPDATE ON BETA-AMYLOID THERAPIES IN CLINICAL DEVELOPMENT

The number of compounds being evaluated in for treatment of AD has grown substantially and now includes more than 60 different compounds [5], with more than 30 of these currently in clinical testing. Most of these agents can be categorized into two general approaches: anti-amyloid approaches and neuroprotective/neurorestorative approaches (Table 9.1). Anti-amyloid approaches include vaccination (both passive and active), beta-secretase inhibitors, gamma-secretase inhibitors or modulators, anti-fibrillization agents, and anti-aggregation agents such as metal chelators. Neuroprotective approaches include antioxidants, anti-inflammatory agents, excitatory neurotransmitter antagonists (e.g., NMDA- and alpha-amino-3-hydroxy-5-methyl-4-isoxazole propionic acid (AMPA)-receptor antagonists), anti-apoptotic agents, and tau-related agents such as GSK3beta inhibitors. A detailed summary of these approaches may be found in a recent review (Salloway). In addition, a number of naturally derived compounds are being tested. Drugs targeting beta-secretase are relative newcomers with most in preclinical evaluation and none having progressed into Phase 3 testing. Later-stage clinical trial results have recently been reported for a number of other agents, and their results from a safety, activity, and efficacy standpoint provide a background and context for considering the design and implementation of clinical trials of β-site APP cleaving enzyme (BACE) inhibitors in the future. In addition, much can be learned from differences in the design and implementation of these studies.

TABLE 9.1 Anti-Amyloid and Neuroprotective Approaches for Treatment of AD (with Selected Examples)

Anti-Amyloid Approaches
    Immunization or passive antibodies (AN1792, bepineuzimab, IV immunoglobulin)
    Gamma-secretase inhibitors/modulators (LY450139, terenfurbil)
    Beta-secretase inhibitors (CTS21166, KMI-429)
    Anti-fibrillization agents (Tramiprosate)
    Statins (atorvastatin, simvastatin)
    PPAR-gamma agonists (rosiglitazone)
    Metal chelating agents (DP-109)
    RAGE-related effects (PF-04494700)
    Oligomer neutralizing agents (AZD-103)
    Other anti-amyloid approaches (DHA, resveratrol)
Neuroprotective approaches (including tau-targeted approaches)
    Nerve growth factors and related therapies (cerebrolysin)
    Antioxidants (vitamins C and E)
    Tau-related approaches (GSK3beta inhibitors, lithium, valproate, methylene blue)
    Anti-inflammatory agents (prednisone, diclofenac, naproxen)
    AMPA-related agents (CX516, LY404187)

PPAR, peroxisome proliferator-activated receptor; RAGE, receptor for advanced glycation end products.

9.2.1 Vaccination Approaches

In preclinical transgenic animal models of AD, both active vaccination with beta-amyloid and passive administration of anti-amyloid antibodies such a bepineuzimab to animals overexpressing human beta-amyloid have shown consistent reduction in brain amyloid, for both soluble and plaque forms [7–11]. These effects on amyloid have been associated with beneficial effects on measures of cognition and memory in animals (such as improved performance in the Morris water maze). Active vaccination with the synthetic beta-amyloid peptide AN1792 (Elan) in patients with AD demonstrated promising clinical effects on rate of decline and decrease in plaque burden [12, 13]. Unfortunately, clinical studies of active immunization with AN1792 were terminated after a subset of AN1792-treated patients developed meningoencephalitis [12]. It has been surmised that such vaccination induces cellular and or humoral immunity against beta-amyloid in the brain that may also be associated with a deleterious proinflammatory response in a subset of susceptible individuals. A recent study examining the long-term effects of immunization found that, while immunization resulted in clearance of amyloid plaques in patients with AD, it did not prevent progressive neurodeneration [14]. These results point out the potential for unexpected safety and efficacy findings as novel approaches are evaluated in the clinic and require that scientists incorporate these findings into theories of AD pathogenesis.

As a consequence of these adverse findings, the focus for a vaccination strategy has shifted toward direct administration of anti-beta-amyloid antibody. Results were reported in 2008 on a Phase 2 study evaluating the safety and preliminary efficacy of a humanized monoclonal antibody against amyloid beta (bepineuzimab,

Elan) [15]. This randomized placebo-controlled multiple ascending dose study was conducted in 234 patients with mild to moderate AD. Four cohorts (plus placebo), received 6 infusions every 3 months over an 18-month period. A number of efficacy and activity measures were assessed throughout treatment, including cognitive and memory tests (ADAS-cog, Neuropsychological Test Battery [NTB], Disability Assessment for Dementia [DAD] Scale, Clinical Dementia Rating Sum of the Boxes [CDR-SB] Scale, Mini-Mental Status Exam [MMSE]), and biomarkers (cerebrospinal fluid [CSF] abeta and tau) and imaging (magnetic resonance imaging [MRI] volumetrics). Patients had a mean age of approximately 70 years, with a baseline MMSE score of 21. Approximately two-thirds were ApoE4 carriers, and over 90% were receiving cholinesterase inhibitors or memantine. While adverse events among bepineuzumab recipients were generally mild to moderate, transient, and not dose-related, 12 (10%) of patients receiving bepineuzumab had vasogenic edema, most detected by MRI, with few or no clinical symptoms. The occurrence of vasogenic edema was dose-related with eight cases occurring at the highest dose (2.0 mg). One patient was treated with steroids for lethargy and confusion. The study did not achieve significance in the primary efficacy end points (ADAS-cog and DAD). However, in post hoc efficacy analyses with adjustment for ApoE4 carrier status, non-dose-related treatment effects were seen in noncarriers on both clinical and MRI measures. Noncarriers showed significantly less brain volume decline than placebo, and phospho-tau levels trended lower in bepineuzumab-treated patients versus placebo-treated patients.

These results were viewed as sufficiently promising by the sponsors to progress to a Phase 3 program in which separate studies are being conducted in ApoE4 carriers and noncarriers. However, there remains significant uncertainty as to whether this passive immunization approach will ultimately prove to be efficacious. From a mechanism standpoint, because immunization approaches target removal of beta-amyloid, and BACE inhibitors target the production of beta-amyloid, results from vaccination approaches may not necessarily apply to BACE inhibitors. Nevertheless, success with the vaccination approach would provide convincing evidence for the validity of the amyloid hypothesis and other approaches targeting amyloid reduction.

9.2.2 Gamma-Secretase Inhibitors/Modulators

Gamma-secretase has been a prominent target for inhibition as an approach toward reducing the production of beta-amyloid, due to its critical role (along with beta-secretase) in the conversion of amyloid precursor protein (APP) into beta-amyloid [16, 17]. Both direct inhibitors and modulators of gamma-secretase activity have been actively pursued. A safety concern related to direct gamma-secretase inhibitors are potential effects on Notch cleavage by gamma-secretase [18, 19]. Notch cleavage is integral to cell differentiation pathways in many organ systems, including the gastrointestinal and lymphoid organs, and genetic knockout of Notch function is lethal in mice. Among the direct inhibitors, most clinical data have published on LY450139 (Eli Lilly), for which Phase 1 data in healthy volunteers and Phase 2 data in AD patients have been published [20–22]. LY450139 is a functional gamma-secretase inhibitor that reduces the rate of formation of beta-amyloid in transgenic mice overexpressing beta-amyloid. In a multicenter, randomized, placebo-controlled trial in 51 patients with mild to moderate AD, patients were randomized to receive LY450139 for a total of 14 weeks in a dose-escalating fashion [22]. The drug appeared to be generally well tolerated; however, there was an excess of adverse events affecting the skin and gastrointestinal (GI) systems among drug recipients, as well as a higher incidence of general symptoms, including somnolence, fatigue, and asthenia. The drug was well absorbed following oral dosing, and drug was detected in CSF. Similar to findings in healthy volunteers, after dosing, a transient decrease over 6 h in plasma beta-amyloid levels of 65% from baseline followed by an increase in levels to greater than baseline over the next 18 h. This biphasic response accompanied by a "rebound" effect has been noted with other gamma-secretase compounds and appears to be due to an increase in gamma-secretase activity when drug levels have declined below a threshold. The significance of these fluctuations in plasma beta-amyloid for changes in CNS levels of beta-amyloid is unclear. No significant reductions were seen in CSF beta-amyloid 1–40 levels; however, there were trends seen in these levels in association with higher drug levels. No significant differences were seen in clinical cognitive measures (ADAS-cog and Alzheimer's Disease Cooperative Study [ADCS]-Activities of Daily Living [ADL] scores), which is not unexpected, given the short trial duration and small numbers of subjects.

The question of whether LY450139 does indeed have an effect on CNS beta-amyloid has recently been addressed using a novel approach measuring the rate of synthesis of beta-amyloid rather than the change in absolute levels in CSF [23]. Bateman et al. have presented results of a method in which nonradioactive C13-labeled leucine is administered in conjunction with study medication, followed by careful and frequent measurement of the ratio of newly labeled beta-amyloid to total beta-amyloid in the CSF to derive a measure of the fractional production rate of newly synthesized beta-amyloid [24]. One potential advantage of this "pulse-chase" approach appears to be a greater ability to detect an inhibition of beta-amyloid in CSF compared with measurement of the total level of beta-amyloid as it shows less intra- and intersubject variability compared with total beta-amyloid levels [25]. Using this approach, they demonstrated that a significant decrease in production of new beta-amyloid in the CSF could be demonstrated following a single oral dose in healthy volunteers [23]. As predicted, there was no significant difference in clearance. There was also a significant correlation between drug levels and decrease in beta-amyloid synthesis. These significant effects were demonstrated with only five subjects per cohort. While this pulse-chase approach remains experimental and has not been extensively evaluated with other beta-amyloid reducing compounds, it provides an appealing option as a potentially useful biomarker to evaluate the CNS pharmacodynamic effects of these compounds.

9.2.3   Beta-Secretase Inhibitors

Although beta-secretase has been identified as a promising drug target, it has proven to be a significant challenge for medicinal chemists to develop potent, selective, nonpeptidic inhibitors of the enzyme capable of crossing both the gut and blood–brain barriers. Thus, limited data have been disclosed on compounds that have entered into clinical testing, and no data have been presented on testing of candidate drugs in AD patients.

CTS21166 (ASP1702) (CoMentis/Astellas) is a potent and selective prototype BACE1 inhibitor for which early human data have been presented in abstract form (International Conference on Alzheimer's Disease, Chicago, 2008). It was developed using structure-based design and showed single-digit nanomolar potency against soluble and cellular BACE1. In mice, rats, and dogs, it showed good oral bioavailability and, in hAPP AD transgenic and wild-type mice, it penetrated the brain and reduced soluble Ab and amyloid plaque. In intravenous and oral toxicological studies in rats and dogs, the compound displayed a good safety profile to support clinical development.

Based upon these promising nonclinical studies, healthy young males were evaluated in two Phase 1 studies. In the first, subjects received single ascending doses of CTS-21166 (up to 225 mg) or vehicle by continuous intravenous infusion. In the second study, subjects received CTS-21166 (200 mg) liquid by oral administration. CTS-21166 was well tolerated up to the maximum intravenous (225 mg) and oral dose (200 mg). Following intravenous infusion, CTS-21166 showed dose-proportional increases in the area under the curve (AUC). Pharmacokinetic profiles across doses showed low intersubject variability. Following oral dosing of CTS-21166 (200 mg) liquid, the bioavailability was 40.5%. A dose-related reduction of plasma beta-amyloid$_{40}$ levels was seen with the maximal reduction of plasma beta-amyloid being greater than 80% of predose basal levels noted 4–8 h after dosing. The reduction was sustained over 72 h with plasma levels slowly returning to baseline. No evidence of plasma rebound in abeta was observed. The EC$_{50}$ for plasma beta-amyoid$_{40}$ reduction based on PK/PD analysis was 21.2 ± 5.9 ng/mL.

In view of the high degree of interest in beta-secretase as a drug development target and the progress reported by many groups with preclinical data, it can be anticipated that the next few years will yield additional potential drug candidates moving into clinical trials.

9.2.4 Other Drugs Targeting Beta-Amyloid Pathway

Large Phase 3 studies were recently completed with two compounds targeting the amyloidogenic pathway. Unfortunately, both failed to demonstrate statistically significant effects on clinical end points.

Tramiprosate (Alzhemed™, Neurochem), is an oral small molecule modification of the amino acid taurine. Its mechanism of action is thought to involve inhibition of fibrillar amyloid production and deposition under the assumption that this would decrease amyloid plaque formation [26]. The drug would not be expected to inhibit production of beta-amyloid. The results of the North American Phase 3 trial in 1,052 AD patients were inconclusive. Apparently, a number of clinical trial conduct issues affected interpretability, including significant variability among the 67 clinical sites. In particular, changes in patients' concomitant treatment with cognitive-enhancing drugs such as cholinesterase inhibitors, memantine, and anti-depressants affected the results for the primary cognitive end points based on neuropsychological testing. Unexpected problems in the control group confounded the interpretation of efficacy. Thirty percent of the control group did not decline in cognition over the 18-month trial period, and a portion of the control group unexpectedly demonstrated a significant improvement in cognition. While the full data from this study has not been published, the results disclosed highlight the challenges in carrying out a large long-term efficacy study in a population as complex as AD.

Tarenflurbil (Flurizan, Myriad) is an oral γ-secretase-modulating agent that showed possible clinical efficacy for the highest dose in patients with mild AD in a Phase 2 trial [27]. The compound belongs to a class of γ-secretase-modulating agents thought to reduce the production of beta-amyloid 1–42, considered by researchers to be the most toxic form of beta-amyloid. A large Phase 3 trial of tarenflurbil with an 18-month treatment period was recently completed [28]. The study enrolled almost 1700 patients across 133 centers in the United States and was the largest such study conducted to date of a disease-modifying approach. On both primary efficacy end points, the ADAS-cog and the ACDS activities of daily living scales, the treatment and placebo showed no significant differences. Importantly, the placebo group declined as predicted, and the trial was adequately powered to detect a meaningful treatment effect. Dropout rates were 33% for placebo and 39% for Flurizan, and the investigators followed the prespecified analysis plan. Thus, the study would have been able to detect a treatment difference if terenflurbil was active and the absence of a treatment effect could not be attributed to inadequate sample size or methodologic issues.

Tarenflurbil may not have been an optimal compound to test this class of drugs. While the compound had shown effects *in vitro* and *in vivo* in mice, data suggest that levels in the human brain may have been inadequate and, in a Phase 1 trial, no significant reductions in plasma and CSF Aβ42 levels of healthy volunteers treated with the highest dose of Flurizan that was then used in the Phase 3 trial [29–31].

These recent results not only highlight the high-risk nature of clinical development of next-generation drugs for AD but also show that it is feasible to conduct large multicenter clinical trials of long duration with low intercenter variability, acceptably low dropout rates, and predictable rates of cognitive decline in a placebo group, allowing for comparisons with active treatment.

9.3 CLINICAL DEVELOPMENT OF BACE INHIBITORS AND OTHER DISEASE-MODIFYING DRUGS

There are a number of challenges that need to be carefully addressed in the clinical development of potential disease-modifying therapies for AD. For companies engaged in research and drug development, whose goals are to develop new drugs in a rapid and cost-efficient manner, the drug development challenge lies in accurately assessing the chances of success at each stage of development, in order to drop drugs unlikely to make it to the marketplace, and to allocate resources and funding for drugs with an increased likelihood of success. An additional challenge, particularly during later stages of development, is the need to address the concerns of regulatory bodies in demonstrating that a novel agent is safe and effective in providing more than symptomatic benefit.

In view of the rapid progress being made in our understanding of the pathogenesis of AD, together with the evolution of thinking on trial designs and use of surrogate biomarkers of activity, and the plethora of drugs now in various stages of development, it is critical that industry, academics, and regulators work closely and collaboratively to define the path forward so that it is clear from the earliest stages of drug development what will be required to get a drug to market that will provide a substantial benefit to patients. A consensus is emerging among opinion leaders and regulators on the major requirements to be met for next-generation treatments for AD.

9.3.1 Early-Phase Clinical Development

The prerequisites for selecting and advancing a potential BACE inhibitor into clinical studies have been focused in three areas: (1) demonstrating safety in a broad toxicology program including multiple-dose toxicity studies; (2) demonstrating penetration of a drug candidate across the blood–brain barrier into the central nervous compartment (CSF and/or brain) in a relevant animal species; and (3) demonstrating effects on brain and CSF levels of beta-amyloid. With respect to safety toxicology, it may be important to evaluate safety following longer dosing periods (e.g., 12 or 24 weeks or longer) prior to initiating human studies in order to obtain early toxicity information that longer dosing periods is not associated with unexpected adverse effects, since it is anticipated that these drugs will be chronically dosed for many years in patients. BACE or its cleavage product, beta-amyloid, is widely distributed in tissues, including platelets, muscle, blood vessels, pancreas, skin, and subcutaneous tissues [32–35]. A potent, systemically administered BACE inhibitor could be expected to inhibit BACE activity throughout the body, and it is unclear whether long-term inhibition may be associated with subtle toxicity as an extension of its pharmacologic activity. In addition, novel small molecule inhibitors need to be carefully screened for potential off-target effects.

It has been challenging to develop BACE inhibitors capable of effectively penetrating into the central nervous compartment [36]. This is partly due to the generally higher molecular weights of specific inhibitors, their physical chemical properties, both of which tend to limit movement across endothelium, as well as the activity of endothelial transporters, such a p-glycoprotein, that very efficiently back-transport compounds out of the central compartment. While these issues can be partly addressed during preclinical studies, clinical data is necessary to confirm penetration into the central nervous system. Unlike assessment of plasma pharmacokinetics, which is straightforward, assessment of drug penetration into the CSF is hampered by the need to perform lumbar punctures with potentially the use of indwelling catheters to provide drug levels at multiple time points. In addition, drug concentrations in the lumbar CSF may not accurately reflect levels in the interstitial fluid in the brain. Since BACE is an intracellular enzyme, levels in the interstitial fluid may not be as relevant as levels intracellularly within neurons.

With these considerations in mind, much can be learned during Phase 1 testing in healthy human subjects. Broadly, the goals during Phase 1 are to: (1) provide an initial assessment of tolerability and safety across a broad range of dose levels and to determine dose-limiting tolerability if feasible; (2) determine basic pharmacokinetic parameters to better understand drug behavior in the blood and body; and (3) utilize this information to narrow down doses for later clinical studies and establish potential dosing regimens. For BACE inhibitors, initial assessment of biologic effects may be made by measuring drug effects on reducing plasma beta-amyloid levels. While changes in plasma beta-amyloid levels suggest the drug is capable of engaging the relevant enzymatic target, and therefore, provides a marker of biologic activity, it does not provide clear-cut indication of activity in the compartment of interest, that is, the brain. Although there can be bidirectional flow of beta-amyloid across the blood–brain barrier, and the concentration of beta-amyloid in the CSF is significantly higher than in blood, the relative contribution of brain/CSF beta-amyloid to overall levels in blood has not been determined [37, 38]. Thus, some indication of activity in the CNS is desirable as a marker of relevant pharmacologic activity.

Such an assessment is feasible during early clinical studies, either in healthy volunteers or AD patients in settings where capabilities are in place to sample CSF. Measurement of changes in levels of CSF beta-amyloid should take into account inter- and intrasubject variability, which can be substantial and requires careful consideration of the number of subjects required to detect a relevant treatment effect. An alternative approach that appears to be more sensitive and less variable is to measure the rate of production of beta-amyloid using essentially a pulse-chase method in which heavy C13-labeled leucine (nonradioactive) is administered intravenously and timed with drug dosing [24]. Samples of CSF taken hourly via in indwelling lumbar catheter are then analyzed for the rate of production (and elimination) of newly C-13 labeled beta-amyloid as a proportion of the total beta-amyloid present. By comparing rates of synthesis from treated and untreated subjects, it is possible to measure the effect of a drug that is expected to inhibit the production of beta-amyloid. This has been used with a gamma-secretase inhibitor, where it has been demonstrated in a small number of healthy subjects that, following single oral doses of LY450139, there is a dose-related reduction in the proportion of newly synthesized beta-amyloid present in the CSF. Similarly, for BACE inhibitors, the pulse-chase approach is also expected to be applicable and relevant. This approach, while very promising, is experimental, and its use has been described with only a single compound to date. In addition, it requires a clinical unit capable of working with indwelling lumbar catheters, as well as specific bioanalytical methods to measure beta-amyloid, and therefore, it is limited to small numbers of subjects and is quite expensive. A further limitation for the use of changes in beta-amyloid levels is the lack of information on how changes in these levels might predict ultimate clinical effects.

9.3.2 Phase 2 Clinical Development

The goals during Phase 2 clinical development are to expand the safety evaluation into the patient population in order to narrow the range of dose levels and regimens that will be tested in Phase 3 pivotal trials, and to obtain safety and activity data sufficient to make a decision as to whether Phase 3 pivotal studies are warranted.

Ideally, this would entail generating efficacy data during Phase 2 that is predictive of clinical efficacy end points required in Phase 3. Data derived from Phase 2 testing are used to determine a number of critical variables in the design of pivotal studies, including selection of the specific patient population (such as stage of disease, genetic status [e.g., APO E4 status]), dose–response relationship and the therapeutic index, and key efficacy end points. In particular, some form of proof-of-concept data is highly desirable to inform decisions regarding continuing development into pivotal studies. In the case of AD, this is particularly a challenge for a number of reasons [39]. Since the next-generation compounds are intended as disease-modifying agents, treatment effects on slowing of disease progression require potentially lengthy (>12–18 months) treatment periods capable of showing a separation in the natural history curves. This entails essentially running a trial resembling a Phase 3 pivotal trial, except it is likely to be underpowered and therefore, runs the significant risk of yielding trends in efficacy that may not reduce uncertainty regarding efficacy. This is the approach taken in the development of bepineuzimab. In such Phase 2 studies, information derived from subset analyses based upon preplanned analyses or post hoc analyses are often used to generate hypotheses that are then incorporated into the pivotal studies. Statistically, this entails making multiple comparisons using small data sets and runs the risk of reaching false-positive conclusions.

Because of these challenges, there is great interest in developing and validating intermediate biomarker measures that might ultimately serve as surrogate markers for clinical efficacy (Table 9.2) [39]. A number of these have been proposed as biomarkers that measure an aspect of the disease considered central to the disease process. These fall into two broad approaches: imaging markers, such as quantitative volumetric MRI and CT scans, functional brain imaging, and amyloid plaque imaging techniques, and biochemical markers, such as CSF beta-amyloid levels and CSF tau levels.

It has been well established that brain size is progressively reduced as dementia progresses in AD, and neuropathological changes first occur in the medial tem-

TABLE 9.2 Outcome Measures for AD Trials

Biomarkers
  Plasma beta-amyloid
  CSF beta-amyloid42[a]
  Volumetric MRI[a]
  FDG PET[a]
  Amyloid PET[a]
  CSF tau/phospho tau[a]
Clinical measures
  ADAS-cog
  ADCS-ADL
  MMSE
  NPI
  Staggered start/stop or slope analysis with cognitive measures*

[a] May provide evidence of disease modification.

poral lobes [40]. From a diagnostic standpoint, structural neuroimaging in AD is focused on detection of medial temporal lobe atrophy, particularly of the hippocampus, parahippocampal gyrus (including the entorhinal cortex) and amygdale [41–43]. Both MR and CT can sensitively measure these parameters, and imaging findings correlate with AD pathology at postmortem. There has been significant progress recently in establishing reliable, reproducible, and sensitive parameters quantifying such changes on MRI and CT that can be potentially implemented across clinical centers for longitudinal studies and clinical trials [44, 45]. Natural history studies have correlated changes in brain volume with clinical progression (rate of medical temporal lobe atrophy in typical aging and AD [46], baseline and longitudinal patterns of brain atrophy in mild cognitive impairment [MCI[patients [47–49], and their use in prediction of short-term conversion of AD (results from Alzheimer's Disease Neuroimaging Initiative [ADNI]). These studies are valuable to determine the natural variability in these quantitative measures and make it possible to predict the expected rate of change in volume over time for a particular population. Changes in brain size assessed with imaging can be closely linked to disease progression and rate of cognitive decline. The eventual establishment of neuroimaging as a validated surrogate marker capable of substituting for measurement of clinical outcomes will require its demonstration in the context of one or more successful treatment trials in which there is a tight link between change on imaging and clinical outcomes following treatment compared with placebo. A reasonable hypothesis could be made that a reduction in the rate of brain shrinkage in a treatment group receiving a BACE inhibitor means that inhibition of the enzyme has beneficially affected secondary downstream important pathogenic events such that the end result is a slowing of neuronal loss. Irrespective of whether volumetric imaging can serve as a validated surrogate biomarker, these data are extremely useful as evidence of meaningful drug activity.

Similarly, changes in other imaging modalities, such as evidence of reductioin in plaque load over time measured by amyloid plaque imaging, would also provide strong biologic evidence for drug activity. Positron emission tomography (PET) imaging studies of amyloid deposition in human subjects with several $A\beta$ imaging agents are currently underway. PET studies of the carbon-11-labeled thioflavin-T derivative Pittsburgh Compound B ($[^{11}C]$PiB) has been extended to include a variety of subject groups including AD, MCI, and healthy controls [50]. The ability to quantify regional $A\beta$ plaque load in the brains of living human subjects has provided a means to begin to apply this technology as a diagnostic agent to detect regional concentrations of $A\beta$ plaques and as a surrogate marker of therapeutic efficacy in anti-amyloid drug trials. A variety of other compounds, including 3′[(18)F]FPIB, [(18)F]FDDNP, [(11)C]SB-13 and [(18)F]F-SB-13 have been developed which have been shown to possess a selective uptake in the brain regions known to have a high beta-amyloid content [51].

Functional magnetic resonance imaging (fMRI) is a noninvasive neuroimaging technique that can be used to study the neural correlates of complex cognitive processes, and the alterations in these processes that occur in the course of neurodegenerative disease [52]. fMRI studies have consistently demonstrated that, compared with cognitively intact older subjects, patients with clinical AD have decreased fMRI activation in the hippocampus and related structures within the medial temporal lobe during the encoding of new memories. More recently, fMRI studies of subjects at risk for AD, by virtue of their genetics or evidence of MCI, have yielded variable results. Some of these studies suggest that there may be a phase of paradoxically increased activation early in the course of prodromal AD. Further studies to validate fMRI in these populations are needed, particularly longitudinal studies to investigate the pattern of alterations in functional activity and the relationship to AD pathology. Compared with volumetric structural imaging and plaque imaging, there is limited data on whether fMRI can be usefully applied as a biomarker for disease-modifying drugs.

While beta-amyloid, total tau (t-tau), and phosporylated tau (p-tau) protein analysis, as assessed in CSF and plasma, have been intensively studied as diagnostic biomarkers for dementia, they have not been as extensively studied as biomarkers of disease severity. Among biochemical markers, CSF t-tau and p-tau, as well as the ratio of these two proteins, are the most widely studied for use as diagnostic aids as well as tracking disease progression [53–56]. Tau binds to microtubules in axons and helps to regulate their assembly and transport. Tau protein undergoes complex regulation, controlled in part by phosphorylation by kinases. Insoluble tau protein is a major component of neurofibrillary tangles in AD and is highly phosphorylated at amino acids at specific sites in the tau sequence. Tau and phosphorylated tau in particular, have emerged as important molecules directly implicated in the pathogenic cascade.

A combination of Abeta42 and t-tau in CSF can discriminate between patients with stable MCI and patients with progressive MCI into AD or other types of dementia with a sufficient sensitivity and specificity [57–59]. Regression analyses demonstrated that pathological CSF (with decreased Abeta42 and and increased tau levels) is a very strong predictor for the progression of MCI into AD.

For compounds expected to affect beta-amyloid, changes in amyloid levels or production are expected as part of its pharmacologic profile. However, it would be potentially very significant if administration of a BACE inhibitor also resulted in changes in tau or phosphor-tau. This could be interpreted as a demonstration of an effect on a downstream parameter considered to be an important marker of AD pathogenesis.

Thus, during Phase 2 evaluation, it is worthwhile to incorporate multiple biomarker end points in addition to clinical cognitive end points. Positive trends across a number of these end points strengthen the data package supporting advancement into Phase 3. Demonstration of effects of a new drug on biomarkers together with clinical effects also support the case that the drug has benefits beyond symptom relief, and an argument can begin to be constructed that the drug is disease modifying.

9.3.3   Phase 3 Clinical Development

The decision to advance a compound from Phase 2 into Phase 3 pivotal trials is a key one from a resource utilization standpoint. From an industry perspective, a Phase 3 clinical trial can be expected to take 3–4 years to carry out, and costs can be expected to range from $100 million to over $200 million dollars per trial depending upon the numbers of patients per arm, duration of treatment, number of dose levels, and extent of end points to be evaluated. At issue also is the fact that access to patients can be potentially limiting, even for trials run internationally, due to the large numbers of drugs moving through the pipeline competing for qualified sites with appropriate patients, and, in the case of BACE inhibitors and other potentially disease-modifying drugs, the likely requirement for limiting enrollment to patients with mild to moderate AD. The long treatment duration of these trials (18 months or more) also means that a patient may only be able to participate in a single trial during the course of their disease, and there may be the need for frequent clinical visits during the trial period that will require a committed caretaker who understands the importance of completing trial participation. Additionally, selection of well-qualified sites with clinical trials experience that have access to adequate numbers of patients can also be limiting. AD trials require significant and dedicated commitment on the part of trial centers, with experienced physicians, study coordinators, neuropsychologists, and ancillary services such as neuroimaging, all working together as a single unit. Clinical sites will need to be selective in which trials they participate in and part of the decision-making process will involve assessing the strength of the data supporting the conduct of Phase 3 trials.

A number of issues need to be carefully considered in the design of Phase 3 trials for BACE inhibitors, including patient population, trial design, duration of therapy, and end points. The selection of the appropriate patient population should take into consideration what has been learned in subset analyses during Phase 2 testing, as well as who will benefit from treatment when the drug is approved and on the market. One important parameter is the stage or severity of disease. For BACE inhibitors and other drugs targeting some aspect of beta-amyloid biology, there is an increasing consensus that the sooner treatment is initiated, the greater the potential benefit. Indeed, some have suggested that once dementia is evident, downstream pathogenic events such as formation of tau-associated tangles and neuronal cell death, as well as inflammatory or oxidative damage may have already been put into play that are no longer responsive to alterations in upstream alterations in beta-amyloid processing. However, this remains speculative. Ideally, it may be desirable to initiate treatment before clinical symptoms are evident or when such symptoms are mild, such as patients with MCI. However, the traditional definition of MCI, which is based largely on cognitive assessment, has been problematic from the standpoint of accurately identifying the pre-dementia patient with underlying Alzheimer's pathology.

Given the significant advances in our understanding of Alzheimer's pathogenesis, a proposal has been made to modify our diagnostic criteria for Alzheimer's type pathology to include findings from relevant biomarkers that are sensitive and specific for AD in addition to cognitive assessment [60]. The National Institute of Neurological and Communicative Diseases and Stroke/Alzheimer's Disease and Related Disorders Association (NINCDS-ADRDA) and the *Diagnostic and Statistical Manual*, Fourth Edition, Text Revision (DSM-IV-TR) criteria for AD are the prevailing diagnostic standards in research; however, they have not been updated to incorporate the tremendous growth of scientific knowledge. As discussed above, a range of reliable biomarkers of AD are now available through structural MRI, molecular neuroimaging with PET, and cerebrospinal fluid analyses. An attempt has been made to incorporate these biomarkers to capture both the earliest stages, before full-blown dementia, as well as the full spectrum of the illness [60]. These new criteria are centered on a clinical core of early and significant episodic memory impairment. They stipulate that there must also be at least one or more abnormal biomarkers among structural neuroimaging with MRI, molecular neuroimaging with PET, and cerebrospinal fluid analysis of amyloid beta or tau proteins. The timeliness of these criteria is highlighted by the many drugs in development that are directed at changing pathogenesis, particularly at the production and clearance of amyloid beta as well as at the hyperphosphorylation state of tau. Validation studies in existing and prospective cohorts are needed to advance these criteria and optimize their sensitivity, specificity, and accuracy. If this revised approach is widely embraced and adopted by clinicians and regulatory bodies, the revised diagnosis of AD will incorporate the tremendous advances in our understanding of the biological bases of the disease. It will also broaden the spectrum of disease to encompass pre-dementia as part of a continuous spectrum of the disease extending into dementia and allow the inclusion of early pre-demented AD (i.e., MCI) into clinical trials.

Information obtained during Phase 2 may suggest that other patient subsets may show different responses to therapy. An unexpected finding seen from the Phase 2 study of passive antibody was the difference in response, both from a safety and efficacy standpoint, among patients who were APOe4 positive or negative.

In terms of trial design, several issues emerge. While the simplest design is a randomized placebo-controlled, parallel arm study, there is interest in incorporating modifications to demonstrate an effect on the underlying disease process, manifested as a change in the rate of decline [61]. In principle, a staggered start or stop design offers the ability to distinguish between symptomatic-only benefits versus disease-modifying benefit by demonstrating that patients treated with an effective disease-modifying drug continue to show a difference in clinical end points against placebo after stopping therapy [62]. An alternative approach is a slope-based analysis, in which frequent end-point assessments taken during treatment show a widening gap between treatment and placebo with longer periods of treatment, indicating that the underlying rate of deterioration has been altered. The practical implementation and analyses from data incorporating these designs are challenging for a number of reasons, including: (1) increasing dropout rates over longer treatment periods, requiring the appropriate statistical handling of missing data; (2) variability in end-point measures with the potential for significant fluctuations in individual perfor-mance over time requiring larger cohort sizes to detect significant mean differences; and (3) drug treatment benefits that may be relatively modest over a 1–2-year period, making it difficult to clearly distinguish differences in slopes on treatment or differ-ences versus placebo off therapy.

The question of duration of treatment is an important one and is determined by competing needs. From the standpoint of maximizing the opportunity to demon-strate a disease-modifying treatment benefit, longer treatment periods can be expected to increase the differences between active and placebo groups. In addition, for a drug that is expected to slow deterioration rather than reverse it, progression in the placebo arm will increase with longer trial duration. However, favoring shorter treatment periods are practical considerations of trial fatigue, increased dropout rates, and the need to keep placebo patients on placebo. Based upon these parameters, current trials for disease-modifying therapies incorporate treatment periods of 12–24 months, with an 18-month treatment period being a reasonable practical compromise.

The selection of appropriate primary and secondary efficacy end points is predicted upon regulatory precedent and requires careful discussion with relevant regulatory bodies. A detailed discussion of the specifics of neuropsychological testing is beyond the scope of this chapter. In general, a new drug for AD must demonstrate clinical benefit on cognitive function, as assessed by two methods: (1) direct evaluation of cognitive function, using a validated instrument, such as the ADAS-cog battery; and (2) clinician/caretaker assessment of overall benefit, such as the CIBIC-plus. The ADAS-cog is a multi-item instrument that has been extensively validated in longitudinal cohorts of AD patients. The ADAS-cog examines selected aspects of cognitive performance, including elements of memory, orientation, attention, reasoning, language, and praxis [63]. The ADAS-cog scoring range is from 0 to 70, with higher scores indicating greater cognitive impairment. Elderly normal adults may score as low as 0 or 1, but it is not unusual for nondemented adults to score slightly higher. Some drawbacks of the ADAS-cog are ceiling and floor effects, limiting its utility in mild and severe patients, and the lack of testing for executive function. As a result, other instruments such as the NTB have been developed and may be incorporated into trials [64].

The CIBIC plus is not a single instrument and is not a standardized instrument like the ADAS-cog [65–67]. Clinical trials for investigational drugs have used a variety of CIBIC formats, each different in terms of depth and structure. In general, the CIBIC plus used is a semi-structured instrument designed to examine four major areas of patient function: general, cognitive, behavioral and activities of daily living. It represents the assessment of a skilled clinician based upon his/her observations at an interview with the patient, in combination with information supplied by a caregiver familiar with the behavior of the patient over the interval rated. The CIBIC plus is scored as a seven-point categorical rating, ranging from a score of 1, indicating "markedly improved," to a score of 4, indicating "no change" to a score of 7, indicating "markedly worse."

These instruments are applicable for either symptomatic only or disease-modifying treatments and may be applied periodically throughout the treatment and follow-up period to monitor for clinical benefit.

9.3.4   Regulatory Considerations

An important regulatory concern among drug developers is the specific claims that will be incorporated into the label for a new AD drug with improved characteristics. There have been efforts to arrive at a regulatory definition of disease modification that can be practically implemented. In the European Union, guidelines have been published focusing on slope analyses as an approach to obtain a disease modification label. In the United States, the FDA has not clearly indicated what approaches could be used. It is possible that some combination of clinical design together with compelling biomarker data could be used to make a case that a therapy is disease modifying.

Some clinical experts have suggested that obtaining disease modification in a regulatory label may not be critical, either from a patient care or commercial perspective [68]. Their view is that the focus instead should be on demonstrating a reasonable, robust, and long-lasting treatment benefit, and patients and doctors will embrace any new therapy with persistent and substantial benefits. However, it seems that formal recognition by regulatory agencies that a new drug provides disease modification would substantially enhance its commercial value by allowing dissemination of information related to it and differentiating it from other compounds.

9.4   FINAL REMARKS

In view of the rapid advances taking place in our scientific understanding of the pathogenesis of AD, together with the tremendous resources being applied by the pharmaceutical industry toward new drugs, as well as the huge unmet need for more effective therapies, there is the need for scientists, drug developers, clinicians, and regulators to find ways to share data, standardize measurements, and conduct multisite biomarker research in such a way that results can be compared side by side. This is particularly important given the number of clinical trials for AD therapies occurring in different parts of the world (Fig. 9.1). Two notable initiatives are laying the groundwork in this direction. One is the ADCS, which has done much to help clinical sites of large multicenter trials standardize appropriate methods and procedures to minimize site variability in addition to supporting the infrastructure of many high-quality clinical research centers [69]. The other is the ADNI, a multi-center

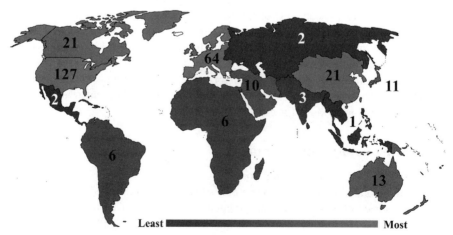

Figure 9.1   Number of clinical trials currently occurring worldwide, adapted from information available at *Clinicaltrials.gov*.

TABLE 9.3   Online Sites with Up-to-Date Resources on AD and Clinical Trials

http://www.nia.nih.gov/Alzheimers/ResearchInformation/ClinicalTrials
http://clinicaltrials.gov
http://www.alz.org/index.asp
http://www.alzforum.org/
http://www.centerwatch.com/clinical-trials
http://www.alzfdn.org/ClinicalTrials/findatrial.html
http://www.alzresearch.org/index.cfm
http://www.adc.ucla.edu/
http://www.alzdiscovery.org/

5-year natural history study run by a public-private consortium [70]. ADNI has focused on areas of common ground to all drug developers in which cooperation and data sharing benefit all participants. In this case, ADNI aims to enable both companies and publicly funded drug developers to define useful neuroimaging biomarkers and methods that will help them as they each subsequently test their proprietary compounds individually.

Finally, it is critically important that patients, their caregivers, and their healthcare providers, are fully informed about the wide range of new potentially groundbreaking therapies that are currently in clinical trials. A number of online sites provide up-to-date information on advances in AD research as well as ongoing clinical studies seeking to recruit qualified patients (Table 9.3).

REFERENCES

1. Maslow, K. 2008. 2008 Alzheimer's disease facts and figures. *Alzheimers Dement* **4**(2):110–133.
2. Blennow, K., de Leon, M.J., Zetterberg, H. 2006. Alzheimer's disease. *Lancet* **368**(9533): 387–403.
3. Terry, A.V., Jr. and Buccafusco, J.J. 2003. The cholinergic hypothesis of age and Alzheimer's disease-related cognitive deficits; Recent challenges and their implications for novel drug development. *J Pharmacol Exp Ther* **306**(3):821–827.
4. Birks, J. 2006. Cholinesterase inhibitors for Alzheimer's disease. *Cochrane Database Syst Rev* (**1**):CD005593.
5. Salloway, S., Mintzer, J., Weiner, M.F., and Cummings, J.L. 2008. Disease-modifying therapies in Alzheimer's disease. *Alzheimers Dement* **4**(2):65–79.
6. Cummings, J.L., Doody, R., and Clark, C. 2007. Disease-modifying therapies for Alzheimer disease. *Neurology* **69**(16):1622–1634.
7. Schenk, D., Barbour, R., Dunn, W. et al. 1999. Immunization with Aβ attenuates Alzheimer's disease-like pathology in the PDAPP mouse. *Nature* **400**:173–177.
8. Janus, C., Pearson, J., and McLaurin, J. 2000. Aβ immunization reduces behavioural impairment and dense-cored plaques in a model of Alzheimer's disease. *Nature* **408**:979–982.
9. Morgan, D. 2005. Mechanisms of Aβ plaque clearance following passive Aβ immunization. *Neurodegen Dis* **2**:261–266.
10. Levites, Y., Smithson, L.A., Price R.W., Dakin, R.S., Yuan, B., Sierks, M.R. et al. 2006. Insights into the mechanisms of action of anti-Aβ antibodies in Alzheimer's disease mouse models. *The FASEB Journal* **20**:2576–2578.

11. Lichtlen, P. and Mohajeri, M.H. 2008. Antibody-based approaches in Alzheimer's resarch; safety, pharmacokinetics, metabolism and analytical tools. *J Neurochem* **104**(4):859–874.
12. Gilman, S., Koller, M., Black, R., Jenkins, L., Griffith, S., Fox, N. et al. 2005. Clinical effects of Aβ immunization (AN1792) in patients with AD in an interrupted trial. *Neurology* **64**:1553–1562.
13. Hock, C., Konietako, U., Streffer, J.R., Tracy, J., Signorell, A., Muller-Tillmanns, B. et al. 2003. Antibodies against beta-amyloid slow cognitive decline in Alzheimer's disease. *Neuron* **38**:547–554.
14. Holmes, C., Boche, D., Wilkinson, D., Yadegarfar, G., Hopkins, V., Bayer, A. et al. 2008. Long-term effects of Aβ 42 immunisation in Alzheimer's disease: follow-up of a randomised, placebo-controlled phase 1 trial. *The Lancet* **372**:216–223.
15. Grundman, M. and Black, R. 2008. Clinical trials of bapineuzumab, a beta-amyloid-targeted immunotherapy in patients with mild to moderate Alzheimer's disease. *Alzheimers Dement* **4**(4, Suppl 2):T166.
16. Wolfe, M.S. and Haass, C. 2001. The role of presenilins in gamma-secretase activity. *J Biol Chem* **276**:5413–5416.
17. Kimberly, W.T. and Wolfe, M.S. 2003. Identity and function of y-secretase. *J Neurosci Res* **74**:353–360.
18. Hartmann, D., Tournoy, J., and Saftig, P. 2001. Implication of APP secretases in notch signaling. *J Mol Neuroscience* **17**:171–181.
19. Micchelli, C.A., Esler, W.P., Kimberly, W.T. et al. 2003. Gamma-secretase/presenilin inhibitors for Alzheimer's disease phenocopy notch mutations in *Drosophila. FASEB J* **17**:79–81.
20. Siemers, M.E., Skinner, M., Dean, M.P., Gonzales, M.C., and Satterwhite, P.J. 2008. Safety, tolerability and changes in amyloid β concentrations after administration of a γ-secretase inhibitor in volunteers. *Clin Neuropharmacol* **28**:126–132.
21. Siemer, M.E., Quinn, J., Kaye, M.J., Farlow, M.M., Porsteinsson, M.A., Tariot, M.P. et al. 2006. The effects of a γ-secretase inhibitor in a randomized study of patients with Alzheimer's disease. *Neurology* **66**:602–604.
22. Fleisher, A.S., Raman, P.R., Siemers, M.E., Becerra, M.L., Clark, M.C., Dean, M.R. et al. 2008. Phase 2 safety trial targeting amyloid β production with a γ-secretase inhibitor in Alzheimer's disease. *Clin Trials* **65**:1031–1038.
23. Bateman, R.J. 2008. Aβ turnover in human subjects. *Alzheimers Dement* **2**:T123–T124.
24. Bateman, R.J., Munsell, L.Y., Morris, J.C., Swarm, R., Tarasheski, K.E., and Holtzman, D.M. 2006. Human anyloid-β synthesis and clearance rates as measured in cerebrospinal fluid in vivo. *Nat Med* **12**:1–6.
25. Bateman, R.J., Wen, G., Morris, J.C., and Holtzman, D.M. 2007. Fluctuations of CSF amyloid-β levels: implications for a diagnostic and therapeutic biomarker. *Neurology* **68**:666–669.
26. Hernandez, S.-M.I., Del Rio, J., Moreno, F., and Avila, J. 2007. Tramiprosate, a drug of potential interest for the treatment of Alzheimer's disease, promotes an abnormal aggregation of tau. *Mol Neurodegener* **2**:17.
27. Wilcock, G., Black, S., Hendrix, S., Zavitz, K., Swabb, E., and Laughlin, M. 2008. Efficacy and safety of tarenflurbil in mild to mederate Alzheimer's disease: a randomised phase II trial. *Lancet Neurol* **7**:483–493.
28. Green, R.C., Schneider, L.S., Hendrix, S.B., Zavitz, K.H., and Swabb, E. 2008. Safety and efficacy of Tarenflurbil in subjects with mild Alzheimer's disease: results from an 18-month multi-center phase 3 trial. *Alzheimers Dement* **2**:T165.
29. Eriksen, J., Sagi, S., Smith, T.W., Das, P., McLendon, D., Ozols, V. et al. 2003. NSAIDs and enantiomers of flurbiprofen target gamma-secretase and lower Abert 42 in vivo. *J Clin Invest* Aug. **112** (3):440–449.
30. Kukar, T., Prescott, S., Eriksen, J., Holloway, V., Murphy, M., Koo, E. et al. 2007. Chronic administration of R-flurbioprofen attenuates learning impariments in transgenic amyloid precursor protein mice. *BMC Neuroscience* **8**:54.
31. Galasko, D., Graff-Radford, N., May, S., Hendrix, S., Cottrel, B.S., Sagi, S. et al. 2007. Safety, tolerability, pharmacokinetics and Abeta levels after short-term administration of R-Flurbiprofen in healthy elderly individuals. *Alzheimer's Disease Association Disorder* Oct.-Dec. **21**(4):292–299.

32. Roher, A.E., Esh, C.L., Kokjohn, T.A., Castano, E., Van Vickle, G.D., Kalback, W.M. et al. 2009. Amyloid beta peptides in human plasma and tissues and their significance for Alzheimer's disease. *Alzheimers Dement* **5**:18–29.

33. Kuo, Y.-M., Kokjohn, T.A., Watson, D.M., Woods, A.S., Cotter, R.J., Sue, L.I. et al. 2000. Elevated Aβ 42 in skeletal muscle of Alzheimer disease suggests peripheral alterations of AβPP metabolism. *Am J Pathol* **156**:797–805.

34. Slemmon, R.J., Painter, C.L., Nadanaciva, S., Catana, F., Cook, A., Motter, R. et al. 2007. Distribution of Aβ peptide in whole blood. *J Chromatogr B* **846**:24–31.

35. Tang, K., Hynan, L.S., Baskin, F., and Rosenberg, R.N. 2006. Platelet amyloid precursor protein processing: a bio-marker for Alzheimer's disease. *J Neurol Sci* **240**:53–58.

36. Moore, K., Zhu, H., Rajapakse, S., Simon, A.J., Pudvah, N.T., Hochman, J.H. et al. 2007. Strategies toward improving the brain penetration of macrocyclic tertiary carbinamine BACE-1 inhibitors. *Bioorg Med Chem Lett* **17**:5831–5835.

37. Kandimalla, K., Curran, G.L., Holasek, S., Gilles, E.J., Wengenack, T., and Podusio, J.F. 2005. Pharmacokinetic analysis of the blood–brain barrier transport of 125 I-amyloid β protein 40 in wild-type and Alzheimer's disease transgenic mice (APP, PS1) and its implications for amyloid plaque formation. *J Pharmacol Exp Ther* **313**:1370–1378.

38. Gierdraitis, V., Sundelof, J., Irizarry, M., Garevik, N., Hyman, B.T., Wahlund, L.-O. et al. 2007. The normal equilibrium between CSF and plasma amyloid beta levels is disrupted in Alzheimer's disease. *Neurosci Lett* **427**:127–131.

39. Cummings, J.L. 2008. Optimizing phase II of drug development for disease-modifying compounds. *Alzheimers Dement* **4**:S15–S20.

40. Braak, H. and Braak, E. 1991. Neuropathological stageing of Alzheimer-related changes. *Acta Neuropathol (Berl)* **82**:239–259.

41. Seab, J., Jagust, W., and Wong, S. 1988. Quantitative NMR measurements of hippocampal antrophy in Alzheimer's disease. *Magn Reson Med* **8**:200–208.

42. Kido, D., Caine, E., and LeMay, M. 1989. Temporal lobe antrophy in patients with Alzheimer's disease: a CT study. *AJNR* **10**:551–555.

43. de Leon, M., George, A., Stylopoulos, L., Smith, G., and Miller, D. 1989. Early marker for Alzheimer's disease: the atrophic hippocampus. *The Lancet* **2**:672–673.

44. Hua, X., Leow, A., Parikshak, N., Lee, S., Chiang, M., Toga, A. et al. 2008. Tensor-based morphometry as a neuroimaging biomarker for Alzheimer's disease: an MRI study of 676 AD, MCI and normal subjects. *Neuroimage* **43**:458–469.

45. Jack, C., Bernstein, M., Fox, N., Thompson, P., Alexander, G., Harvey, D. et al. 2008. The Alzheimer's disease neuroimaging initiative (ADNI); MRI methods. *J Magn Reason Imaging* **27**:685–691.

46. Jack, C., Petersen, R., and Xu, Y. 1998. Rate of medial temporal lobe atrophy in typical aging and Alzheimer's disease. *Neurology* **51**:993–999.

47. Petersen, R., Jack, C., and Xu, Y. 2000. Memory and MRI-based hippocampal volumes in aging and AD. *Neurology* **54**:581–587.

48. Fox, N.C., Crum, W.R., Scahill, R.I. et al. 2001. Imaging of onset and progression of Alzheimer's disease with voxel-compression mapping of serial magnetic reasonance images. *The Lancet* **358**:201–205.

49. Misra, C., Fan, Y., Davatzikos, C. 2009. Baseline and longitudinal patterns of brain antrophy in MCI patients, and their use in prediction of short-term conversion of AD: results from ADNI. *Neuroimage* **44**:1415–1422.

50. Mathis, C., Lopresti, B., and Klunk, W. 2007. Impact of amyloid imaging on drug development in Alzheimer's disease. *Nucl Med Biol* **34**:809–822.

51. Henriksen, G., Yousefi, G., Drzezga, A., and Wester, H. 2008. Development and evaluation of compounds for imaging of beat-amyloid plaque by means of positron emission tomography. *Eur J Nucl Med Mol Imagining* **35**:S75–S81.

52. Sperling, R. 2007. Functional MRI studies of associative encoding in normal agind, mild cognitive impairment, and Alzheimer's disease. *Ann N Y Acad Sci* **1097**:146–155.

53. Vandermeeren, M., Mercken, M., and Vanmechelenk, E. 1993. Detection of tau proteins in normal and Alzheimer's disease cerebrospinal fluid with a sensitive sandwich enzyme-linked immuno. *J Neurochem* **61**:1828–1834.

54. Motter, R., Vigo-Pelfrey, C., and Kholodenko, D. 1995. Reduction of beta-amyloid peptide-42 in the cerebrospinal fluid of patients with Alzheimer's disease. *Ann Neurol* **38**:643–648.

55. Arai, H. and Terajima, M.M. 1995. Tau in cerebrospinal fluid; a potential diagnostic marker in Alzheimer's disease. *Ann Neurol* **38**:649–652.

56. Andreasen, N., Vanmechelen, E., and Van de Voorde, A. 1998. Cerebrospinal fluid tau protein as a biochemical marker for Alzheimer's disease; a community ased follow up study. *J Neurol Neurosurg Psychiatry* **64**:298–305.

57. Galasko, D., Chang, L., and Motter, R. 1998. High cerebrospinal fluid tau and low amyloid beta42 levels in clincial diagnosis of Alzheimer disease and relation to apoliopoprotein E genotype. *Arch Neurol* **55**:937–945.

58. Hulstaert, F., Blennow, K., and Ivanoiu, A. 1999. Improved discrimination of AD patients using beta-amyloid and tau levels in CSF. *Neurology* **52**:1555–1562.

59. Sunderland, T., Linker, G., and Mirza, M. 2003. Decreased beta amyloid1-42 and increased tau levels in cerebrospinal fluid of patients with Alzheimer's disease. *JAMA* **289**:2094–2103.

60. Dubois, B., Geldman, H., Jacova, C., Dekosky, S.T., Barberger-Gateau, P., Cummings, J. et al. 2007. Research criteria for the diagnosis of Alzheimer's disease; revising the NINCDS-ADRDA criteria. *The Lancet* **6**:734–746.

61. Cummings, J. 2006. Challenges to demonstrating disease-modifying effects in Alzheimer's disease clinical trials. *Alzheimers Dement* **2**:263–271.

62. Parkinson Study Group. 2004. A controlled, randomized, delayed-start study of rasagiline in early Parkinson's disease. *Arch Neurol* **61**:561–566.

63. Mohs, R., Knopman, D., Petersen, R., Ferris, S., Ernesto, C., Grundman, M. et al. 1997. Development of cognitive instruments for use in clinical trials of antidementia drugs: additions to the Alzheimer's disease assessment scale that broadens its scope: the Alzehimer's disease cooperative study. *Alzheimer's Disease Assoc Disord* **11**:S13–S21.

64. Harrison, J., Psychol, C., Minassian, S., Jenkins, L., Black, R., Koller, M. et al. 2007. A neuropsychological test battery for use in Alzheimer disease clinical trials. *Arch Neurol* **64**:1323–1329.

65. Leber, P. 1990. *Guidelines for the Clinical Evaluations of Antidementia Drugs*. Washington, DC: Food & Drug Administration.

66. Scheider, L. and Olin, J.D. 1997. Validity and reliability and the Alzheimer's disease cooperative study-clinical global impressions of change. *Alzheimer's Disease Assoc Disord* **11**:S22–S32.

67. Knopman, D.K., Gracon, S., and Davis, C. 1994. The clinicians interview-based impression (CIBI): a clinicians global change rating scale in Alzheimer's disease. *Neurology* **44**:2315–2321.

68. Doody, R.S. 2008. We should not distinguish between symptomatic and disease-modifying treatment in Alzheimer's disesase drug development. *Alzheimers Dement* **4**:S21–S25.

69. Morris, J., Ernesto, C., Schafer, K., Coats, M., Leon, S., Sano, M. et al. 1997. Clinical dementia rating training and reliability and reliability in mullticenter studies: the Alzheimer's disease cooperative study experience. *Neurology* **48**:1508–1510.

70. Misra, C., Fan, Y., and Davatzikos, C. 2008. Baseline and longitudinal patterns of brain atrophy in MCI patients, and their use in prediction of short-term conversion to AD: results from ADNI. *Neuroimage* **44**:1415–1422.

FUTURE STRATEGIES FOR DEVELOPMENT OF NOVEL BACE INHIBITORS: ANTI-APP β-SITE ANTIBODY AND APP BINDING SMALL MOLECULE APPROACHES FOR ALZHEIMER'S DISEASE

Beka Solomon,[1] Michal Arbel-Ornath,[1] Clare-Peters Libeu,[2] and Varghese John[2]

[1]Department of Molecular Microbiology & Biotechnology, George S. Wise Faculty of Life Sciences, Tel-Aviv University, Tel Aviv, Israel and [2]Buck Institute for Age Research, Novato, CA

10.1 INTRODUCTION

Alzheimer's disease (AD) is a progressive neurodegeneration and is the most common form of dementia in the elderly. The disease is characterized by a massive cell loss of mainly cholinergic neurons, deposition of fibrillar amyloid-β (Aβ) peptides as senile plaques, and intracellular accumulation of hyperphosphorylated tau as neurofibrillary tangles [1].

Although AD pathogenesis is complex and remains unclear, the accumulation of Aβ is considered to be the earliest event in a complex cascade, which eventually leads to neurodegeneration, as seen in compelling genetic and biochemical evidence [2]. The amyloid cascade hypothesis [2–5] states that overproduction of Aβ, or failure to clear this peptide, leads to AD primarily through amyloid deposition, which is presumed to be involved in neurofibrillary tangles formation, neuronal dysfunction, and microglia activation, all of which characterize AD affected brain tissues [6–9].

BACE: Lead Target for Orchestrated Therapy of Alzheimer's Disease, Edited by Varghese John
Copyright © 2010 John Wiley & Sons, Inc.

Considering the causative role of Aβ in AD etiology, novel therapeutic strategies that lower Aβ levels or prevent the formation of the neurotoxic Aβ species are predicted to stop or slow down the progression of neurodegeneration in AD. Indeed, the major focus over the last decade has been to inhibit brain Aβ production and aggregation, to increase parenchymal Aβ clearance, and to interfere with Aβ-induced cell death. Research clarifying the metabolic pathways that regulate Aβ production from its precursor protein amyloid precursor protein (APP) has revealed that the secretases that produce Aβ may be good therapeutic targets since inhibition of either β- or γ-secretase limits Aβ production. The fact that β-secretase initiates APP processing, and thus serves as the rate-limiting step in production of Aβ, have attracted efforts from many research groups aimed at the enzyme inhibition. The discovery of β-site APP cleaving enzyme (BACE1), which has been discussed in detail in Chapter 2, has prompted it as a main target for AD drug development. Indeed, over the last 7 years, several inhibitors were reported to reduce Aβ levels in plasma and/or brain of AD transgenic mice models (for review, see Reference 10), one of which has recently completed Phase I clinical trials (for more details, see Chapter 9).

Along with the development of BACE1 inhibitors and the generation of its knockout mice, accumulating data raise some concerns regarding a total inhibition of the enzyme, as it shares the processing of other substrates with immunological and neurological functions. Additionally, other enzymes, including cathepsin B, were shown to serve as β-secretase, cleaving APP at the same β-site [11].

In order to overcome some of the drawbacks that may arise from BACE1 inhibition, we developed a novel approach to inhibit Aβ production via antibodies against the β-secretase cleavage site of APP. These antibodies bind both wild-type and Swedish mutated APP expressed in transgenic mice brain tissues and do not bind any form of Aβ peptides. Administration of these antibodies to the cells condition media [12] and to a transgenic (Tg) mice model of AD resulted in a considerable decrease in intracellular Aβ levels (Arbel et al., manuscript in preparation). The relevance of intraneuronal accumulation of mainly Aβ42 as an early event in AD pathogenesis suggests that this approach may be applicable as a novel therapeutic strategy in AD treatment.

Here we review several aspects of BACE1 as a candidate for drug discovery, the subcellular trafficking of Aβ production, and performance of anti β-site antibodies in cellular and animal models of AD. We also briefly review the status of developing APP binding molecules as an approach to inhibition of cleavage of β-site of APP.

10.2 β-SECRETASE: DISCOVERY, FUNCTION, AND INHIBITORS

After more than 10 years of intense investigation, four independent teams of researchers have each identified the same protein, considered to be β-secretase, BACE [13–16]. Although BACE1 acts on APP as β-secretase to generate Aβ peptides [13–16], it is not clear whether this is its normal physiological task.

BACE1 is a 501 amino acid transmembrane aspartyl protease consisting of two active site motives at amino acids 93–96 and 289–292 in the lumenal domain, each containing the highly conserved sequence of aspartic proteases DT/SGT/S (reviewed in Reference 17). At the amino acid level, BACE shows <30% sequence identity with human pepsin family members. BACE was also shown to exhibit all the known properties of β-secretase [13]. Tissue culture and animal studies indicated that β-secretase is expressed in all tissues but is expressed at highest levels in the brain. BACE cleaves APP mainly at the amino terminus of the Aβ peptide domain and is widely expressed in different organs, including the brain and in various cell types [18]. A second human homolog, identified shortly after BACE1 identification, sharing 64% similarity at the amino acid sequence, termed BACE2, is expressed in the heart, kidney, and placenta, but less in the brain, making BACE1 the major β-secretase in the brain [19]. To date, the physiological role of BACE2 remains unknown, but it seems that the enzyme does not have a pivotal role in APP processing and thus is not considered a target for AD therapeutics.

The discovered structural and physiological characteristics of BACE1 have rapidly promoted it as a prime target for drug discovery in AD [11]. This strategy was further supported by studies showing that Aβ levels of BACE1-deficient mice were reduced by more than 90% [18, 20, 21]. Moreover, initial behavioral analysis of BACE1-deficient mice showed no obvious deficits in neurological and physiological functions [21].

Developing specific BACE1 inhibitors and evaluating their efficacy *in vivo* has been difficult, partly because there appears to be a nonlinear relationship between decreased BACE1 activity *in vivo* and reduction of Aβ levels in the brain. Studies using heterozygous BACE1 knockout animals have shown that a 50% decrease in BACE1 activity leads to a much smaller decrease (~15%) of brain Aβ levels [22].

A further difficulty is the low brain penetration of most inhibitors due to the fact that many are substrates for P-glycoprotein, a plasma membrane protein that actively extrudes a wide range of amphiphilic and hydrophobic drugs from cells, which is important in preventing the accumulation of several drugs in the brain. Moreover, as peptidomimetics of the β-cleavage site, BACE1 inhibitors are, therefore, as large as predicted by the crystal structure of the BACE1 active site. Moreover, APP is poorly cleaved by BACE1 because its amino acid sequence around the BACE1 cleavage site does not fit with the substrate specificity of BACE1 determined by *in vitro* experiments (reviewed in Reference 23). In the Madin-Darby canine kidney (MDCK) cell line, a system to study polarized sorting mechanisms of proteins, most of BACE1 is sorted to the apical surface where very little APP is observed [24]. Instead, APP undergoes sorting to the opposite, basolateral side, suggesting that APP is not the major physiological substrate of BACE1.

In addition, BACE1 inhibitors will have to be highly selective for BACE1 to minimize interference with other aspartic protease, namely pepsin, cathepsin D, cathepsin E, napsin A, and renin. Potential BACE1 inhibitors will also need to spare BACE2, which shares high homology levels with BACE1 and is expressed in the peripheral organs rather than in the brain because of their antagonistic functions.

Emerging data have showed the involvement of BACE1 in the proteolytic processing of other proteins, two of which share distinct importance with immunological function: the P-selectin glycoprotein ligand-1 [25], which mediates leukocyte adhesion and the sialyl-transferase ST6Gal I [26], an enzyme that is secreted after cleavage and is involved in regulating immune responses. The interaction of a sialyl-alpha2,6 galactose residue, which is synthesized solely by ST6Gal I, with a B cell-specific lectin, CD22/Siglec-2, is important for B cell function [26]. It is notable that mice deficient in some glycosylation enzymes that appear to grow normally show subtle neurological abnormalities with increasing age; glycosphingolipid-deficient mice show lethal audiogenic seizures induced by a sound stimulus. In this regard, it is important to note that a possible immunological phenotype in BACE1 knockout mice might have been overlooked, since these animals have not yet been challenged immunologically. BACE1 was also shown to be involved in processing of APP homologue, APLP2. The levels of APLP2 proteolytic products were decreased in BACE1-deficient mice and were increased in BACE1-overexpressing mice [27]. A study utilizing BACE1 knockout mice suggested type III neuregulin1 (NRG1), an axonally expressed factor that is required for glial cells development and myelination, as a novel substrate for BACE1 cleavage. The authors thus postulated that BACE1 is required for peripheral nerve myelination, probably via processing of type III NRG1 [28].

Findings that 4-month-old BACE1 knockout mice had mild deficits in a task that assesses spatial memory [29] suggest that chronic reduction in BACE1 activity could impact learning and memory. Moreover, utilizing APP/PS1 double transgenic mice, as well as BACE1-deficient mice, suggests that BACE1 and APP processing are critical for cognitive, emotional, and synaptic function [30].

Importantly, cathepsin B inhibitors were recently shown to improve mice performance in Morris Water Maze paradigm and to lower cerebral Aβ levels *in-vivo*. Aβ reduction was associated with decrease in sAPPβ levels, suggesting that these inhibitors could modulate β-secretase activity. Aβ-mediated reduction via cathepsin B inhibitors was restricted to transgenic models expressing wild-type APP [31]. These results demonstrate that other protease inhibitors could also modulate the β-secretase activity.

The findings reviewed above, describing other native substrates of BACE1 besides APP and other proteases that could modulate APP processing in a similar manner, suggest that strategies using anti β-site antibodies or small molecules that bind to APP and interfere with β-secretase activity are therapeutically very attractive and with potential for enhanced safety profile.

10.3 GENERATION OF Aβ PEPTIDES VIA THE ENDOCYTIC PATHWAY

Over the past few years, cell biological studies support the view that Aβ is generated intracellularly from the endoplasmic reticulum (ER) [32] to the trans-Golgi network (TGN) and the endosomal–lysosomal system [33]. In neurons, APP metabolism releasing the Aβ peptide occurs at all sorting stations. Regarding the Aβ species generated in the different neuronal compartments, the long form of Aβ (Aβ42) is produced in the ER/cisGolgi and at or near the cell surface, and the short form of

Aβ (Aβ40) is produced in the TGN/endosomal compartment and also at or near the cell surface (reviewed in Reference 34).

The generation of both Aβ40 and Aβ42 in endosomes is well established [32, 35–37]. Antibody uptake and biotinylation studies showed that most of the cell surface-located APP is reinternalized into early endosomal compartments from where it can be recycled back to the cell surface, or can be retrieved later to endosomal/lysosomal compartments and/or to the TGN [38, 39]. Mutagenesis of the internalization signal of APP reduced both Aβ40 and Aβ42 secretion [33], and expression of the dominant negative dynamin mutant that prevents endocytosis in the transfected cell lines decreased ratios of secreted Aβ42/Aβ40 for these APP constructs [35]. Within the secretory and endocytic pathways, BACE1 shares major trafficking routes with its protein substrate APP. Cell models using chimeric forms of APP that retain APP in the ER, or direct APP trafficking to the lysosome or cell surface, indicate that production of Aβ40 occurs mainly in the endocytic pathway, while Aβ42 is produced both in the ER/cis-Golgi apparatus and in the endocytic pathway [37]. Production of Aβ in Chinese hamster ovary (CHO) cells involves internalization of APP from the cell surface [40], as deletion of the cytoplasmatic tail of APP significantly decreases cleavage by β-secretase. These experiments confirmed that Aβ could be derived through processing of APP endocytosed from the cell surface in addition to the secretory pathway [40]. Full-length APP can be internalized from the cell surface and targeted to endosomes and lysosomes, where COOH-terminal fragments containing the entire Aβ sequence have been detected.

Recent morphological evidence from living cells reinforces the hypothesis that APP–BACE1 interactions occur at the cell surface and early endosomes. There is a strong and previously unemphasized interaction at the cell surface where APP and BACE1 dramatically co-localize and then appear to be internalized together into early endosomes [41]. The majority of cell surface APP and BACE1 were internalized after 15 min, but they remained strongly co-localized in the early endosomal compartment where fluorescence resonance transfer (FRET) analysis demonstrated continued close interaction [41]. By contrast, at later time points, almost no co-localization or FRET were observed in lysosomal compartments. To determine whether the APP–BACE1 interaction on cell surface and endosomes contributed to Aβ synthesis, the labeled cell surface APP demonstrated detectable levels of labeled Aβ within 30 min. Taken together, these data confirm close APP–BACE1 interaction at the early endosomes, and highlight the cell surface as an additional potential site for APP–BACE1 interaction.

Here we propose a new approach to limit BACE1 activity, which exploits the interaction of APP and BACE1 at the cell surface prior to their internalization into the early endosomes [41]. This new approach is based on β-secretase cleavage of APP itself rather than inhibiting the entire enzyme activity (Fig. 10.1).

10.4 GENERATION OF ANTI-APP β-SITE ANTIBODIES

The β-secretase cleavage site, which resides between amino acids 666–673 of APP770 (corresponding to the amino acid sequence ISEVKMDA), is highly con-

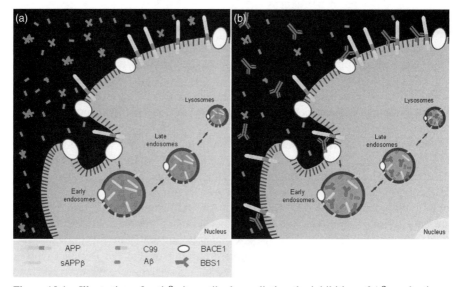

Figure 10.1 Illustration of anti β-site antibody mediating the inhibition of Aβ production via the endocytic pathway. (a) Aβ peptides are generated by two pathways: the secretory and the endocytic pathways, after which the generated peptides are either secreted or degraded in the cell. For simplicity purposes, only the endocytic pathway of Aβ production is illustrated. Accordingly, cell surface APP molecules, which are in close interaction with BACE1 molecules, are internalized into the early endosomes where the acidic pH favors BACE1 cleavage. The immediate product of BACE1 cleavage, C99, is further cleaved by γ-secretase to release Aβ peptides, which in turn can be either secreted or degraded in the cell. (b) The addition of BBS1, anti-APP β-site antibody, results in APP binding on the surface, flowing co-internalization of both APP and the antibody into the early endosomes. Within the endosomes, antibody binding is speculated to interfere with BACE1 cleavage and thus restrict Aβ production. In such a scenario, both the immediate products of BACE1 cleavage, soluble APPβ and C99, and Aβ levels are reduced. Since Aβ peptides are generated inside the cell, inhibition of its generation will be reflected in both the intra- and extracellular Aβ pools. The production of Aβ through the secretory pathway is not illustrated for simplicity purposes. (See color insert.)

served through evolution, while the double Swedish mutation localized at the same site exhibits the sequence NL instead of KM (amino acids 670,671 of APP770). To generate the antibodies against APP β-site, we chose the peptides that mimic the half-Swedish mutation chimeric peptide in which M670L mutation was introduced (multiple antigen peptide [MAP] – [ISEVKLDA]$_8$). The one amino acid substitution, using MAP displaying half-Swedish mutated APP β-site, enabled the generation of a high antibody titer against both the wild-type and Swedish mutated β-sites in BALB/C mice in a short period of time (6 weeks) [12]. The MAP system, first described in 1988 [42], is based on a small immunologically inert core molecule of radially branching lysine dendrites onto which a number of peptide antigens are anchored. The MAP system method was shown to be beneficial for producing high-titer anti-peptide antibodies [43, 44] and synthetic peptide vaccines [42]. Sera fractions consisting of anti-β-site polyclonal antibodies were collected and mice with the highest antibody levels were sacrificed and their spleens used for preparation of monoclonal antibodies (mAbs). A series of mAbs was obtained, and mAb BBS1 (blocking β-site 1), which showed the higher affinity in binding MAP expressing the wild-type β-site sequence, was chosen for further analysis. Anti-β-site polyclonal and mAbs were characterized for their ability to bind full-length APP and to interfere with APP processing and, thus, with Aβ production.

10.5   ANTIBODY INTERFERENCE WITH Aβ PRODUCTION IN CELLULAR MODEL

The effect of APP β-site antibodies, both polyclonal and monoclonal, on APP processing was evaluated in CHO cells stably transfected with wild-type human APP751 isoform (kindly provided by Professor D. Selkoe, Harvard Medical School, Boston, MA). The polyclonal antibodies were also examined for their ability to interfere with Swedish mutated APP processing by using CHO cells stably expressing Swedish mutated human APP695 isoform (kindly provided by Dr. C. Eckman, Mayo Clinic, Jacksonville, FL).

10.5.1   Polyclonal Antibodies

In the wild-type APP cellular model, the addition of purified polyclonal antibodies against APP β-site to the cells condition media for 24 h led to approximately 40% reduction in secreted Aβ levels. Intracellular Aβ levels, analyzed after 5 days incubation with the antibodies, were reduced by 50% in comparison with the basal Aβ levels. Purified nonimmune sera, used as the negative control, did not produce any change in Aβ levels within the secreted and intracellular Aβ pools.

A similar experiment was performed using the Swedish APP expressing cells; however, the effect of anti-β-site polyclonal antibodies was quite minor, reaching about 10% reduction in secreted Aβ levels and 7% reduction in intracellular Aβ levels [12].

These results are in accordance with the fact that the Swedish APP-mutated β-site is of higher affinity to BACE1 and thus a higher proportion of APP molecules are processed during maturation in the ER and trans-Golgi apparatus via the secretory pathway [45, 46]. Indeed, the substrate turnover rate (Kcat) of BACE was shown to be 10-fold higher in the presence of a short peptide carrying the Swedish mutation than in the presence of the wild-type peptide [47]. Since antibody mediated inhibition of β-secretase cleavage mainly affects cell surface APP molecules, their effect could hardly be noticed in this cellular system.

10.5.2   mAb BBS1

A thorough *in vitro* characterization of the APP β-site mAb was previously published [12]. Anti-APP β-site mAb, BBS1, showed high affinity binding of the MAP displaying eight copies of the wild-type APP β-site with an estimated dissociation constant (K_D) of 1.165 nM. The immunocomplex was found to remain 95% stable

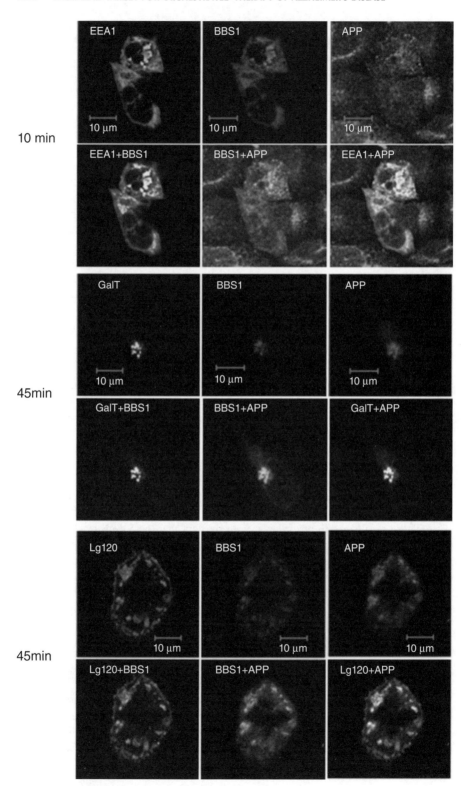

within pH 5, the optimal pH for β-secretase activity which occurs in the early endo-somes. The antibody ability to bind APP β-site in the context of full-length APP was demonstrated by Western blot and immunofluorescence using CHO cells over-expressing wild-type human APP, as well as by immunohistochemistry of brain sections from human APP transgenic mice model. By utilizing brain sections from two different lines of APP transgenic mice, we were able to demonstrate antibody ability to bind both wild-type and Swedish mutated APP β-sites. Conversely, despite the presence of the first two amino acid residues of Aβ within the immunogen used to generate this mAb, BBS1 does not bind any form of Aβ peptides.

Since most β-secretase activity is localized within intracellular compartments, we tested antibody ability to co-internalize into the cell with APP after binding at the cell surface at different time points. For that purpose, we transiently transfected the wild-type APP expressing cells with fluorescent resident proteins of either the early endosomes (EEA1), lysosomes (Lg120), or the Golgi apparatus (GalT). Twenty-four hours post transfection, we added the antibody to the condition media at different time points after which cells were fixed, permeabilized, and antibody presence was detected with fluorescent anti-mouse IgG antibodies. BBS1 was rapidly internalized into the cell and could be detected in the early endosomes after very short intervals. At longer intervals (from 10 min and onward), antibody was visualized in the early endosomes of an increasing number of cells in each field and its levels within the early endosomes were elevated with time. From 15 min incuba-tion and onward, BBS1 antibody could be detected in the lysosomes, with a more profound staining after 45 min. Antibody presence in the Golgi apparatus could be detected only after 45 min incubation (Fig. 10.2). Antibody trafficking suggests receptor-mediated internalization and trafficking through the endocytic pathway, as was expected knowing that APP is internalized into the early endosomes via clathrin-coated pits [48].

Once administered in the growing media of cells overexpressing wild-type APP, BBS1 reduced the extra- and intracellular Aβ levels. The secreted Aβ levels were reduced by about 20% compared with the basal levels after short intervals (from 3 to 12 h). Interestingly, after 5 days incubation with the antibody, the intracel-lular Aβ levels were dramatically reduced (estimated as 50% reduction) in compari-son with the basal intracellular Aβ levels. The levels of C99, the direct product of APP cleavage by BACE, were reduced by 20% after a 4-h treatment with BBS1 and

---

Figure 10.2 BBS1 internalization and trafficking in CHO cells overexpressing APP. Mammalian expression vectors consisting of either EEA1, Lg120, or GalT fused to eGFP, were used to label the early endosomes, lysosomes, and Golgi apparatus, respectively. Twenty-four hours post transfection, BBS1 antibody was administered to the growing media and incubated at 37°C for different intervals. Cells were then fixed and permeabilized and anti-mouse secondary antibody conjugated to Cy3 (red) was added to follow BBS1 localization. Anti-APP carboxy terminal antibody followed by secondary antibody conjugated to Cy5 (purple) was used to detect APP localization. Cell labeling was visualized using LSM-510 Zeiss confocal microscope and a co-localization software. The bottom panels at each time point represent merged images as indicated. Bars = 10 μm. (See color insert.)

were in accordance with the decrease in secreted Aβ levels at short intervals. Notably, antibodies directed to the amino terminal of APP have failed to produce such an effect, both with the extra- and intracellular Aβ pools. Importantly, BBS1 incubation did not harm the cells' viability as determined by 3-(4,5-dimethylthiazol-2-Yl)-2,5-diphenyltetrazolium bromide (MTT) reduction assay [12].

To examine whether inhibition of BACE1 activity resulted in increased α-secretase cleavage of APP, soluble α-APP levels were quantified by Western blot after 24 and 48 h of incubation with BBS1 antibody. Soluble α-APP levels were not affected by antibody treatment. The fact that inhibition of β-secretase activity did not lead to accelerated α-cleavage of APP supports former studies suggesting the existence of two distinct APP pools: raft-resident APP molecules that are mainly cleaved by β-secretase and APP outside rafts that are mainly subjected to α-secretase cleavage [49]. In addition, a recent report by the V. Lee research group, utilizing both BACE1 and TACE (α-secretase) inhibitors, showed that under normal conditions, despite having a similar trans-Golgi localization, these two proteases do not compete for APP and thus inhibition of BACE1 did not alter sAPPα levels and vice versa [50].

10.6 ANTIBODY INTERFERENCE WITH Aβ PRODUCTION IN ANIMAL MODELS

Swedish mutated APP β-site serves better for β-secretase cleavage and is mainly cleaved through the secretory pathway and, as demonstrated with the polyclonal antibodies, cellular systems expressing Swedish mutated APP were not affected by the treatment, suggesting that the animal model must consist of the wild-type APP β-site. To date, we have performed three *in vivo* studies: (1) intracranial infusion of BBS1 to a non-transgenic mice model with induced Aβ levels; (2) systemic, 2-month antibody administration to London mutated transgenic mice; (3) chronic, 6-month antibody administration to Tg2576 – safety study. Manuscripts summarizing the first two studies are currently being prepared for publication and thus will be briefly reviewed. The third study, mainly focused on safety issues, was previously published [51].

10.6.1 Intracranial Infusion of BBS1 to a Non-Transgenic Mice Model with Induced Aβ Levels

In order to demonstrate the *in vivo* feasibility of our approach, we used a non-transgenic mice model with induced Aβ levels [52]. Accordingly, neprilysin inhibitor thiorphan is infused into the mouse left ventricle and induces reversible deposition of endogenous murine Aβ. In contrast to the existing transgenic mice models that show enhanced production of Aβ peptide, the thiorphan infusion model represents an impaired Aβ clearance and is thought to be more relevant to sporadic AD cases in which Aβ degradation was shown to be impaired [53–55]. Additionally, the high soluble Aβ levels induced in this model are in contrast to the transgenic models in which most of the Aβ is aggregated. Our data from cellular models suggest a differential effect of BBS1 between the secreted and intracellular Aβ levels. Considering that most intracellular Aβ is soluble (from monomers to low molecular weight oligomers), this model provides an opportunity to evaluate the effect of these antibodies in the brain-soluble fraction.

Co-infusion of BBS1 antibody and thiorphan into the left ventricle of male C57BL wild-type mice led to a dramatic reduction in total Aβ levels, both in the intracellular and extracellular enriched fractions within the brain-soluble fraction, estimated as 60% and 89% reduction, respectively. Of note, despite the induced Aβ levels, these mice neither develop any behavioral abnormalities nor do they develop any other Aβ-associated neuropathologies such as astrocytes and microglia activation.

10.6.2   Systemic, 2-Month Antibody Administration to London Mutated Transgenic Mice

To investigate BBS1 treatment efficacy while administered through the peritoneum, we used female transgenic mice expressing the London mutated APP (V717I) under the regulation of thy-1 promoter on an FVB × C57BL background (reMYNDInc., Leuven, Belgium) [56]. The antibody was administered at 2-week intervals for 2 months after which mice nonspatial memory was assessed prior to sacrifice. Mice treated with BBS1 showed a positive trend of improved memory throughout training compared with saline-treated mice in the probe test in terms of time and frequencies. Insoluble Aβ42 and Aβ40 levels in treated animals were reduced by 25% and 40%, respectively. Membrane-associated Aβ oligomers were reduced by 26% in the treated animals. Serological analysis further supported these results, demonstrating a 40% reduction in the area occupied by the amyloid dense core and about 30% reduction in intracellular Aβ accumulation within the hippocampal neurons in animals treated with the antibody. Similar to the results in the cellular model, BBS1 treatment led to about 20% reduction in soluble APPβ levels without altering the levels of sAPPα. Importantly, no further microglia and astrocyte activation was observed as a result of antibody treatment.

10.6.3   Chronic 6-Month Antibody Administration to Tg2576 – Safety Study

The two described studies were highly valuable in demonstrating the feasibility and efficacy of antibodies against APP β-site. Although some of the current immunotherapies investigated in clinical trials employ Aβ antibodies that bind endogenous APP, we performed an additional study that mainly focuses on assessing the possible adverse effects that may result from a chronic administration of BBS1, which is an anti-APP antibody. Since BBS1 was shown to bind both wild-type and Swedish mutated APP molecules, we used the most widely available transgenic mice, Tg2576, which overexpress human Swedish mutated APP, to evaluate the safety of a chronic BBS1 treatment. As previously mentioned, the Swedish mutated APP is not the most suitable model to test methodologies aimed at interfering with β-secretase activity, since APP in this model is mainly cleaved through the secretory pathway rather than the endocytic pathway. However, most of the available transgenic mice express

Swedish mutated APP, and recent results from studies that evaluate the positive effect of BACE inhibitors were performed with these mice [57]. Accordingly, two doses of the antibody were tested in comparison to a saline-treated group. Immunizations were initiated at 6 months of age prior to the appearance of plaques, and were continued for a 6-month period in which mice were immunized at 14-day intervals. At the age of sacrifice, behavioral deficits, plaque pathology, reactive astrocytes, and microglia already existed [51].

During the 6 months of treatment, mice from all three treatment groups gained weight in similar percentages, suggesting that no side effects or inconvenience resulted from the antibody treatment. The levels of proinflammatory cytokines TNF-α and IL-1β in the plasma did not differ among the three treatment groups. Similarly, brain levels of IL-1β did not differ among the three treatment groups, while the levels of the anti-inflammatory cytokine IL-10 were elevated. Blood and urine biochemistry tests, including kidney functions, were normal, indicating no internal organ failure. These results were also supported by normal morphology of liver, kidney, and spleen tissues, as observed by the gross-anatomy organ examination. Further histological evaluation of the kidneys showed no abnormalities.

Since the BBS1 antibody does not bind Aβ plaques and is rapidly internalized into the cell after APP binding, microglia activation characterizing Aβ-specific antibodies was not expected. We evaluated the levels of microglia activation using F4/80 staining in three distinct areas: dentate gyrus, hippocampus hilus, and parietal cortex. A significant and dose-dependent decrease in microglia staining was observed in the treated groups compared with the saline-treated group. Glial fibrillary acidic protein (GFAP) staining for reactive astrocytes did not show any difference between the three treatment groups. We further performed CD3 staining of brain sections to evaluate the possibility of T-cells penetrating the brain parenchyma. No T-cells were detected in any of the sections analyzed.

Accumulating evidence suggests that immunotherapies against Aβ lead to hemorrhages within brain blood vessels because clearance of Aβ from the tissue to the capillaries damages their integrity [58, 59]. Since the BBS1 antibody does not bind Aβ, soluble peptides, or plaques, we speculated that this antibody would not induce hemorrhages in the brains of the immunized transgenic animals. Importantly, the number of microhemorrhages was significantly lower in the BBS1-high-dose treated group compared with the phosphate buffer solution (PBS)-treated animals. Notably, very few hemorrhages were evident in this strain of transgenic mice at the age of euthanasia (12 months). As was predicted, passive intraperitoneal administration of BBS1 antibody to this mice model did not lead to a significant reduction in insoluble brain Aβ levels. This data was in accordance with the unchanged C99/APP ratios in these mice.

10.7 IDENTIFICATION OF APP BINDING SMALL MOLECULES THAT BLOCK β-SITE CLEAVAGE OF APP

Small molecules that bind APP and inhibit BACE cleavage have the potential to be specific and effective inhibitors of the aberrant processing of APP – much like the anti-APP antibody approach. These molecules represent noncompetitive substrate-specific inhibitors of BACE. Furthermore, such small molecule inhibitors can be optimized for potency and potentially developed to be brain permeable and orally bioavailable. Like the β-site antibody, these small molecules would be specific for cleavage of APP and would not affect other substrates processed by BACE [25–27].

In a previous work from Merck and company [60], a novel series of benzofuran-containing compounds such as molecule **1** (Fig. 10.3) were reported to bind to APP and inhibit Aβ production. These small molecules were shown to be micromolar inhibitors of BACE cleavage of APP (IC$_{50}$ ~ 11 μM) but had no direct effect on BACE itself as they did not inhibit the processing of the commonly used BACE peptidic substrate P$_5$-P$_5'$. Using surface plasmon resonance, compound **1** was shown to bind APP with a micromolar binding affinity. These results demonstrate the possibility of developing compounds that can bind APP and inhibit Aβ production, as a novel therapeutic approach for AD.

In order to identify potent and effective compounds based on this approach for development as preclinical candidates, it is important to set up a rapid screening paradigm for such inhibitors. One such approach which is being developed at the Buck Institute involves assays using the DELFIA technology [61] and soluble ectodomain of APP$_{695}$ (eAPP, residues 19–624) for identification of small molecules that can bind APP. Compounds identified from such screens would then be evaluated for their inhibition of the processing of APP to Aβ. The high-throughput dissociation-enhanced lanthanide fluorescent immunoassay (DELFIA)-based assay enables screening of large small molecule libraries for APP binding. Lead molecules identified from such a screening paradigm would be optimized for potency and bioavailability toward identification of preclinical candidates for AD. At the Buck Institute, we have cohorts of PDAPP AD mouse model and non-transgenics that will be used in the evaluation of these mouse models for *in vivo* efficacy.

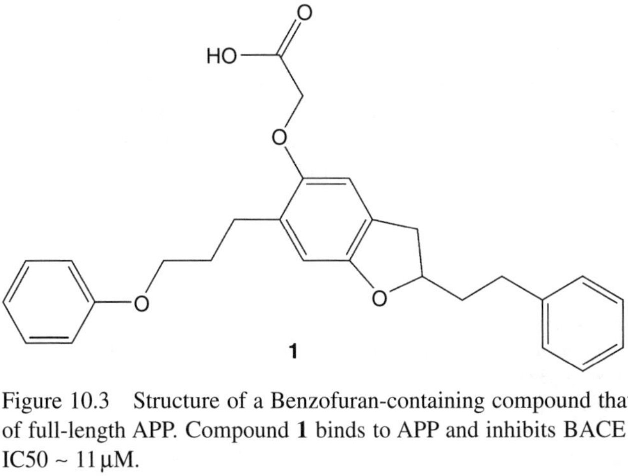

Figure 10.3 Structure of a Benzofuran-containing compound that blocks BACE cleavage of full-length APP. Compound **1** binds to APP and inhibits BACE cleavage of APP with a IC50 ~ 11 μM.

10.8   FINAL REMARKS

In light of the ongoing debate regarding which species is the villain inducing neuronal and synaptic loss in AD, a logical way to intervene with the amyloid cascade is to interfere with Aβ production and partially restrict it, resulting probably with lower levels of all the aforementioned species. Considering previously described drawbacks involved in BACE1 inhibition [11, 13], the approaches reviewed here serve as an attractive alternative specifically aimed at inhibiting β-secretase activity, leaving the native function of BACE1 toward its other substrates unharmed.

The importance of limiting intracellular Aβ formation at early stages of AD development is emphasized in many studies [62]. It is likely that the reduction in total Aβ levels need not be complete in order to implicate a beneficial effect if preventive therapy can be initiated. In AD caused by most mutations in APP, PS1, or PS2, the levels of Aβ42 are increased by as little as 30% [63]. Such an elevation can result in the onset of AD 30–40 years earlier than typical late-onset AD cases. By inference, it is likely that reducing the total Aβ levels by 30%, or effecting similar selective reductions in the highly pathogenic Aβ42, may delay the development of AD to such an extent that it is no longer a major health-care problem. In view of this data, the ability of BBS1 antibody to reduce intracellular and extracellular Aβ levels, demonstrated in cellular and animal models, may be even more relevant in preventing neuronal dysfunction and thus be used as a prophylactic therapeutic for AD. Similarly, compounds that bind APP and modulate BACE cleavage would like the APP β-site antibodies to be specific and effective in inhibiting Aβ production and as a novel therapy for AD.

ACKNOWLEDGMENTS

We wish to express our great gratitude to Gilad Sivan for his contribution to the antibody trafficking experiments, Idan Rakover for his contribution to the tg2576 study, Dr. Maria Becker, Dr. Vered Lavie, Myra Gartner, Nurit Chimovitz, and Polina Rabinovich-Toidman for their assistance with the London mutated transgenic mice study. Finally, we wish to acknowledge Mrs. Faybia Margolin for manuscript proofreading and the members of our laboratory for helpful discussions. We acknowledge the support of the Bredesen Laboratory and members of the Alzheimer's Drug Discovery Network (ADDN) at the Buck Institute in the development of the screening assays for APP binding molecules and in the production of eAPP.

REFERENCES

1. Selkoe, D.J. 2001. Alzheimer's disease: genes, proteins, and therapy. *Physiol Rev* **81**:741–766.
2. Hardy, J. and Allsop, D. 1991. Amyloid deposition as the central event in the aetiology of Alzheimer's disease. *Trends Pharmacol Sci* **12**:383–388.
3. Selkoe, D.J. 1996. Amyloid beta-protein and the genetics of Alzheimer's disease. *J Biol Chem* **271**:18295–18298.
4. Hardy, J. 1997. Amyloid, the presenilins and Alzheimer's disease. *Trends Neurosci* **20**:154–159.

5. Hardy, J. and Selkoe, D.J. 2002. The amyloid hypothesis of Alzheimer's disease: progress and problems on the road to therapeutics. *Science* **297**:353–356.

6. Busciglio, J., Lorenzo, A., Yeh, J., and Yankner, B.A. 1995. Beta-amyloid fibrils induce tau phosphorylation and loss of microtubule binding. *Neuron* **14**:879–888.

7. Gotz, J., Probst, A., Spillantini, M.G., Schafer, T., Jakes, R., Burki, K., and Goedert, M. 1995. Somatodendritic localization and hyperphosphorylation of tau protein in transgenic mice expressing the longest human brain tau isoform. *Embo J* **14**:1304–1313.

8. Lewis, J., Dickson, D.W., Lin, W.L., Chisholm, L., Corral, A., Jones, G., Yen, S.H., Sahara, N., Skipper, L., Yager, D., Eckman, C., Hardy, J., Hutton, M., and McGowan, E. 2001. Enhanced neurofibrillary degeneration in transgenic mice expressing mutant tau and APP. *Science* **293**:1487–1491.

9. Hardy, J., Duff, K., Hardy, K.G., Perez-Tur, J., and Hutton, M. 1998. Genetic dissection of Alzheimer's disease and related dementias: amyloid and its relationship to tau. *Nat Neurosci* **1**:355–358.

10. Ghosh, A.K., Gemma, S., and Tang, J. 2008. Beta-secretase as a therapeutic target for Alzheimer's disease. *Neurotherapeutics* **5**:399–408.

11. Hook, V., Toneff, T., Bogyo, M., Greenbaum, D., Medzihradszky, K.F., Neveu, J., Lane, W., Hook, G., and Reisine, T. 2005. Inhibition of cathepsin B reduces beta-amyloid production in regulated secretory vesicles of neuronal chromaffin cells: evidence for cathepsin B as a candidate beta-secretase of Alzheimer's disease. *Biol Chem* **386**:931–940.

12. Arbel, M., Yacoby, I., and Solomon, B. 2005. Inhibition of amyloid precursor protein processing by beta-secretase through site-directed antibodies. *Proc Natl Acad Sci U S A* **102**:7718–7723.

13. Vassar, R., Bennett, B.D., Babu-Khan, S., Kahn, S., Mendiaz, E.A., Denis, P., Teplow, D.B., Ross, S., Amarante, P., Loeloff, R., Luo, Y., Fisher, S., Fuller, J., Edenson, S., Lile, J., Jarosinski, M.A., Biere, A.L., Curran, E., Burgess, T., Louis, J.C., Collins, F., Treanor, J., Rogers, G., and Citron, M. 1999. Beta-secretase cleavage of Alzheimer's amyloid precursor protein by the transmembrane aspartic protease BACE. *Science* **286**:735–741.

14. Sinha, S., Anderson, J.P., Barbour, R., Basi, G.S., Caccavello, R., Davis, D., Doan, M., Dovey, H.F., Frigon, N., Hong, J., Jacobson-Croak, K., Jewett, N., Keim, P., Knops, J., Lieberburg, I., Power, M., Tan, H., Tatsuno, G., Tung, J., Schenk, D., Seubert, P., Suomensaari, S.M., Wang, S., Walker, D., Zhao, J., McConlogue, L., and John, V. 1999. Purification and cloning of amyloid precursor protein beta-secretase from human brain. *Nature* **402**:537–540.

15. Yan, R., Bienkowski, M.J., Shuck, M.E., Miao, H., Tory, M.C., Pauley, A.M., Brashier, J.R., Stratman, N.C., Mathews, W.R., Buhl, A.E., Carter, D.B., Tomasselli, A.G., Parodi, L.A., Heinrikson, R.L., and Gurney, M.E. 1999. Membrane-anchored aspartyl protease with Alzheimer's disease betasecretase activity. *Nature* **402**:533–537.

16. Hussain, I., Powell, D., Howlett, D.R., Tew, D.G., Meek, T.D., Chapman, C., Gloger, I.S., Murphy, K.E., Southan, C.D., Ryan, D.M., Smith, T.S., Simmons, D.L., Walsh, F.S., Dingwall, C., and Christie, G. 1999. Identification of a novel aspartic protease (Asp 2) as beta-secretase. *Mol Cell Neurosci* **14**:419–427.

17. Citron, M. 2002. Beta-secretase as a target for the treatment of Alzheimer's disease. *J Neurosci Res* **70**:373–379.

18. Cai, H., Wang, Y., McCarthy, D., Wen, H., Borchelt, D.R., Price, D.L., and Wong, P.C. 2001. BACE1 is the major beta-secretase for generation of Abeta peptides by neurons. *Nat Neurosci* **4**:233–234.

19. Bennett, B.D., Babu-Khan, S., Loeloff, R., Louis, J.C., Curran, E., Citron, M., and Vassar, R. 2000. Expression analysis of BACE2 in brain and peripheral tissues. *J Biol Chem* **275**:20647–20651.

20. Luo, Y., Bolon, B., Kahn, S., Bennett, B.D., Babu-Khan, S., Denis, P., Fan, W., Kha, H., Zhang, J., Gong, Y., Martin, L., Louis, J.C., Yan, Q., Richards, W.G., Citron, M., and Vassar, R. 2001. Mice deficient in BACE1, the Alzheimer's beta-secretase, have normal phenotype and abolished betaamyloid generation. *Nat Neurosci* **4**:231–232.

21. Roberds, S.L., Anderson, J., Bas, G., Bienkowski, M.J., Branstetter, D.G., Chen, K.S., Freedman, S.B., Frigon, N.L., Games, D., Hu, K., Johnson-Wood, K., Kappenman, K.E., Kawabe, T.T., Kola, I., Kuehn, R., Lee, M., Liu, W., Motter, R., Nichols, N.F., Power, M., Robertson, D.W., Schenk, D., Schoor, M., Shopp, G.M., Shuck, M.E., Sinha, S., Svensson, K.A., Tatsuno, G., Tintrup, H., Wijsman,

J., Wright, S., and McConlogue, L. 2001. BACE knockout mice are healthy despite lacking the primary beta-secretase activity in brain: implications for Alzheimer's disease therapeutics. *Hum Mol Genet* **10**:1317–1324.

22. Pangalos, M.N., Jacobsen, S.J., and Reinhart, P.H. 2005. Disease modifying strategies for the treatment of Alzheimer's disease targeted at modulating levels of the beta-amyloid peptide. *Biochem Soc Trans* **33**:553–558.

23. Dewachter, I. and Van Leuven, F. 2002. Secretases as targets for the treatment of Alzheimer's disease: the prospects. *Lancet Neurol* **1**:409–416.

24. Capell, A., Meyn, L., Fluhrer, R., Teplow, D.B., Walter, J., and Haass, C. 2002. Apical sorting of beta-secretase limits amyloid beta-peptide production. *J Biol Chem* **277**:5637–5643.

25. Lichtenthaler, S.F., Dominguez, D.I., Westmeyer, G.G., Reiss, K., Haass, C., Saftig, P., De Strooper, B., and Seed, B. 2003. The cell adhesion protein P-selectin glycoprotein ligand-1 is a substrate for the aspartyl protease BACE1. *J Biol Chem* **278**:48713–48719.

26. Kitazume, S., Tachida, Y., Oka, R., Kotani, N., Ogawa, K., Suzuki, M., Dohmae, N., Takio, K., Saido, T.C., and Hashimoto, Y. 2003. Characterization of alpha 2,6-sialyltransferase cleavage by Alzheimer's beta-secretase (BACE1). *J Biol Chem* **278**:14865–14871.

27. Pastorino, L., Ikin, A.F., Lamprianou, S., Vacaresse, N., Revelli, J.P., Platt, K., Paganetti, P., Mathews, P.M., Harroch, S., and Buxbaum, J.D. 2004. BACE (beta-secretase) modulates the processing of APLP2 in vivo. *Mol Cell Neurosci* **25**:642–649.

28. Willem, M., Garratt, A.N., Novak, B., Citron, M., Kaufmann, S., Rittger, A., DeStrooper, B., Saftig, P., Birchmeier, C., and Haass, C. 2006. Control of peripheral nerve myelination by the beta-secretase BACE1. *Science* **314**:664–666.

29. Ohno, M., Sametsky, E.A., Younkin, L.H., Oakley, H., Younkin, S.G., Citron, M., Vassar, R., and Disterhoft, J.F. 2004. BACE1 deficiency rescues memory deficits and cholinergic dysfunction in a mouse model of Alzheimer's disease. *Neuron* **41**:27–33.

30. Laird, F.M., Cai, H., Savonenko, A.V., Farah, M.H., He, K., Melnikova, T., Wen, H., Chiang, H.C., Xu, G., Koliatsos, V.E., Borchelt, D.R., Price, D.L., Lee, H.K., and Wong, P.C. 2005. BACE1, a major determinant of selective vulnerability of the brain to amyloid-beta amyloidogenesis, is essential for cognitive, emotional, and synaptic functions. *J Neurosci* **25**:11693–11709.

31. Hook, V.Y., Kindy, M., and Hook, G. 2008. Inhibitors of cathepsin B improve memory and reduce beta-amyloid in transgenic Alzheimer disease mice expressing the wild-type, but not the Swedish mutant, beta-secretase site of the amyloid precursor protein. *J Biol Chem* **283**:7745–7753.

32. Koo, E.H. and Squazzo, S.L. 1994. Evidence that production and release of amyloid beta-protein involves the endocytic pathway. *J Biol Chem* **269**:17386–17389.

33. Perez, R.G., Soriano, S., Hayes, J.D., Ostaszewski, B., Xia, W., Selkoe, D.J., Chen, X., Stokin, G.B., and Koo, E.H. 1999. Mutagenesis identifies new signals for beta-amyloid precursor protein endocytosis, turnover, and the generation of secreted fragments, including Abeta42. *J Biol Chem* **274**:18851–18856.

34. Nixon, R.A., Mathews, P.M., and Cataldo, A.M. 2001. The neuronal endosomal-lysosomal system in Alzheimer's disease. *J Alzheimers Dis* **3**:97–107.

35. Chyung, J.H. and Selkoe, D.J. 2003. Inhibition of receptor-mediated endocytosis demonstrates generation of amyloid beta-protein at the cell surface. *J Biol Chem* **278**:51035–51043.

36. Perez, R.G., Squazzo, S.L., and Koo, E.H. 1996. Enhanced release of amyloid beta-protein from codon 670/671 "Swedish" mutant beta-amyloid precursor protein occurs in both secretory and endocytic pathways. *J Biol Chem* **271**:9100–9107.

37. Soriano, S., Chyung, A.S., Chen, X., Stokin, G.B., Lee, V.M., and Koo, E.H. 1999. Expression of beta-amyloid precursor protein-CD3gamma chimeras to demonstrate the selective generation of amyloid beta(1-40) and amyloid beta(1-42) peptides within secretory and endocytic compartments. *J Biol Chem* **274**:32295–32300.

38. Huse, J.T., Pijak, D.S., Leslie, G.J., Lee, V.M., and Doms, R.W. 2000. Maturation and endosomal targeting of beta-site amyloid precursor protein-cleaving enzyme. The Alzheimer's disease beta-secretase. *J Biol Chem* **275**:33729–33737.

39. Walter, J., Fluhrer, R., Hartung, B., Willem, M., Kaether, C., Capell, A., Lammich, S., Multhaup, G., and Haass, C. 2001. Phosphorylation regulates intracellular trafficking of beta-secretase. *J Biol Chem* **276**:14634–14641.

40. Koo, E.H., Squazzo, S.L., Selkoe, D.J., and Koo, C.H. 1996. Trafficking of cell-surface amyloid beta-protein precursor. I. Secretion, endocytosis and recycling as detected by labeled monoclonal antibody. *J Cell Sci* **109**(Pt 5):991–998.

41. Kinoshita, A., Fukumoto, H., Shah, T., Whelan, C.M., Irizarry, M.C., and Hyman, B.T. 2003. Demonstration by FRET of BACE interaction with the amyloid precursor protein at the cell surface and in early endosomes. *J Cell Sci* **116**:3339–3346.

42. Tam, J.P. 1988. Synthetic peptide vaccine design: synthesis and properties of a high-density multiple antigenic peptide system. *Proc Natl Acad Sci U S A* **85**:5409–5413.

43. Wang, C.Y., Looney, D.J., Li, M.L., Walfield, A.M., Ye, J., Hosein, B., Tam, J.P., and Wong-Staal, F. 1991. Long-term high-titer neutralizing activity induced by octameric synthetic HIV-1 antigen. *Science* **254**:285–288.

44. Posnett, D.N., McGrath, H., and Tam, J.P. 1988. A novel method for producing anti-peptide antibodies. Production of site-specific antibodies to the T cell antigen receptor beta-chain. *J Biol Chem* **263**:1719–1725.

45. Haass, C., Lemere, C.A., Capell, A., Citron, M., Seubert, P., Schenk, D., Lannfelt, L., and Selkoe, D.J. 1995. The Swedish mutation causes early-onset Alzheimer's disease by beta-secretase cleavage within the secretory pathway. *Nat Med* **1**:1291–1296.

46. Thinakaran, G., Teplow, D.B., Siman, R., Greenberg, B., and Sisodia, S.S. 1996. Metabolism of the "Swedish" amyloid precursor protein variant in neuro2a (N2a) cells. Evidence that cleavage at the "beta-secretase" site occurs in the Golgi apparatus. *J Biol Chem* **271**:9390–9397.

47. Gruninger-Leitch, F., Schlatter, D., Kung, E., Nelbock, P., and Dobeli, H. 2002. Substrate and inhibitor profile of BACE (beta-secretase) and comparison with other mammalian aspartic proteases. *J Biol Chem* **277**:4687–4693.

48. Nordstedt, C., Caporaso, G.L., Thyberg, J., Gandy, S.E., and Greengard, P. 1993. Identification of the Alzheimer beta/A4 amyloid precursor protein in clathrin-coated vesicles purified from PC12 cells. *J Biol Chem* **268**:608–612.

49. Ehehalt, R., Keller, P., Haass, C., Thiele, C., and Simons, K. 2003. Amyloidogenic processing of the Alzheimer beta-amyloid precursor protein depends on lipid rafts. *J Cell Biol* **160**:113–123.

50. Kim, M.L., Zhang, B., Mills, I.P., Milla, M.E., Brunden, K.R., and Lee, V.M. 2008. Effects of TNFalpha-converting enzyme inhibition on amyloid beta production and APP processing in vitro and in vivo. *J Neurosci* **28**:12052–12061.

51. Rakover, I., Arbel, M., and Solomon, B. 2007. Immunotherapy against APP beta-secretase cleavage site improves cognitive function and reduces neuroinflammation in Tg2576 mice without a significant effect on brain Abeta levels. *Neurodegener Dis* **4**(5):392–402.

52. Dolev, I. and Michaelson, D.M. 2004. A nontransgenic mouse model shows inducible amyloid-beta (Abeta) peptide deposition and elucidates the role of apolipoprotein E in the amyloid cascade. *Proc Natl Acad Sci U S A* **101**:13909–13914.

53. Yasojima, K., Akiyama, H., McGeer, E.G., and McGeer, P.L. 2001. Reduced neprilysin in high plaque areas of Alzheimer brain: a possible relationship to deficient degradation of beta-amyloid peptide. *Neurosci Lett* **297**:97–100.

54. Cook, D.G., Leverenz, J.B., McMillan, P.J., Kulstad, J.J., Ericksen, S., Roth, R.A., Schellenberg, G.D., Jin, L.W., Kovacina, K.S., and Craft, S. 2003. Reduced hippocampal insulin-degrading enzyme in late-onset Alzheimer's disease is associated with the apolipoprotein E-epsilon4 allele. *Am J Pathol* **162**:313–319.

55. Maruyama, M., Higuchi, M., Takaki, Y., Matsuba, Y., Tanji, H., Nemoto, M., Tomita, N., Matsui, T., Iwata, N., Mizukami, H., Muramatsu, S., Ozawa, K., Saido, T.C., Arai, H., and Sasaki, H. 2005. Cerebrospinal fluid neprilysin is reduced in prodromal Alzheimer's disease. *Ann Neurol* **57**:832–842.

56. Moechars, D., Gilis, M., Kuiperi, C., Laenen, I., and Van Leuven, F. 1998. Aggressive behaviour in transgenic mice expressing APP is alleviated by serotonergic drugs. *Neuroreport* **9**:3561–3564.

57. Chang, W.P., Koelsch, G., Wong, S., Downs, D., Da, H., Weerasena, V., Gordon, B., Devasamudram, T., Bilcer, G., Ghosh, A.K., and Tang, J. 2004. In vivo inhibition of Abeta production by memapsin 2 (beta-secretase) inhibitors. *J Neurochem* **89**:1409–1416.

58. Wilcock, D.M., Rojiani, A., Rosenthal, A., Subbarao, S., Freeman, M.J., Gordon, M.N., and Morgan, D. 2004. Passive immunotherapy against Abeta in aged APP-transgenic mice reverses cognitive

deficits and depletes parenchymal amyloid deposits in spite of increased vascular amyloid and microhemorrhage. *J Neuroinflammation* **1**:24.

59. Morgan, D. 2005. Mechanisms of A beta plaque clearance following passive A beta immunization. *Neurodegener Dis* **2**:261–266.
60. Espeseth, A.S., Xu, M., Huang, Q., Coburn, C.A., Jones, K.L., Ferrer, M., Zuck, P.D., Strulovici, B., Price, E.A., Wu, G., Wolfe, A.L., Lineberger, J.E., Sardana, M., Tugusheva, K., Pietrak, B.L., Crouthamel, M.C., Lai, M.T., Dodson, E.C., Bazzo, R., Shi, X.P., Simon, A.J., Li, Y., and Hazuda, D.J. 2005. Compounds that bind APP and inhibit Abeta processing in vitro suggest a novel approach to Alzheimer disease therapeutics. *J Biol Chem* **280**:17792–17797.
61. Inglese, J., Samama, P., Patel, S., Burbaum, J., Stroke, I.L., and Appell, K.C. 1998. Chemokine receptor–ligand interactions measured using time-resolved fluorescence. *Biochemistry* **37**: 2372–2377.
62. Ohyagi, Y. 2008. Intracellular amyloid beta-protein as a therapeutic target for treating Alzheimer's disease. *Curr Alzheimer Res* **5**:555–561.
63. Scheuner, D., Eckman, C., Jensen, M., Song, X., Citron, M., Suzuki, N., Bird, T.D., Hardy, J., Hutton, M., Kukull, W., Larson, E., Levy-Lahad, E., Viitanen, M., Peskind, E., Poorkaj, P., Schellenberg, G., Tanzi, R., Wasco, W., Lannfelt, L., Selkoe, D., and Younkin, S. 1996. Secreted amyloid beta-protein similar to that in the senile plaques of Alzheimer's disease is increased in vivo by the pre-senilin 1 and 2 and APP mutations linked to familial Alzheimer's disease. *Nat Med* **2**:864–870.

AFTERWORD

Ruth Abraham
Israel

A lifetime of memories exists in constellation all through the brain, but without a reliable system of retrieval, they'll sit dormant forever

—David Shenk

INTRODUCTION

Observed from the outside, Alzheimer's disease (AD) patients drawing on paper or shaping clay into pots or figures, might appear to be involved in nothing more than pleasant busy-time activity. However, when taking part in an art therapy session, the patient is exposed to more than that, the very least of which is an opportunity to express bottled-up feelings such as anger and sadness. As the disease progresses, there is a large loss of neuronal connections, and what is demonstrated through artwork is the activation of existing, dormant connections, compensating for the loss of language, logical and sequential thought processes.

AD patients are increasingly isolated, lonely, and marginalized, in many ways rendered invisible. The confirmation that they continue to exist in a social fabric is enhanced by attentive listening, understanding, and feedback from the therapist. Sharing memories and feelings through the language of art compensates for the diminishing capacity to communicate through words.

AD patients tend to suffer from lack of initiative, are often listless, and lack confidence. As they lose their language skills, they are assailed by the anxiety of not being able to communicate and of not being understood. When he sits in the large common rooms of facilities, the AD patient can often be seen dozing, staring into space, or fiddling purposelessly with objects. In the art room, that same patient becomes fully engaged, touching upon early memories, making color choices specifically to their taste, making significant marks on the page. Creative acts such as these are a source of rich pleasure, something that AD patients progressively lack in their lives. I have witnessed noticeable physiological changes during the sessions; there is often a marked decrease in agitation and breathing becomes deeper and calmer. Valuable research could be done taking objective measures of general health both before and after the session, such as blood pressure levels, heart rate, and respiratory rate, in an attempt to ascertain physiological changes occurring as a result of the creative involvement.

BACE: Lead Target for Orchestrated Therapy of Alzheimer's Disease, Edited by Varghese John
Copyright © 2010 John Wiley & Sons, Inc.

235

One of the defining criteria of any therapy is that it results in sustained improvement beyond the actual therapy session. This necessitates insight, memory, and subsequent internalization. Since AD patients are considered unable to learn, in the sense of absorbing and retaining new information, the question arises whether art therapy could be defined as a therapy for them. In my book, *When Words Have Lost Their Meaning: Alzheimer's Patients Communicate Through Art* (Greenwood Publication, 2005), I have shown that the art productions of many of the patients, even in the advanced stages of dementia, did improve over time, meaning there was a learning and internalization process. The participants acquired greater skill, used the materials more efficiently, made more considered choices, and their use of color became richer.

ARTWORK AS A MEASURE OF THE PROGRESSION OF AD

Pictures painted by AD patients have been thought of as X-rays of the declining mind. For instance, the portraits of Utermohlen, http://www.37signals.com/svn/posts/81-william-utermohlens-self-portraits, are a documentation of the way AD impacted on the painterly skills of this talented artist. As the dementia progressed, the images lost their complexity, clarity, and depth, an indication of cortical deterioration. On the other hand, the art of many AD patients, who had not painted in the past, displayed minor but definitive improvements over time. As these patients attempted to recollect memories and struggled to communicate through images, color, design, and patterning, it is possible to assume that new neuronal transmissions were being activated; new connections, absent at the start of the process, were being rewired. The investigation of these subtle changes occurring in the art of AD patients might shine light on the power of art activity to stimulate greater retrieval capability in the brain.

In this section, there are a number of artworks by AD patients at differing stages of the disease. While the details of the images may have some correlation to the declining state of the mind, each of the pictures below served differing needs of the individual patient. The use of specific art material helped them express current emotions. In all of these cases, their work improved during the period they took part in the art therapy sessions.

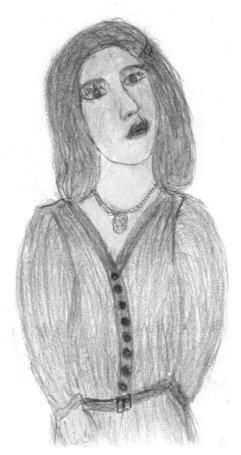

Image 1   Sheila used sharp pointed pencil crayons to create many pictures of women. The small repetitive hatched lines with which she painstakingly filled areas of the dress, skin, and hair, were a means to calm her compulsive tendencies and agitated state (mild cognitive impairment). (See color insert.)

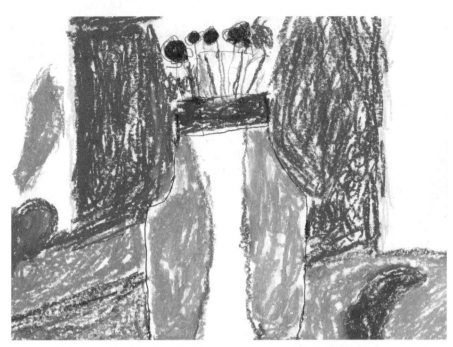

Image 2   Bella filled pages with colorful patterns, many of them taking on the form of flowers which she so loved. Continuing to draw even in her home where her caregivers provided her with pages and crayons, the art became a significant consolation in her more isolated condition. The art helped her focus and quieted her obsessional questions and wandering (moderate stage dementia).

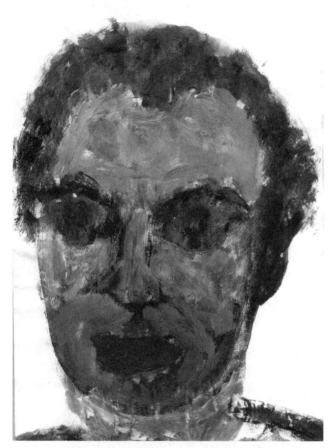

Image 3   Joe was struggling with severe paranoia which he portrayed in the glaring eyes
of this portrait. A mild mannered man, he repeatedly used the art to express anger and fear
that lay hidden behind his unemotional facade. The rich layering of liquid paint (gouache)
and dramatic use of color lends expressive power to the work (moderate stage dementia).
(See color insert.)

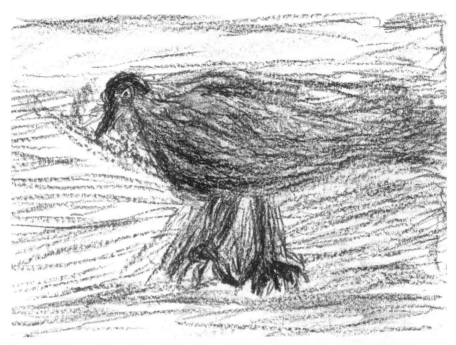

Image 4   Myron chose oil pastel, drawing repeated parallel lines to create this bird, an image of flight and movement. The work was done with energy and determination, surprising in a man who was almost mute, and for many of the initial sessions, had been a passive observer (late stage dementia).

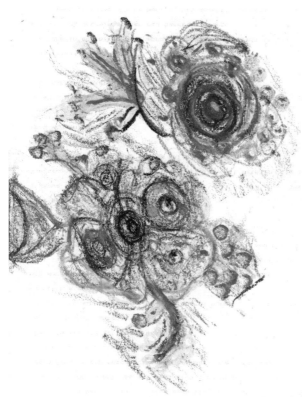

Image 5   This is Alice's attempt to copy a still life. It was a great achievement, given that her perception of figure and ground was already seriously impaired. She made joyful use of oil pastel to create many colorful works (late stage dementia). (See color insert.)

INDEX

AD (Alzheimer's disease)
  Aβ therapies in clinical development,
    98–199
    β-secretase, 201–202
    drugs, 202–203
    early-phase, 204–205
    γ-secretase modulators, 200–201
    phase 2, 205–208
    phase 3, 208–211
    regulatory phase, 211–212
    vaccination, 199–200
  alternative model, 7–9
  animal testing, 45, 199
    canines, 163–167
    mice, 7, 161–163, 188
    nonhuman primates, 167–168
  as cellular dependence inbalance, 3–4
  clinical and physiological hallmarks, 36
  defined, 36, 177, 217
  preclinical testing, 159–169
  projected growth of, by 2050, 1, 197
  as state of altered dependence, 6
  structural abnormalities, 15
ADAM
  -9, 37
  -10, 1, 37
  -17, 37
ADAS-cog (Alzheimer's Disease
    Assessment Scale-cog), 197, 200, 211
ADCS (Alzheimer's Disease Cooperative
    Study), 201, 212
ADME (adsorption, distribution,
    metabolism, excretion), 35, 177–193
  optimized, 180–188
    GlaxoSmithKline, 184–188
    Merck, 181–184
  in vivo efficiency, 188–193
ADNI (Alzheimer's Disease Neuroimaging
    Initiative), 207, 212–213

adsorption, distribution, metabolism,
    excretion. See ADME
AIDS, 29, 178
Alzheimer's disease. See AD
Alzheimer's Disease Assessment Scale-cog.
    See ADAS-cog
Alzheimer's Disease Cooperative Study.
    See ADCS
Alzheimer's Disease Neuroimaging
    Initiative. See ADNI
Amgen, 20, 88
amyloid cascade, 217
angiotensinogen, 22
antibody
  anti-APP β-site, 221–223
  interference, 223–226
    in animal models, 226–228
    nontransgenic mice, 226–227
    Tg2576, 227–228
    transgenic mice, 227
  mAb 6E10, 24
  mAb 22C11, 24
  mAb BBS1, 223–226
  monoclonal, 223
  polyclonal, 223
AP (aspartyl protease), 18, 21, 123
  AA, 37–38
  AD, 37–38
  Asp2. See BACE
  catalytic mechanism, 39–40
  classification, 37–38
  inhibition, 41–42
  kinetic mechanism, 40–41
  memapsin 1. See BACE2
  memapsin 2. See BACE
  obstacles to inhibitors development, 29
  presenilin, 123–124
  substrate specificity, 42–45
apoptosis, 3

BACE: Lead Target for Orchestrated Therapy of Alzheimer's Disease, Edited by Varghese John
Copyright © 2010 John Wiley & Sons, Inc.

APP (β-amyloid precursor protein), 1, 3–4, 15–17, 159, 160, 180, 218. *See also* MBP; mutation
  695-residue variant, 14, 23, 221, 227
  751-residue variant, 16
  770-residue variant, 36, 221–222
  APLP1, 42
  APLP2, 220
  C83, 15, 18, 22–23
  C89, 37
  C99, 5, 37, 159
  mutations, 9
  neo, 4
  N-terminal, 5, 131, 159
  processing, 36–37
  residues 657–664 of human, 4
  sAPPα, 5, 7, 20, 24, 159, 226, 227
  sAPPβ, 2, 4, 5, 9, 20, 24, 25, 220
  small molecules that block β-site cleavage, 228–229
  Swedish (Sw), 16, 20, 22, 43, 51, 138, 218, 223, 225, 226–228
    EVNL/DAEF, 70
    KM-NL, 23–25
  Type I, 16
  wild type (Wt), 20, 22, 43, 218, 220, 225
aromatics (2EWY), 139
Asp2. *See* BACE1
asparagine
  132, 19
  151, 19
  202, 19
  333, 19
Astellas Pharma, 72
Astex Therapeutics, 108, 144
  Library of Available Substances, 149
AstraZeneca, 108
ATLAS (Astex Therapeutics Library of Available Substances), 149
atrophy, dentate gyral, 5
Automated Ligand Identification System, 75

BACE (β-site APP cleaving enzyme), 1, 36, 159, 177, 219, 229. *See also* enzyme
  1, 218–219, 220, 221, 226
  2, 219
    memapsin 1, 24, 29, 37
  Asp2, 23, 24, 25, 123

assay
  biological, 35–55
  enzyme, 53
  inhibitors screening, 50–53
  protein, 54–55
cleavage
  caspace cleavage, and neuronal trophic dependence, 4–5
  dependence receptors, and AD pathology, 5–9
  as a molecular switching mechanism, 2–3
  downstream pathways, 5
  γ-, 16, 20
  inhibitors, 59–94
  assay strategies, 45–46
  memapsin 2, 18, 26, 123
  preparation, 126–135
    in *E.coli*, 129–130
    soluble derivitives, 127–128
  protein overview, 18–21
  structure, 38–39
  validation of, 27
Bateman, R. J., 201
Baxter, E. W., 131
BBB (blood–brain barrier), 125, 160–161, 166–167, 177–180, 205
benzyl carbamates (2HIZ), 139
bepineuzimab, 206
β-amyloid precursor protein. *See* APP
β-site APP cleaving enzyme. *See* BACE
Biacore, 108
biomarkers, 15–16, 206–207
blood–brain barrier. *See* BBB
bond
  Ala-Thr, 16
  Arg-Arg, 18
  Asp-Ala, 70
  Asp–Lys, 24
  Asp-Thr/Ser-Gly, 18, 23
  Ile-Ala, 72–73
  Lys-Leu, 24, 37
  Met-Asp, 16
  Phe-Ala, 24, 37
  Phe-Phe, 24, 37
  Phe-Val, 19
  Tyr-Glu, 16
  Val-Ile, 16
  Val-Met, 72–73
bridge, disulfide, 26

Bristol-Myers Squibb (BMS), 85–87
Bruinzeel, W., 128
Buck Institute, 229

CAA (cerebrovascular amyloid
    angiopathy), 166–167
Caenorhabditis elegans, 2, 23
Caflisch, A., 145
calculated molar refractivity. See CMR
caspase
  apical, 3
  -6, 1, 5, 7
  -8, 1, 3–4, 7
  -9, 3
cDNA
  2256 bp, 20
cell
  COS-7 APP751, 25
  death
    factors inducing programmed, 2
    neuronal, 7
  MDCK, 219
  Neuro-2A, 24
  neuroblastoma
    IMR-32, 24
  Schwann, 28
  SH-SY5Y APP695, 23
central nervous system. See CNS
cerebral hemorrhagic syndrome, 9
cerebrospinal fluid. See CSF
cerebrovascular amyloid angiopathy. See
    CAA
chemistry, computational, 47, 116,
    125–126, 145
  affinity binding predictions, 146
  brain penetration modeling, 147–148
  protonation states and impact, 148
  selectivity assessment, 146–147
  virtual screening
    combination, 149–150
    fragment-based, 149
    ligand-based, 148–149
Chinese hamster ovary. See CHO
CHO (Chinese hamster ovary), 128, 221
chromosome 11q23–24, 23
CIBIC (Clinician's Interview Based
    Impression of Change-plus), 197,
    211
Clinician's Interview Based Impression of
    Change-plus. See CIBIC

CMR (calculated molar refractivity),
    186–187
CNS (central nervous system), 28,
    205
collagen, types I and IV, 6
CoMentis, 72, 94, 192
CoMentis/Astellas, 202
computerized tomography. See CT
crystallization, 125–126, 127
CSF (cerebrospinal fluid), 206, 208–210
CT (computerized tomography), 206

D664A, 5
Dab, 6
DAD, 200
DCC (detected in colorectal cancer),
    2–3
DELFIA technology, 229
detected in colorectal cancer. See DCC
disease modification, 198
DR6 (death receptor 6), 4–5
Drosophila, 51–52
DSM-IV-TR criteria, 209
dysfunction, synaptic, 2

Elan, 21–22, 59–70
Eli Lilly, 72–74
endoplasmic reticulum (ER). See ER
endothiapepsin, 118
enzyme. See also BACE
  alkaline phosphatase (AP), 49–50
  Asp1, 23, 24, 51
  Asp3, 23
  Asp4, 23
  Asp664, 5
  CYP3A4, 168
  glycosylation, 220
  liver cytochrome P450
    CYP3A4, 178, 190
  pepsin, 26
  renin, 29
  sialyl-transferase ST6Gal I, 220
EPSP (excitatory postsynaptic potential), 5
ER (endoplasmic reticulum), 220–221
Escherichia coli (E. coli), 21, 26, 108, 127,
    129–130, 131
EST (expressed sequence tag), 23
  AA136368, 26
  AA207232, 26
  R55398, 26

excitatory postsynaptic potential. *See*
EPSP
expressed sequence tag. *See* EST

Fe65, 6
FEP (free-energy perturbation), 146
FlexX, 148
Pharm, 148
fluorescence resonance transfer. *See* FRET
Flurbiprofen, 124
Flurizan, 203
fMRI (functional magnetic resonance
imaging), 207–208
free-energy perturbation. *See* FEP
FRET (fluorescence resonance
transfer), 49, 221
F-spondin, 6
functional magnetic resonance imaging. *See*
fMRI

GlaxoSmithKline, 80–82
glycosylation, 127
N-linked, 19
glypican, 6
Golgi/endoplasmic reticulum, 18, 25. *See
also* TGN

HBA (H-bond acceptors), 81
H-bond acceptors. See HBA
HE (hydroxyethylene) isostere, 70, 74, 80,
136, 136–137, 180
HEA (hydroxyethylamine) isostere, 61,
85–86, 87–88, 136, 136–137, 180
HEK293 (human embryonic kidney)
cells, 20–21, 51, 59, 108, 128
clone, 23–24
high-pressure liquid chromatography. *See*
HPLC
high-throughput screening. *See* HTS
HMC (hydroxymethylcarbonyl
isostere), 88–89
HPLC (high-pressure liquid
chromatography), 44, 47, 50
HTS (high-throughtput screening), 35, 59,
77, 90, 107, 143, 180
hydroxyethylamine isostere. *See* HEA
hydroxyethylene isostere. *See* HE
hydroxymethylcarbonyl isostere. *See*
HMC
hypertension, 29, 178

hypomyelination, 28
hypothesis, amyloid cascade, 1

IL-R2 (interleukin-1 receptor II), 45
imaging. *See also* CT; fMRI; MRI; PET
amyloid plaque, 207
inhibition
competitive, 41
noncompetitive, 42
uncompetitive, 42
inhibitors
acetamide, 88
aminoquinolines to
aminopyridines, 112–116
anti-amyloid, 198
assay
capture (CA), 48
chemiluminescence (CL), 49–50
electrochemiluminescence
(ECL), 49–50
fluorescence polarization (FP),
48–49
fluorescence resonance transfer, *See*
FRET
HPLC, 50
strategies, 46–48
time-resolved-FRET (TR-FRET), 49
BACE, 197–213
novel, 217–230
BACE1, 160–161
benzamide, 88
biophysical, 108–110
Compound 1, 109–110
Compound 2, 109
Compound 3, 110–111
Compound 4, 111
Compound 5, 111, 181–183
Compound 6, 111, 181
Compound 7, 111, 183
Compound 8, 111–112
TC-1, 183, 190–191
Compound 9, 116, 183
Compound 10, 116, 184
Compound 11, 116
Compound 12, 116
(GSK188909), 186, 188–189
Compound 13, 116–117, 184–186
Compound 14, 116–117, 184
Compound 15, 117, 187
Compound 16, 118

Compound 17, 118
Compound 18, 118
Compound 19, 118
Compound 20, 118–119
Compound 71, 77–77
Compound 86, 83
Compound 87, 83–84
Compound 90, 85
Compound 91, 86–87
Compound 93, 86
Compound 94, 87
Compound 97 (NB-544), 87
Compound 98 (NB-533), 87
Compound 108 (KMI-429), 89
Compound 109 (KMI-758), 89
Compound 110 (KMI-1283), 89
Compound 111 (WY-25105), 90–91
Compound 115 (WY-24454), 90–91
Compound 120 (WY-258131), 92–93
CTS-21166, 29, 72, 192
CTS-21166 (ASP1702), 202
fragment screening
    advantages and disadvantages, 107
    approaches, 107–121
    rules, 107
GF120918, 189, 191–192
glutamic acid, 139
GRL-8234, 71
GSK188909, 81
hydrazones, 111–112
identified, 110
imidazolidinone 89, 84
isocytosines to dihydroisocysteines,
    117–119
isophthalimide, 86
Kunitz, 16
LY-450139, 124, 200–201, 205
macrocyclic, 61–62
morpholine, 74
neuroprotective, 198
nonpeptidomimetic, 141–142
    acylguanidines, 143
    carbenimines, 142–143
    dihydroaminoquinazolines, 144–145
OM-99, 111
OM-99-2, 70–71, 108, 139, 146, 148,
    180
oxirane, 88
peptidomimetics, 135–138
    piperazinone/imidazodinone, 141

    piperidine, 141
    pyrrolidine, 141
phenyureas, 111
piperidine, 74, 82–83
piperizinone 88, 84
prodrug HEA, 61–63
pyridone, 88
pyrrolidine, 74, 82–83, 86
renin, 138
structure-based drug design,
    123–151
tertiary carbinamine, 167–168
    TC-1, 168
tyramines, 116–117
WAY-258131, 192
interdependence, synaptic element, 7
interleukin-1 receptor II. See IL-R2
isophthalate (2IQG), 139
isostere. See HE; HEA; HMC; TSI

KAI1, 6
kinase, tyrosine, 2
Kyoto Pharmaceutical University/University
    of Tokyo, 88

laminin, 6–7
lanthanides, 49
LIE (linear interaction energy), 146
ligand, trophic, 3
Limongelli model, 148–149
linear interaction energy. See LIE
lipoprotein receptor-related protein. See
    LRP
long-term potentiation. See LTP
loss
    neuronal, 2, 160
    synaptic, 2
LRP (lipoprotein receptor-related
    protein), 45
LTP (long-term potentiation), 5

magnetic resonance imaging. See MRI
maltose-binding protein. See MBP
MAP system, 222–225
MBP (maltose-binding protein). See also
    APP
    Aβ, 3, 5, 9, 15–16, 16–17, 20, 159
        1–40, 16
        1–42, 1, 16
        amyloidogenicity, 16–17

MBP (maltose-binding protein) (*cont'd*)
  as "antitrophin," 6
  derivation of, 1
  -40, 16, 221
  -42, 16, 218, 220–221, 230
  C-26, 21
  C-83, 15, 18, 22–23
  C-89, 20
  C-99, 20, 21
  C-125, 21, 22
  multimerization, Aβ-induced, 5
MC (Monte Carlo) simulations, 146
MCI (mild cognitive impairment), 1
MD (molecular dynamics), 146
memapsin 2. *See* BACE1
Merck, 74–80, 229
methionine 35, 4
mice
  knockout, 27–28
  PDAPP transgenic, 28, 161–163
Michaelis-Menten model, 40–41
mild cognitive impairment. *See* MCI
MMSE, 200
molecular dynamics. *See* MD
Monte Carlo simulations. *See* MC
MRI (magnetic resonance imaging), 200, 206, 210
mutation. *See also* APP
  affecting Aβ processing, 9
  Arctic, 9
  D664A, 7

National Center for Biotechnology
    Information. *See* NCBI
NCBI (National Center for Biotechnology
    Information), 26
neoepitope, 4
NeoGenesis, 75
neogenin, 2–3
neophobia. *See* LTP
netrin, 7
  -1, 6
neurodegeneration, 2–3, 199
neurons, cholinergic, 217
Neuropsychological Test Battery. *See*
    NTB
neurotransmitters, 7
  acetylcholine, 197
  cholinesterase, 197
NINCDS-ADRDA criteria, 209

NMR, 107
Novartis, 87–88
NRG1 (type III neuregulin1), 220
NTB (Neuropsychological Test
    Battery), 200

Oklahoma Medical Research Foundation
    (OMRF), 25–26, 70–72
oligodendrocytes, 28
1FKN, 140
oxyacetamide, 143

p21-activated kinase. *See* PAK
PAK, 5
Patched, 3
PDB (protein data bank), 131
PDGF-B (platelet-derived growth
    factor-B), 5
peptide
  Aβ, 36, 217, 220–221. see APP
  AICD, 7
  AN1792, 199
  biomarkers, 15
  C31, 9
  GLTNIKTEE ISEISY-EVEFRWKK, 44,
    50
  Jcasp, 9
  LB83190, 51–52
  LB83192, 51–52
  LB83202, 51–52
  p3, 7
  P10-P4' (Stat-Val), 22
  SEISY-EVEFRWKK, 44, 50
peripheral nervous system. *See* PNS
permeability glycoprotein. *See* P-gp
PET (positron emission tomography), 207,
    210
P-gp (permeability glycoprotein), 29
Pharmacia, 22–25
Pharmacia (Pfizer), 59–70
pharmacokinetic profile. *See* PK
PK (pharmacokinetic profile), 177
plaques, neuritic, 15, 36, 159, 199, 217
platelet-derived growth factor-B. *See*
    PDGF-B
PNS (peripheral nervous system), 28
pockets
  binding
    S2 and S4, 139–140
    S1-S4, 142

S3, 143
specificity, 131–136
    S1, 138
    S3, 135, 138–139
positron emission tomography. *See* PET
presenilin-1, 2
prime side, and specificity pockets,
    140–141
protease
    aspartyl, 219. *See* AP
        renin, 146–147
    cathepsin B, 218, 220
    cathepsin D (Cat-D), 18, 23, 25, 61,
        74–75, 123, 139, 146–147, 219
    cathepsin E, 139, 219
    cysteine, 21
    HIV-, 22, 25, 29, 63, 123, 160, 178
        Ritonavir, 191
    insulin-degrading enzyme, 37
    Lopinavir, 178
    metallo, 21
    napsin A, 219
    neprilysin, 37
    nexin-II, 16
    pepsin, 22, 123, 219
    peptidyl peptidases, 124
    renin, 22, 25, 63, 74–75, 160, 123, 178,
        219
        Aliskiren, 178
    serine, 21
protein, 15
    Aph1, 37, 44, 123
    Aph2, 44
    cytoskeletal tau, 160
    flexibilty, 145–146
    hyperphosphorylated microtubule binding
        tau, 4, 36
    natural, as BACE substrate, 46
    neuregulin-1 (NRG1), 28, 45
    nicastrin, 37, 123
    Notch, 124, 200
    Pen2, 37, 123
    phosporylated tau (p-tau), 208
    presenilin, 37, 123, 160
    P-selectin glycoprotein ligand-1, 220
    tau (t-tau), 208
    Type I transmembrane, 18
protein data bank. *See* PDB
proteoglycan, heparan sulfate, 6
P-selectin glycoprotein ligand 1. *See* PSGL-1

PSGL-1 (P-selectin glycoprotein ligand 1),
    45
Ptc, 2–3
pulse-chase, 205
pyridyl (2HM1), 139
pyrrolidinones (2VIZ), 139

radical, sulfuranyl, 4
receptor
    axon guidance
        DCC, 9
    death 6. see DR6
    "dependence," 2
    insulin, 4
    neurotrophin
        p75NTR, 9
Research Collaboratory for Structural
    Bioinformatics, 131
residue
    α-, 9
    Ala, 26
    Arg, 19, 44, 61, 129, 135, 139, 141,
        146–147
    Asn, 23, 25, 44
    Asp, 21, 22–23, 25, 36–37, 42, 114–116,
        116, 118–119, 143, 144, 145, 146, 148
        664, 3, 7
        protonated and nonprotonated, 39
    β-, 9
    γ-, 9, 18, 24
    Gln, 138
    Glu, 18–19, 22, 36–37, 44, 134, 139
    Glu11, 51
    Gly, 19, 44, 116, 137
    Gyl, 134
    Ile, 44, 138, 140, 149
    Leu, 21–22, 129, 135, 138, 142
    Lys, 22–23, 134
    major, 1
    Met, 21, 22, 36, 44, 61
    Nle, 44
    Phe, 44, 116, 138, 149
    Pro, 141
    Ser, 19, 26, 44, 135, 143, 145
    Sta, 22
    Thr, 18–19, 26, 44, 84, 135, 139, 140, 143
    Trp, 138, 149
    Tyr, 22, 36, 116, 134, 138, 139, 141,
        143, 144, 146
    Val, 18, 21, 44, 140

RET, 2–3
retraction, neurite, 2, 5, 7
Roche compound collection, 108, 116
"rule of five," 125

SAR (structure-activity relationships), 126,
    180
SBDD (structure-based drug design), 125
Schering Plough, 82–85
secretase
    α-, 1, 16, 37, 159, 226
    β-, 16–20, 36–37, 123, 124–125, 159,
        160, 177, 201–202, 218, 218–220,
        221–222, 225, 226. *See* BACE
    BACE, 220
    γ-, 37, 123–125, 159–160, 200–201, 218.
        See also BACE
sequence
    Arg-His5-Asp-Ser-Gly-Tyr10-Glu-Val-
        His-His-Gln, 22
    Asn-Leu, 16
    DT/SGT/S, 219
    EVNF-EVEF, 51
    Gly-Tyr-Glu-Val, 43
    Ile-Ser-Glu-Val-Lys-Met-Asp1-Ala-Glu-
        Phe-Arg-His, 22
    ISY-EV, 51
    Leu-Val-Phe-Phe-Ala-Glu-Asp, 24
    Lys-Met-Asp-Ala, 43
    SEVKM-DAEFR, 138
    SEVNL-DAEFR, 138
6-sialyltransferase. *See* ST6Gal1
SmithKlein Beecham (SKB), 25
Sonic hedgehog, 3
ST6Gal1 (6-sialyltransferase), 45
Stokes shifts, 49
structure-activity relationships. *See* SAR
structure-based drug design. *See* SBDD
sugar, O-linked, 19
sulfones (2VIY), 139
sultams (2VIJ), 139
Sunesis, 77
surface plasmon resonance, 107–108, 116,
    117

T18H9.2, 23
TACE. *See* secretase, α-
tangles, intracellular neurofibrillary, 15, 36,
    159–160
    hyperphosphorylated tau, 217

Tarenflurbil, 203
Terminal Fragment
    C-, 131
    83, 24–25
    99, 24–25
    N-, 28
Tessier-Lavigne, 5
TGN (trans-golgi network), 125, 220–221.
    See also Golgi/endoplasmic
        reticulum
therapies
    donepazil, 197
    galantamine, 197
    memantine, 197
    rivastigmine, 197
thermodynamic integration. *See* TI
TI (thermodynamic integration), 146
Tramiprosate, 202–203
trans-golgi network. *See* TGN
transition-state isostere. *See* TSI
transport defects, axonal, 2
triplets
    AVE, 44
    EVD, 44
    EVE, 44
    TSI (transition-state isostere), 72–73, 76,
        80, 136. *See also* HE; HEA
    aminoethylenes, 136
    statine, 136, 180
2VJ9, 140
type III neuregulin1. *See* NRG1

Unc5H2 (uncoordinated gene 5 homologue
    2), 2–3
uncoordinated gene 5 homologue 2. *See*
    Unc5H2

vapor diffusion experiment, 131
Vertex pharmacophore, 148–149
VGSC (voltage-gated sodium
    channels), 44–45
voltage-gated sodium channels. *See*
    VGSC

Wyeth, 90–94

X-ray crystallography, 45, 107–108, 111,
    116, 119, 130–135, 144